Psychiatric-Mental Health Nurse Practitioner Program Companion and Board Certification Exam Review Workbook

Trae Stewart

Psychiatric-Mental Health Nurse Practitioner Program Companion and Board Certification Exam Review Workbook

Springer

Trae Stewart
PsychMatters LLC
Las Vegas, NV, USA

ISBN 978-3-031-60896-4 ISBN 978-3-031-60894-0 (eBook)
https://doi.org/10.1007/978-3-031-60894-0

This Springer imprint is published by the registered company Springer Nature Switzerland AG
The registered company address is: Gewerbestrasse 11, 6330 Cham, Switzerland

To all past, current, and future Psychiatric-Mental Health Nurse Practitioners (PMHNPs), this book is dedicated to you. Your commitment to improving the lives of individuals and communities through compassionate, evidence-based care is an inspiration. May this companion guide you on your journey toward becoming a skilled and knowledgeable advocate, leader, and healthcare provider to those with mental illnesses.

Preface

Mental health has paramount importance in the context of an individual's holistic well-being. It plays a vital role in enabling people to lead satisfying and meaningful lives, while maintaining a positive state of mind. Unfortunately, the reality is that a substantial number of individuals across the globe face significant challenges in accessing necessary psychiatric care. The World Health Organization (WHO) estimates that approximately one in four individuals will experience a mental health disorder at some point in their lives. This alarming statistic emphasizes the magnitude and impact of mental health conditions on global disability rates (McGorry et al. 2022; Mongelli et al. 2020).

Despite the prevalence of mental health disorders, there exists a shortage of psychiatric healthcare providers, particularly in underserved and rural areas. This shortage can be attributed primarily to the inadequate availability of mental health professionals, like psychiatrists, nurse practitioners, psychologists, and social workers. Global statistics illustrate that the average ratio of mental health workers per 100,000 population stands slightly above 4.5, but this figure varies significantly across different regions worldwide. For instance, in sub-Saharan Africa, a region grappling with numerous health challenges, the ratio drops significantly, reaching a concerning 0.5 mental health workers per 100,000 population. In sharp contrast, high-income countries boast a more favorable ratio of mental health workers, with approximately 18 mental health workers per 100,000 population (APA 2013; Alfakeh 2021; AlSalem et al. 2020; Anbesaw et al. 2024; Kovács-Tóth et al. 2021).

The scarcity of psychiatric care is particularly severe in rural areas, where access to mental health services is limited due to a lack of providers. The United States is a prime example, with its vast geographical landscape and approximately 20% of its population residing in rural areas. Surprisingly, these regions are home to only 10% of the nation's mental health providers. As a result, individuals living in rural areas often endure long waiting times for appointments and encounter significant difficulties when attempting to access specialized care. These challenges affect their ability to receive the necessary treatment (APA 2013; Brouwers 2020; Keeley 2021; Solmi et al. 2022).

Beyond the shortage of mental health professionals, various notable barriers hinder individuals from accessing the care they require. The presence of stigma surrounding mental illness remains a pervasive issue, preventing many individuals from seeking the treatment and support they need. The fear of judgment and discrimination leaves people feeling isolated and reluctant to discuss their mental health challenges, which only exacerbates their conditions. Additionally, the lack of insurance coverage and high out-of-pocket costs pose significant financial obstacles for individuals seeking mental health services. Consequently, many choose to forgo treatment, leading to the deterioration of their mental health and overall well-being.

To effectively combat the shortage of psychiatric care providers and enhance access to mental health treatment, a variety of potential solutions can be implemented. One promising approach involves increasing funding for mental health services, thereby attracting and retaining more professionals in the field. By investing in training programs and providing financial incentives to encourage individuals to pursue careers in mental health, it is possible to alleviate the shortage and ensure an adequate workforce to meet the demand. One such training opportunity is for Psychiatric-Mental Health Nurse Practitioners (PMHNPs).

Another viable solution lies in the expanded use of technology, particularly telepsychiatry and teletherapy, to reach individuals in underserved areas. These approaches allow for convenient and accessible mental health treatment from the comfort of one's home. By leveraging this technology, it becomes feasible to increase the number of people who can access care, ultimately bridging the gap in mental health services. Telepsychiatry and teletherapy also eliminate geographical barriers, enabling individuals in remote areas to receive high-quality mental health treatment and support.

Furthermore, improving insurance coverage for mental health services plays a crucial role in reducing financial barriers. This includes expanding programs like Medicaid and other insurance initiatives to encompass mental health services, ensuring that individuals have the financial means to seek treatment without facing exorbitant costs. Additionally, increasing the number of mental health providers who accept insurance will enhance affordability and make care more attainable for individuals in need, further breaking down the financial obstacles that prevent people from accessing the necessary care.

Addressing the shortage of psychiatric care providers and improving access to mental health treatment is a complex challenge that necessitates a comprehensive approach. However, by implementing a combination of strategies, including increasing funding, leveraging technology, improving insurance coverage, and expanding the role of non-psychiatric healthcare professionals in mental healthcare, it becomes possible to enhance access to care for individuals worldwide. By doing so, we can ensure that everyone has the opportunity to receive the treatment they need to maintain their mental health and overall well-being, thus contributing to the creation of a healthier and happier society (Beck et al. 2020; Fulginiti et al. 2021; Hyland et al. 2021; Jakovljevic et al. 2020; Keeley 2021; McGorry et al. 2022; Newcomb et al. 2020; World Health Organization 2021, 2022).

Role of Psychiatric-Mental Health Nurse Practitioners (PMHNPs)

PMHNPs occupy a crucial and vital role within the healthcare system, delivering essential mental health services to individuals across all age groups. As advanced practice registered nurses (APRNs), PMHNPs undergo rigorous and extensive graduate-level education and clinical training in psychiatric-mental health nursing. They possess the expertise, skills, and knowledge to diagnose and effectively treat various mental health conditions utilizing a diverse array of evidence-based therapeutic interventions.

As a PMHNP student, you've embarked on a noble and impactful career path dedicated to making a meaningful difference in the lives of individuals grappling with mental health conditions. Your journey thus far has been marked by extensive clinical training and education, equipping you with the necessary skills and knowledge to provide compassionate and effective care to those in need. Now, as you stand on the precipice of taking the PMHNP board certification exam, a blend of excitement and nervous anticipation naturally arises within you.

The PMHNP board certification exam represents a pivotal milestone in your professional journey. It has been designed to rigorously assess your expertise, abilities, and competence as a PMHNP. This comprehensive examination covers a broad spectrum of topics ranging from assessment and diagnosis to treatment planning, interventions, and ethical and legal considerations. Administered by the reputable American Nurses Credentialing Center (ANCC), this exam stands as an essential requirement for achieving PMHNP certification.

Recognizing the escalating prevalence and significance of mental health concerns in society and the ever-increasing demand for highly qualified and competent PMHNPs, it is imperative to provide aspiring practitioners with unfailing access to dependable, cutting-edge resources that will effectively prepare them for the challenging certification exam. The book *Psychiatric-Mental Health Nurse Practitioner Program Companion and Board Certification Exam Review Workbook* emerges as a direct and concrete response to this pressing need.

Given that the certification exam encompasses an extensive and vast spectrum of topics, navigating the complex study process can undoubtedly become overwhelmingly daunting for many. However, this text successfully provides a highly effective roadmap, enabling individuals to effectively breakdown and deconstruct the vast material into easily digestible and comprehensible segments, thereby facilitating a more efficient and tailored approach to learning.

By encouraging learners to focus on mastering one critical topic at a time, the program companion and workbook optimizes the learning experience and greatly enhances knowledge retention. Moreover, the text boasts a plethora of learning resources that are tailored to accommodate and effectively cater to diverse learning styles and preferences. Ultimately, this approach empowers aspiring PMHNPs to effectively engage and connect with the material in a truly personal and profound manner.

With this unparalleled, comprehensive, and cutting-edge approach, aspiring PMHNPs can confidently embark on their path with an unwavering sense of assurance, security, and self-assuredness, knowing that they possess the unparalleled and unrestricted resources that are vital for their inevitable success. The text is their ultimate companion in achieving their dreams and making a significant difference in the lives of individuals struggling with mental health issues.

Target Audiences for the Book

1. Current PMHNP students:

   For current PMHNP students, this comprehensive text serves as an indispensable companion throughout their entire academic journey. Its content is meticulously aligned with the PMHNP scope of practice, ensuring an enriched and holistic educational experience. By providing comprehensive coverage of the most vital exam content, this workbook empowers students to delve deeper into their studies. Through its interactive activities, students can actively reinforce their learning, apply their knowledge to real-world situations, and identify specific areas that require further exploration and focus. With this invaluable tool in their hands, PMHNP students can rest assured that they are well-prepared for the challenges of both clinical practice and the rigorous certification exam, thus setting the stage for a successful and fulfilling career in psychiatric-mental health nursing.
2. Recent graduates of PMHNP programs preparing for the ANCC board certification exam:

   Recent graduates of PMHNP programs are at a crucial juncture as they embark on their journey towards preparing for the widely respected and rigorous ANCC board certification exam. Acquiring certification as a PMHNP involves a comprehensive assessment of one's knowledge and skills in this specialized field. In recognition of the significance of this milestone, this workbook provides a lifeline of unparalleled support during this critical period of exam preparation. Delving into this review of exam content, recent PMHNP graduates gain access to interactive tools that enable them to assess their understanding, identify areas of strength and weakness, and focus their efforts accordingly. By actively engaging with the material, graduates not only build unwavering confidence, but they also deepen their knowledge and hone their abilities, thus ensuring a remarkable level of preparedness for success on the certification exam. This invaluable resource facilitates the seamless transition from the academic realm to professional practice as fully certified and capable PMHNPs.
3. Instructors and program leaders in PMHNP programs:

   The pivotal role of instructors and program leaders in PMHNP programs is immeasurable, and it has an immense impact in shaping the educational experiences of aspiring PMHNPs. Within this profound context, this workbook serves as a resource to support and aid these highly esteemed and respected educators.

Instructors adeptly and masterfully incorporate this exceptional workbook into their curriculum to enrich classroom instruction, invigorate discussions, and flawlessly harmonize and synchronize student learning outcomes with the highest and most exacting standards of accreditation. Instructors can effectively foster an environment that encourages deep and profound engagement and simultaneously assess student comprehension, retention, and progress. This resource acts as a catalyst and substantially elevates the caliber and effectiveness of teaching in PMHNP programs, holistically preparing students for the formidable and intellectually rigorous academic challenges and demanding and intricate professional requirements that lie ahead, thus ensuring the highest standards of excellence, proficiency, and competence in the distinguished field of psychiatric-mental health nursing.

4. Practicing PMHNPs seeking ongoing professional development:

   For seasoned Practicing PMHNPs, the pursuit of ongoing professional development manifests as a fundamental and integral component and lies at the very core and essence of maintaining clinical excellence and delivering optimal care to the esteemed patients. In recognition of this undeniable and crucial imperative, this workbook emerges as an indispensable, readily accessible, and unparalleled resource for these practitioners. Seasoned PMHNPs can continuously expand their extensive knowledge base, refine and polish their already exemplary and exceptional skills, and stay abreast and attuned to research, diagnostics, and novel and pioneering treatment modalities. This commitment to unceasing and continuous professional growth and development ultimately translates into significantly and measurably improved patient care, consistently elevated positive outcomes, and an unwavering dedication to upholding the highest, most exacting standards of psychiatric-mental health nursing care, unrelentingly placing the esteemed patients and their well-being at the forefront of clinical practice.

Book Contents

The *Psychiatric-Mental Health Nurse Practitioner Program Companion and Board Certification Exam Review Workbook* caters to PMHNP students, program leaders, faculty, and practicing PMHNPs, providing valuable resources for educational, clinical, and professional development endeavors. Whether embarking on educational journeys, refining clinical skills, or seeking teaching support, this workbook empowers individuals to become knowledgeable and compassionate PMHNPs. Below are brief descriptions of each chapter in the book.

Roles, Regulations, and Scope of Practice: This chapter offers an in-depth exploration of the multifaceted roles and responsibilities of PMHNPs. It delves into the scope of practice regulations. Detailed discussions on PMHNPs' evolving roles in various healthcare settings and their impact on patient care are presented.

Theories and Frameworks: Foundational to PMHNPs' practice, this chapter delves into psychological theories and frameworks. It explores the biopsychosocial model, trauma-informed care, recovery-oriented practice, and contemporary paradigms shaping psychiatric-mental health nursing.

Ethics and Legal Principles: Navigating complex ethical and legal terrains, this chapter equips PMHNPs with essential concepts. Discussions cover ethical principles, confidentiality, informed consent, duty to report, and malpractice prevention, ensuring high standards of care and professional conduct.

Anatomy and Physiology of the Brain and Nervous System: Vital for PMHNPs, this chapter provides an in-depth understanding of the brain and nervous system's anatomy and physiology. It explores the central nervous system's structure, neurotransmitters, and their roles in mental health and illness, enhancing diagnostic and treatment skills.

Assessment and Diagnosis Fundamentals: Focusing on competent assessment and accurate diagnosis, this chapter equips PMHNPs with comprehensive skills. Topics include psychiatric history-taking, mental status examination, and differential diagnosis, integrating evidence-based guidelines and diagnostic criteria.

Psychopharmacology: Indispensable for PMHNPs, this chapter delves into psychopharmacological management of psychiatric disorders. It covers psychotropic medications, mechanisms of action, side effect profiles, medication selection, titration, monitoring, and strategies for addressing adherence challenges.

Mood Disorders: A significant aspect of psychiatric-mental health nursing, this chapter extensively explores mood disorders. Topics include major depressive disorder, bipolar disorders, diagnostic criteria, pathophysiology, and evidence-based treatments, enabling holistic care provision.

Anxiety Disorders and Obsessive-Compulsive Disorder: Prevalent and impactful conditions, anxiety disorders and obsessive-compulsive disorder (OCD), receive a comprehensive examination here. Assessment, diagnosis, and evidence-based treatment modalities are explored for generalized anxiety disorder, panic disorder, phobias, and OCD.

Schizophrenia, Psychosis, and Delusions: Addressing unique challenges, this chapter provides an in-depth analysis of schizophrenia and related psychotic disorders. Topics include assessment, diagnosis, early intervention, evidence-based pharmacological and psychosocial treatments, and managing multifaceted needs.

Neurocognitive Disorders and Geriatric Mental Health: Navigating challenges posed by neurocognitive disorders, this chapter focuses on assessment, diagnosis, and evidence-based interventions. Providing care to older adults with cognitive impairments, it emphasizes person-centered approaches and caregiver support.

Substance-Related and Addictive Disorders: Demanding specialized expertise, substance-related and addictive disorders are extensively covered. Topics include assessment, diagnosis, evidence-based treatments, integrated care approaches, and addressing the interplay between mental health and substance use.

Personality Disorders: Presenting unique challenges, personality disorders receive an extensive examination. Topics include borderline, narcissistic, and antisocial personality disorders, covering diagnostic criteria, etiology, and evidence-based treatments.

Child/Adolescent Neurodevelopmental and Psychiatric Disorders: Addressing specialized care for children and adolescents, this chapter explores a range of conditions. Topics include ADHD, autism spectrum disorder, disruptive mood dysregulation disorder, assessment, diagnosis, and evidence-based interventions.

Sleep-Wake Disorders: Significantly impacting mental health, sleep-wake disorders are comprehensively examined. Topics include evidence-based treatments and emphasizing the importance of sleep hygiene and behavioral interventions.

Sexual Dysfunctions, Gender Dysphoria, and Paraphilic Disorders: Requiring sensitive care, sexual dysfunctions, gender dysphoria, and paraphilic disorders are explored. Topics include assessment, diagnosis, evidence-based treatments, gender-affirming care, and addressing sexual dysfunctions.

Trauma, Somatization, Violence, and Forensics: Addressing profound implications for mental health, trauma and violence are comprehensively examined. Topics include trauma-informed care, somatic symptom disorders, forensic psychiatry, assessment strategies for trauma survivors, and evidence-based interventions.

Individual, Group, and Family Therapies: Essential components of practice, therapeutic interventions are extensively covered. Topics include individual, group, and family therapies, psychotherapies, therapeutic techniques, and application of evidence-based modalities.

Culturally Competent Care: Imperative for patient-centered care, cultural competence is emphasized. Topics include cultural considerations, respecting individual values, beliefs, and traditions, ensuring culturally sensitive care provision.

Public Health, Biostatistics, and Research Foundations: Integral to evidence-based practice, public health principles and research foundations are explored. Topics include biostatistics, research methodologies, critical appraisal of research findings, and their application in mental healthcare.

Leadership, Advocacy, Policy, and Quality Improvement: Shaping the future of practice, leadership, advocacy, policy, and quality improvement are extensively covered. Topics include roles and responsibilities of PMHNPs as leaders and advocates, policy issues affecting mental health, and enhancing patient outcomes through quality improvement.

Appendix A: Crunch Time Review: Offering a condensed yet comprehensive review, this section assists students in final exam preparations. It serves as a high-yield resource for reinforcing knowledge and identifying areas requiring further review.

Appendix B: PMHNP Interview Questions: Tailored for graduates and practicing PMHNPs, this section provides commonly asked interview questions. Detailed responses and tips empower individuals to navigate the job-seeking process with confidence.

How to Use This Book

For students embarking on this challenging path, thoroughly comprehending the well-organized structure of the *Psychiatric-Mental Health Nurse Practitioner Program Companion and Board Certification Exam Review Workbook* is absolutely essential. The workbook is intelligently organized into chapters that align seamlessly with the major content areas of the PMHNP certification exam, facilitating comprehensive coverage of all the vital topics, including assessment, diagnosis, treatment planning, interventions, and ethical and legal considerations.

Each chapter commences with an introduction that adeptly highlights the importance, purpose, and critical key concepts that will be examined and explored in the forthcoming chapter. This information serves as a foundational schema, upon which students can expertly scaffold and seamlessly integrate new knowledge and invaluable information throughout the duration of their program and during the highly critical and intense exam review stage.

To genuinely maximize the boundless potential for active learning, students are strongly advised to diligently read, comprehensively study, and genuinely understand all the material, employing effective note-taking techniques, highlighting significant passages and key points, and actively engaged discussions with peers and mentors to deepen their understanding, foster greater retention, and ultimately enhance the overall learning experience. Actively engaging with the interactive activities interspersed throughout the workbook serves as a poignant means to expertly reinforce key concepts, meaningfully apply the acquired knowledge in practical and highly realistic scenarios, and astutely identify both strengths and areas that necessitate further deliberate focus and improvement.

Embracing effective time management strategies is key to the entire preparation process. This aspect necessitates and demands students to create a highly detailed and personalized study schedule that effectively accounts for all other critical aspects of their busy and demanding lives, allocate dedicated and focused study time each and every single day, and systematically break down the expansive and multifaceted material into easily manageable and digestible segments. By setting realistic and attainable goals, tracking personal progress throughout the entire preparation journey, and consistently staying highly organized, students can successfully and proactively sustain both motivation and focus, especially during potentially challenging and overwhelming moments.

Lastly, it is absolutely vital, and should be viewed as an integral component of the entire exam preparation process, to wholeheartedly prioritize personal health and overall well-being. Promoting nurturing important habits such as obtaining sufficient rest, consistently maintaining a balanced and nourishing dietary regimen, and seamlessly incorporating regular and invigorating physical activity into the already bustling routine serves as a deeply empowering and palpable means to effectively sustain personal energy levels, conscientiously maintain crystal-clear focus, substantially diminish and alleviate the debilitating impact of unnecessary stress and anxiety, and ultimately facilitate and ensure optimal performance during the pivotal PMHNP certification exam.

For professional and dedicated instructors, facilitating student learning is undeniably critical. Instructors are highly encouraged to enthusiastically utilize the companion workbook as a comprehensive and indispensable resource to expertly guide student learning throughout the duration of their esteemed PMHNP program. Instructors may integrate the various chapters and carefully crafted interactive activities that are featured within the workbook into the overarching curriculum, effectively underscoring key concepts, creating invaluable opportunities for students to actively apply the acquired knowledge, and ultimately fostering greater depths of understanding.

Instructors should supplement their classroom instruction by assigning relevant chapters and targeted activities as both pre-class readings and challenging homework assignments. Further they can assign a set of practice exercises in class sessions to facilitate dynamic and enriching conversations, monitor comprehension and retention levels, and astutely pinpoint any areas of potential confusion or gaps in understanding that require immediate attention and further review. Demonstrating genuine care and offering additional support to each student is required in the transformational instructional process.

Accompanying Springer Nature Flashcard App

In conjunction with the *Psychiatric-Mental Health Nurse Practitioner Program Companion and Board Certification Exam Review Workbook*, learners will have access to the highly innovative Springer Nature Flashcard App. This incredible app was designed to complement your book-based study and preparation journey. By utilizing this user-friendly app, you will be equipped with a dynamic tool that offers not only portability but also an efficient method to reinforce your knowledge, assess your learning, and effortlessly identify any areas that may require further review.

With an extensive collection of almost 2,000 thoughtfully crafted multiple-choice questions, the flashcard app covers all the key concepts, terms, pharmacology, therapeutic approaches, and critical standards of practice that are absolutely essential for mastering the PMHNP board certification exam. These comprehensive flashcards have been expertly organized into easily navigable categories that correspond to the chapters of the accompanying book. This feature allows you to tailor your study sessions to specifically focus on certain topics or alternatively access all the areas for a more comprehensive review.

Each flashcard presents you with an engaging question and a selection of possible answers. However, the true beauty of this app lies in the fact that the correct answer will only be revealed after you submit your own selection. This design facilitates active recall and provides you with the invaluable opportunity to self-assess your understanding. Furthermore, you have the ability to mark specific cards that you find particularly challenging, allowing you to conveniently revisit and reinforce your understanding of those topics as needed. This targeted study method is guaranteed to greatly enhance your learning experience. In addition to its incredible educational features, the app also diligently keeps track of your progress, offering you invaluable insights into your strengths and any areas in which you might need to direct more effort.

To truly make the most of the Springer Nature Flashcard App, it is recommended that students dedicate regular, short sessions to reviewing the flashcards. By incorporating these active recall sessions into your study routine, you will solidify your understanding and embed the knowledge even deeper into your memory. This technique has been proven to be particularly effective for preparing for the high-stakes environment of the certification exam. One of the greatest advantages of the app is its seamless integration into your daily life. Regardless of whether you find yourself between clients, commuting, or simply have a spare moment, the app effortlessly fits into your busy schedule, providing you with a highly convenient and powerful tool to help you succeed on the PMHNP board certification exam. Embrace this exceptional opportunity to enhance your learning experience and take yet another transformative step towards becoming a certified PMHNP.

Good Luck!

Las Vegas, NV, USA Trae Stewart

References and Resources

AlSalem M, Alamri R, Hejazi S. Nonpsychiatric healthcare professionals' attitudes toward patients with mental illnesses in Makkah city, Saudi Arabia: a cross-sectional study. Neuropsychiatr Dis Treatm. 2020;16:341–8. https://doi.org/10.2147/NDT.S236148.

American Psychiatric Association. Diagnostic and statistical manual of mental disorders. 5th ed. 2013. https://doi.org/10.1176/appi.books.9780890425596.

Anbesaw T, Asmamaw A, Adamu K, Tsegaw M. Mental health literacy and its associated factors among traditional healers toward mental illness in Northeast, Ethiopia: a mixed approach study. PLoS One. 2024;19(2):e0298406. https://doi.org/10.1371/journal.pone.0298406.

Beck JS, Lundwall RA, Gabrielsen T, Cox JC, South M. Looking good but feeling bad: "Camouflaging" behaviors and mental health in women with autistic traits. Autism. 2020;24(4):809–21. https://doi.org/10.1177/1362361320912147.

Brouwers EPM. Social stigma is an underestimated contributing factor to unemployment in people with mental illness or mental health issues: position paper and future directions. BMC Psychol. 2020;8(1):36. https://doi.org/10.1186/s40359-020-00399-0.

Fulginiti A, Rhoades H, Mamey MR, Klemmer C, Srivastava A, Weskamp G, Goldbach JT. Sexual minority stress, mental health symptoms, and suicidality among LGBTQ youth accessing crisis services. J Youth Adolesc. 2021;50(5):893–905. https://doi.org/10.1007/s10964-020-01354-3.

Hyland P, Vallières F, Cloitre M, Ben-Ezra M, Karatzias T, Olff M, et al. Trauma, PTSD, and complex PTSD in the Republic of Ireland: prevalence, service use, comorbidity, and risk factors. Soc Psychiatry Psychiatr Epidemiol. 2021;56(4):649–58. https://doi.org/10.1007/s00127-020-01912-x.

Jakovljevic M, Bjedov S, Jaksic N, Jakovljevic I. COVID-19 pandemia and public and global mental health from the perspective of global health security. Psychiatr Danub. 2020;32(1):6–14. https://doi.org/10.24869/psyd.2020.6.

Keeley B. The State of the World's Children 2021: On my mind—promoting, protecting and caring for children's mental health. 2021. https://www.unicef.org/lac/en/reports/state-of-the-worlds-children-2021-on-my-mind.

Kovács-Tóth B, Oláh B, Papp G, Szabó IK. Assessing adverse childhood experiences, social, emotional, and behavioral symptoms, and subjective health complaints among Hungarian adolescents. Child Adolesc Psychiatry Mental Health. 2021;15(1):1–12. https://doi.org/10.1186/s13034-021-00365-7.

McGorry PD, Mei C, Chanen A, Hodges C, Alvarez-Jimenez M, Killackey E. Designing and scaling up integrated youth mental health care. World Psychiatry. 2022;21(1):61–76. https://doi.org/10.1002/wps.20938.

Mongelli F, Georgakopoulos P, Pato MT. Challenges and opportunities to meet the mental health needs of underserved and disenfranchised populations in the United States. Focus. 2020;18(1):16–24. https://doi.org/10.1176/appi.focus.20190028.

Newcomb ME, Hill R, Buehler K, Ryan DT, Whitton SW, Mustanski B. High burden of mental health problems, substance use, violence, and related psychosocial factors in transgender, non-binary, and gender diverse youth and young adults. Arch Sex Behav. 2020;49(2):645–59. https://doi.org/10.1007/s10508-019-01533-9.

Solmi M, Radua J, Olivola M, Croce E, Soardo L, Salazar de Pablo G, et al. Age at onset of mental disorders worldwide: large-scale meta-analysis of 192 epidemiological studies. Mol Psychiatry. 2022;27(1):281–95. https://doi.org/10.1038/s41380-021-01161-7.

World Health Organization. Guidance on community mental health services: promoting person-centred and rights-based approaches. World Health Organization; 2021. https://iris.who.int/handle/10665/341648.

World Health Organization. World mental health report: transforming mental health for all. World Health Organization; 2022. https://iris.who.int/handle/10665/356119.

Contents

About the Author

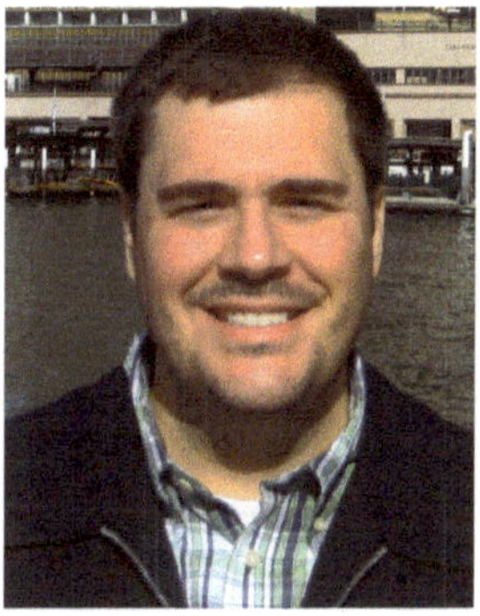

Trae Stewart, PhD, MPH, MSN, MS, MN, PMHNP-BC boasts an illustrious career, marked by his tenure as a professor at esteemed institutions such as Texas State University and the University of Central Florida. Prior to his academic pursuits, Dr. Stewart honed his skills as a Behavioral Health RN in the dynamic environment of an acute psychiatric unit at the Cleveland Clinic. His passion for nursing education led him to serve as faculty at the University of Colorado, Anschutz Medical Campus.

With a commitment to global health, Dr. Stewart has lent his expertise to consultancy projects spanning across diverse regions, including Palestine, Afghanistan, East Africa, Australia, New Zealand, and Chile, as a distinguished Fulbright Specialist. His contributions to the field are evident through his extensive publication record, comprising over 50 peer-reviewed journal articles, book chapters, and books. He has served as a question item writer/reviewer for the NCLEX. Dr. Stewart's dedication has been recognized with prestigious teaching, research, and service awards throughout his career.

Dr. Stewart's academic journey is characterized by a remarkable breadth of knowledge, underscored by his academic achievements. He holds a PhD in International Development and Intercultural Education from the University of Southern California, an MPH in Environmental Health from Texas A&M University, and two Master's degrees in Nursing from Case Western Reserve University. Additionally, he earned an MS in Forensic Psychology from Arizona State University.

Currently, Dr. Stewart channels his expertise as a Board Certified Psychiatric-Mental Health Nurse Practitioner, providing compassionate care to clients in private practice. His multifaceted background and unwavering dedication to the field continue to shape the landscape of psychiatric-mental health nursing.

Abbreviations

5-HT	5-Hydroxytryptamine
AA	Alcoholics anonymous
AANP	American Association of Nurse Practitioners
ABA	Applied behavior analysis
ACA	Affordable Care Act
ACE	Adverse childhood experiences
ACEI	Angiotensin-converting enzyme inhibitor
ACEN	Accreditation Commission for Education in Nursing
ACO	Accountable Care Organizations
ACT	Assertive community treatment
ACTH	Adrenocorticotropic hormone
ADA	American Diabetes Association
ADHD	Attention Deficit Hyperactivity Disorder
ADLs	Activities of Daily Living
AE	Adverse effect
AI	Appreciative inquiry
AI/AN	American Indian/Alaska Native
AIMS	Abnormal Involuntary Movement Scale
ALP	Alkaline phosphatase
ALS	Amyotrophic lateral sclerosis
ALT	Alanine transaminase
AMPA	Alpha-amino-3-hydroxy-5-methyl-4-isoxazolepropionic acid
AN	Anorexia nervosa
ANC	Absolute neutrophil count
ANCC	American Nurses Credentialing Center
ANOVA	Analysis of Variance
ANS	Autonomic nervous system
APA	American Psychiatric Association
APNA	American Psychiatric Nurses Association
APOE	Apolipoprotein E
APRN	Advanced Practice Registered Nurse
ASD	Autism spectrum disorder
ASPD	Antisocial personality disorder
ASQ	Ages and Stages Questionnaires

AST	Aspartate transaminase
AUDIT	Alcohol Use Disorders Identification Test
BAC	Blood alcohol concentration
BDD	Body dysmorphic disorder
BDI	Beck depression inventory
BE	Binge eating disorder
BiPAP	Bilevel positive airway pressure
BMI	Body mass index
BMP	Basic metabolic panel
BN	Bulimia nervosa
BPD	Borderline personality disorder
BPSD	Behavioral and psychological symptoms of dementia
BSDS	Bipolar Spectrum Diagnostic Scale
BUN	Blood urea nitrogen
CAGE	Cut down, Annoyed, Guilty, Eye-opener
CAM	Confusion Assessment Method
CARF	Commission on Accreditation of Rehabilitation Facilities
CBC	Complete blood count
CBT	Cognitive-behavioral therapy
CBT-I	Cognitive behavioral therapy for insomnia
CCNE	Commission on Collegiate Nursing Education
CD	Conduct disorder
CDC	Centers for Disease Control and Prevention
CDI	Children's Depression Inventory
CFI	Cultural Formulation Interview
CINA	Clinical Institute Narcotic Assessment
CIWA	Clinical Institute Withdrawal Assessment
CMP	Comprehensive metabolic panel
CN	Cranial nerve
CNM	Certified Nurse Midwife
CNP	Certified Nurse Practitioner
CNS	Central nervous system
COA	Coenzyme A
COMT	Catechol-*O*-methyltransferase
COPD	Chronic obstructive pulmonary disease
COWS	Clinical Opiate Withdrawal Scale
CPAP	Continuous positive airway pressure
CPR	Cardiopulmonary resuscitation
CPS	Child protective services
C-PTSD	Complex post-traumatic stress disorder
CQI	Continuous quality improvement
CRAFFT	Car, Relax, Alone, Forget, Friends, Trouble
CRNA	Certified registered nurse anesthetist
CSF	Cerebrospinal fluid
C-SSRS	Columbia Suicide Severity Rating Scale

CT	Computed tomography
CVA	Cerebrovascular accident
CXR	Chest X-ray
CYP	Cytochrome P450
DATA	Drug Addiction Treatment Act
DBA	Depression and bipolar support alliance
DBT	Dialectical behavior therapy
DEA	Drug Enforcement Administration
DI	Diabetes insipidus
DID	Dissociative identity disorder
DKA	Diabetic ketoacidosis
DLB	Dementia with Lewy bodies
DLPFC	Dorsolateral prefrontal cortex
DMDD	Disruptive mood dysregulation disorder
DSM	Diagnostic and Statistical Manual of Mental Disorders
DT	Delirium tremens
ECT	Electroconvulsive therapy
ED	Emergency department
EEG	Electroencephalogram
EHR	Electronic health record
EKG	Electrocardiogram
EMDR	Eye movement desensitization and reprocessing
ENS	Enteric nervous system
EPDS	Edinburgh Postnatal Depression Scale
EPS	Extrapyramidal symptoms
ERP	Exposure and response prevention
FAS	Fetal alcohol syndrome
FASD	Fetal alcohol spectrum disorder
FDA	Food and Drug Administration
FFS	Fee-for-service
FMR-1	Fragile X mental retardation-1
FNSD	Functional neurological symptom disorder
GABA	Gamma-aminobutyric acid
GAD	Generalized anxiety disorder
GBMI	Guilty but mentally ill
GDS	Geriatric Depression Scale
GERD	Gastroesophageal reflux disease
GFR	Glomerular filtration rate
GGT	Gamma-glutamyl transferase
GRADE	Grading of Recommendations, Assessment, Development, and Evaluation
HA	Headache
HAM-A	Hamilton Rating Scale for Anxiety
HAM-D	Hamilton Depression Rating Scale
HBM	Health belief model

HDL	High-density lipoprotein
HEADDS	Home, Education/Employment, Activities, Drugs, Depression, Safety
HEENT	Head, Eyes, Ears, Nose, Throat
HIPAA	Health Insurance Portability and Accountability Act
HITECH	Health Information Technology for Economic and Clinical Health Act
HIV	Human immunodeficiency virus
HPA	Hypothalamic-pituitary-adrenal
HPTA	Hypothalamic-pituitary-thyroid-adrenal
HSDD	Hypoactive sexual desire disorder
HSV	Herpes simplex virus
IADL	Instrumental activities of daily living
IBR	Interest-based relational approach
IBS	Irritable bowel syndrome
ICD	International Statistical Classification of Diseases and Related Health Problems
INR	International normalized ratio
IPV	Intimate partner violence
IRB	Institutional Review Board
IRT	Image rehearsal therapy
LACE	License, Accreditation, Certification, and Education
LADLS	Lawton Instrumental Activities of Daily Living Scale
LBD	Lewy body dementia
LDL	Low-density lipoprotein
LFT	Liver function tests
LGBTQI	Lesbian, Gay, Bisexual, Transgender, Queer, Intersex
LSD	Lysergic acid diethylamide
MADRS	Montgomery-Asberg Depression Rating Scale
MAO	Monoamine oxidase
MAOI	Monoamine oxidase inhibitors
MAT	Medication-assisted treatment
MDA	Mood Disorders Association
MDD	Major depressive disorder
MDQ	Mood Disorder Questionnaire
MEG	Magnetoencephalography
MHPAEA	Mental Health Parity and Addiction Equity Act
MI	Motivational interviewing
MMSE	Mini-Mental State Examination
MoCA	Montreal Cognitive Assessment
MP	Metabolic panel
MPA	Medroxyprogesterone acetate
MRI	Magnetic resonance imaging
MS	Multiple sclerosis
N/V	Nausea/vomiting
NAC	*N*-Acetylcysteine
NACNS	National Association of Clinical Nurse Specialists

NAMI	National Alliance on Mental Illness
NCD	Neurocognitive disorders
NDRI	Norepinephrine-dopamine reuptake inhibitor
NGRI	Not guilty by reason of insanity
NHTSA	National Highway Traffic Safety Administration
NIDA	National Institute on Drug Abuse
NIMH	National Institute of Mental Health
NMDA	*N*-Methyl-D-aspartate
NMHA	National Mental Health Association
NMS	Neuroleptic malignant syndrome
NNRTI	Non-nucleoside reverse transcriptase inhibitors
NP	Nurse practitioner
NREM	Non-rapid eye movement
NSAID	Nonsteroidal anti-inflammatory drug
OCD	Obsessive-compulsive disorder
OCPD	Obsessive-compulsive personality disorder
ODD	Oppositional defiant disorder
OR	Odds ratio
OSA	Obstructive sleep apnea
PAD	Psychiatric advance directives
PANDAS	Pediatric autoimmune neuropsychiatric disorders associated with streptococcal infections
PCHM	Patient-centered medical homes
PCP	Primary care physician
PDD	Persistent depressive disorder
PDE-5	Phosphodiesterase-5
PDSA	Plan-Do-Study-Act
PE	Physical examination
PET	Positron emission tomography
PHI	Protected health information
PHQ-9	Patient Health Questionnaire 9
PICOT	Population, Intervention, Comparison, Outcome, Time
PLM	Periodic Limb Movement
PMDD	Premenstrual dysphoric disorder
PMHNP	Psychiatric-mental health nurse practitioner
PNS	Peripheral nervous system
PSD	Polysubstance dependence
PSG	Polysomnography
PTSD	Post-traumatic stress disorder
QI	Quality improvement
RAS	Reticular activating system
RCT	Randomized controlled trial
REM	Rapid eye movement
REMS	Risk evaluation and mitigation strategy
RPR	Rapid plasma reagin

SAD	Seasonal affective disorder
SARI	Serotonin antagonist and reuptake inhibitors
SBIRT	Screening, Brief Intervention, and Referral to Treatment
SCN	Suprachiasmatic nucleus
SE	Side effect
SFT	Solution-focused therapy
SIADH	Syndrome of inappropriate antidiuretic hormone
SJS	Stevens-Johnson syndrome
SLE	Systemic lupus erythematosus
SLUM	Saint Louis University Mental Status Exam
SMART	Specific, Measurable, Achievable, Relevant, Time-bound
S-MAST	Short Michigan Alcoholism Screening Test
SNRI	Serotonin-norepinephrine reuptake inhibitors
SNS	Somatic nervous system
SOC	Standard of care
SPARI	Serotonin partial agonist and reuptake inhibitor
SPECT	Single photon emission computed tomography
SSD	Somatic symptom disorder
SSRI	Selective serotonin reuptake inhibitors
STI	Sexually transmitted infection
SUD	Substance use disorder
TBI	Traumatic brain injury
TCA	Tricyclic antidepressants
TD	Tardive dyskinesia
TF-CBT	Trauma-focused cognitive behavioral therapy
TIP	Treatment Improvement Protocol
TKI	Tyrosine kinase inhibitor
TMS	Transcranial magnetic stimulation
TQM	Total quality management
TSH	Thyroid-stimulating hormone
TURP	Transurethral resection of the prostate
UA	Urinalysis
UTI	Urinary tract infection
VNS	Vagus nerve stimulation
VTA	Ventral tegmental area
WHO	World Health Organization
WKS	Wernicke-Korsakoff syndrome
WPATH	World Professional Association for Transgender Health
Y-BOCS	Yale-Brown Obsessive-Compulsive Scale
YMRS	Young Mania Rating Scale

Roles, Regulations, and Scope of Practice

1

Test your learning and check your understanding of this book's contents: use the "Springer Nature Flashcards" app to access questions.

To use the app, please follow the instructions below:

1. Go to https://flashcards.springernature.com/login
2. Create a user account by entering your e-mail address and assigning a password.
3. Use the following link to access your SN Flashcards set: ▶ https://sn.pub/62J0Ar

If the link is missing or does not work, please send an e-mail with the subject "SN Flashcards" and the book title to customerservice@springernature.com

Nurse practitioners (NPs) are advanced practice registered nurses (APRNs) who have completed advanced education and clinical training beyond their initial nursing education. They play a vital role in the healthcare system, providing high-quality, patient-centered care to individuals and families across the lifespan. Understanding the roles and responsibilities of NPs is important for both healthcare professionals and patients, as it can help to ensure that patients receive the appropriate level of care and that NPs are able to practice to the full extent of their education and training.

Nurse practitioners are regulated at both the state and national levels. Each state has its own board of nursing that sets the guidelines for NP practice, including the specific duties and responsibilities that NPs are authorized to perform. At the national level, NPs are also regulated by professional organizations such as the American Association of Nurse Practitioners (AANP) and the National Association of Clinical Nurse Specialists (NACNS). These organizations provide guidelines and standards for NP practice, as well as resources and support for NPs to continue their education and professional development.

The scope of practice for NPs varies depending on the specific role and specialty, as well as the state in which they practice. In general, NPs are trained to assess,

T. Stewart, *Psychiatric-Mental Health Nurse Practitioner Program Companion and Board Certification Exam Review Workbook*,
https://doi.org/10.1007/978-3-031-60894-0_1

diagnose, and manage acute and chronic health conditions, as well as to provide preventive care and health education. They may work in a variety of settings, including primary care clinics, hospitals, and specialty practices, and may collaborate with other healthcare professionals such as physicians and nurses to provide comprehensive care to patients. NPs are also able to prescribe medications and order diagnostic tests, within the scope of their practice and according to state laws and regulations. Overall, the roles, regulations, and scope of practice of NPs play a crucial role in ensuring that patients receive high-quality, patient-centered care.

Nurse practitioners should understand their roles, guiding regulations, and scope of practice to provide proper treatment and practice within the limits of their education and training. In this chapter, we will explore the various roles, regulations, and scope of practice of NPs, including the specific duties they can perform and the settings in which they work.

1. Match each of the nurse practitioner core competencies with its description. Then, provide an example of each competency specific to PMHNP practice

Core competency	Description	Example in PMHNP practice
_____Scientific foundations	A. Emphasizes ethical principles, legal standards, and moral norms in healthcare. It involves making principled decisions in practice	
_____Leadership	B. Involves continuously questioning clinical practice for improvement and integrating evidence into care	
_____Quality	C. Encompasses the use of information technology in healthcare and the ability to find, evaluate, and use information effectively	
_____Practice inquiry	D. Refers to the ability to influence policy, advocate for patients, and lead changes to improve health outcomes	
_____Technology and information literacy	E. Refers to the ability to practice autonomously in providing safe, high-quality care. Includes decision-making and accountability	
_____Policy	F. Understanding and influencing policies affecting health care at various levels, including organizational, local, and federal	
_____Health delivery system	G. Focuses on improving healthcare quality and patient safety through evidence-based practice and quality improvement measures	
_____Ethics	H. Involves understanding and integrating scientific principles underpinning healthcare. Covers knowledge of biophysical, psychological, and analytical sciences	
_____Independent practice	I. Involves the understanding of the healthcare system and its impact on patient care, including organizational structures and healthcare economics	

2. By whom was the nurse practitioner role first introduced? Where?

3. What are the four APRN roles identified by the License, Accreditation, Certification, and Education (LACE) model?

   1. ______________________________
   2. ______________________________
   3. ______________________________
   4. ______________________________.

4. The ______________________________ offers the only PMHNP board certification examination as of 2023.

5. What two organizations offer accreditation of nurse practitioner programs?

   1. ______________________________
   2. ______________________________

6. The ______________________ and the ______________ ______________ have legal authority to grant practice authority to nurse practitioners.

7. What does the Nurse Practice Act within a particular state cover?

8. Developed with a physician colleague, a __________________ ________ defines practice oversight and drug prescription scope for nurse practitioners within certain states.

9. When a state agency permits an individual to engage in professional practice, it is known as ______________________.

10. ______________________ ensures a minimum level of professional competence. Completing a degree program is one step in this process.

11. Professional board examinations are a step in __________________ ________, wherein an individual proves that they have met minimum standards for practice.

12. The ______________________________ is the professional organization that certifies PMHNPs as of 2023.

13. The PMHNP's scope of practice is the same from state to state.

    TRUE FALSE

14. The ____ define the quality and type of practice that a PMHNP should provide to patients, at a minimally acceptable level. These expectations are legally enforceable.

15. ____ is the agreement that verbal or written client information will not be disclosed unless a release of information has been signed.

16. What are 5 instances when a PMHNP may disclose patient information?

    1. ____
    2. ____
    3. ____
    4. ____
    5. ____

17. What are a patient's four rights under HIPAA?

    1. ____
    2. ____
    3. ____
    4. ____

18. The ____ incentivizes the use of electronic health records.

19. What qualifies an individual <18 years old as an emancipated minor?

20. What 5 pieces of information must be shared with a patient in order to qualify as informed consent?

    1. ____
    2. ____
    3. ____
    4. ____
    5. ____

21. What are the different professional roles in which a PMHNP might engage?

22. The ______________________________ approves and regulates medications and medical devices.

23. The ______________________________ regulates controlled substances at the federal level.

24. The ______________________________ tracks public health trends, aggregates data, and publishes mandates for public health and safety.

25. What is the purpose of the Affordable Care Act (2010)?

26. What are 4 assurances for patients under the ACA?

    1. ______________________________
    2. ______________________________
    3. ______________________________
    4. ______________________________

27. Name 3–5 circumstances for which a PMHNP will receive a disciplinary action.

    1. ______________________________
    2. ______________________________
    3. ______________________________
    4. ______________________________
    5. ______________________________

28. Each state's Nurse Practice Act delineates a PMHNP's ______________ ______________. This explains who is able to provide what care and where.

29. The ______________________________ is an official reference explicitly stating the rights and privileges regarding the type of practice. It further defines nurse practitioner roles and actions, identifies competencies assumed by members of the profession, guides professional practice judgment, reflects expectations of care, can be used to legally describe the profession's work, and may contain specific practice protocols and actions when a deviation occurs.

30. To what does "an NP with full practice authority" refer to?

1.1 Answers and Explanations to Chapter Activities

1.

Core competency	Example in PMHNP practice
____H______Scientific foundations	A PMHNP applying knowledge of psychopharmacology to tailor medication plans for patients with mood disorders
______D______Leadership	Leading a team to implement new protocols for patient safety in a psychiatric unit
_____G______Quality	Implementing a new patient monitoring system to reduce incidents of self-harm in inpatient care
______A______Practice inquiry	Researching the latest treatment modalities for PTSD and incorporating them into practice
______C______Technology & information literacy	Utilizing telehealth platforms to provide care to remote or underserved populations
______F______Policy	Advocating for policy changes to improve access to mental health services in rural areas
______I______Health delivery system	Working with community health organizations to develop integrated care models for mental health
_____B______Ethics	Addressing ethical dilemmas in patient confidentiality and informed consent in psychiatric settings
_____E______Independent practice	Operating a private practice where the PMHNP independently manages patient care and treatment plans

2. Drs. Loretta Ford and Henry Silver; University of Colorado.
3. Certified Registered Nurse Anesthetist (CRNA), Certified Nurse Midwife (CNM), Clinical Nurse Specialist (CNS), Certified Nurse Practitioner (CNP).
4. American Nurses Credentialing Center (ANCC).
5. Commission on Collegiate Nursing Education (CCNE), Accreditation Commission for Education in Nursing (ACEN).
6. State legislatures.
7. The Nurse Practice Act covers the use of the nurse practitioner title, what is considered advanced practice, laws covering scope, credentialing requirements, disciplinary action, and required collaborations for practice.
8. Collaborative agreement.
9. Licensure.
10. Credentialing.
11. Certification.
12. American Nurses Credentialing Center (ANCC).
13. FALSE.
14. Standards of practice.
15. Confidentiality.
16. Intent to harm, information shared with client attorneys or the courts, insurance records, reporting publicly surveilled diseases, and mandated reporting of abuse.
17. To be educated about HIPAA, access their own medical records, request amendments to their health information within their records, and require permission to disclose their information.
18. Health Information Technology for Economic and Clinical Health Act (HITECH).

19. An individual <18 years old may be considered an emancipated minor if they are married, a parent, or living independently from family.
20. Diagnosis and prognosis, description and purpose of the intervention, risks of treatment, outcomes of not undergoing treatment, and alternatives to the proposed intervention.
21. Research/scholarship, mentoring, advocacy, policy-making, case management, direct care, risk assessment, and management.
22. Food and Drug Administration (FDA).
23. Drug Enforcement Administration (DEA).
24. The Centers for Disease Control and Prevention (CDC).
25. The 2010 Affordable Care Act (ACA) aims to expand health insurance coverage through Medicaid expansion and Health Insurance Marketplaces, increase quality and efficiency, lower costs by coordinating treatment, end insurance discrimination by eliminating preexisting conditions bias, and improve health outcomes through prevention and wellness programs.
26. Allows dependent children to remain covered under their parents, insurance until age 26

    - Prohibits the rejection by insurance companies for preexisting conditions.
    - Employers are penalized if they choose not to provide health insurance to their employees.
    - Individuals are penalized if they fail to purchase health insurance.

27. Practicing without a license or proper collaboration or supervision.

    - Fraud.
    - Falsification of records, inaccurate records, and incomplete records.
    - Deviation from standards of care.
    - Failure to apply appropriate nursing judgment.

28. Scope of practice.
29. Nurse Practice Act.
30. "An NP with full practice authority" is a Nurse Practitioner (NP) who can work without physician supervision. They can independently provide healthcare services within their education, training, and certification. State rules vary, but full practice authorization may include prescribing controlled medications, interpreting diagnostic tests, and managing patient care. In some states, NPs have full practice authority, reflecting a trend toward increasingly autonomous positions in response to primary care provider shortages. It aims to increase access to care, optimize NP skills and training, and fill healthcare gaps, especially in underprivileged areas.

References and Resources

American Association of Nurse Practitioners. (2020). Standards for practice for the nurse practitioner. https://www.aanp.org/advocacy/advocacy-resource/position-statements/standards-of-practice-for-nurse-practitioners.

American Association of Nurse Practitioners. (n.d.). State practice environment. https://www.aanp.org/advocacy/state/state-practice-environment.

American Association of Nurse Practitioners (AANP) (2015). Use of terms such as mid-level provider and physician extender. https://www.aanp.org/advocacy/advocacy-resource/position-statements/use-of-terms-such-as-mid-level-provider-and-physician-extender.

American Nurses Association. Nursing: scope and standards of practice. 3rd ed. Silver Spring, MD: American Nurses Association; 2015.

American Psychiatric Association, editor. Diagnostic and statistical manual of mental disorders: DSM-5-TR. 5th ed. American Psychiatric Association Publishing; 2022.

American Psychiatric Nurses Association (APNA). Expanding Mental Health Care Services in America: The Pivotal Role of Psychiatric-Mental Health Nurses. An Informational Report Prepared by The American Psychiatric Nurses Association; 2019. https://www.apna.org/files/public/Resources/Workforce_Development_Report_Final_Draft_6_25.pdf.

Birch K, Ling A, Phoenix B. Psychiatric nurse practitioners as leaders in behavioral health integration. J Nurse Pract. 2021;17:112–5. https://doi.org/10.1016/j.nurpra.2020.09.001.

Buppert C. Nurse practitioner's business practice and legal guide. 7th ed. Jones & Bartlett Learning; 2021.

Carranza AN, Munoz PJ, Nash AJ. Comparing quality of care in medical specialties between nurse practitioners and physicians: a systematic review. J Am Assoc Nurse Pract. 2020;33(3):184–93.

Johnson K, Vanderhoef D, Magrath N. Psychiatric-mental health nurse practitioner review and resource manual. American Nurses Credentialing Center, American Nurses Association; 2020.

Kumar A, Kearney A, Hoskins K, Iyengar A. The role of psychiatric mental health nurse practitioners in improving mental and behavioral health care delivery for children and adolescents in multiple settings. Arch Psychiatr Nurs. 2020;34:275–80. https://doi.org/10.1016/j.apnu.2020.07.022.

Muench U, Fraze TK. The future of behavioral health-harnessing the potential of psychiatric mental health nurse practitioners. JAMA Netw Open. 2022;5(7):e2224365. https://doi.org/10.1001/jamanetworkopen.2022.24365.

U.S. Department of Health and Human Services. (n.d.). Health insurance portability and accountability act (HIPAA). https://www.hhs.gov/hipaa/index.html.

U.S. Drug Enforcement Administration. (n.d.). The controlled substances act. https://www.dea.gov/drug-information/csa.

Zakhari R. The psychiatric-mental health nurse practitioner certification review manual. Springer Publishing Company; 2021.

Notes:

Notes:

2 Theories and Frameworks

Test your learning and check your understanding of this book's contents: use the "Springer Nature Flashcards" app to access questions using ▶ https://sn.pub/62J0Ar.

To use the app, please follow the instructions in Chap. 1.

Theories and frameworks are important tools for nurse practitioners to understand and apply (Leininger 1991). They provide a structured approach to understanding complex phenomena and can guide decision-making and action (Rogers 1970).

Theories and frameworks in nursing organize understanding and address complicated phenomena, inform intervention and practice development, and support research and evaluation. A nurse practitioner may employ a health behavior change theory (Prochaska and DiClemente 1982) to create a program to help patients adopt healthier lifestyles. A pain management approach can assist patients using pharmaceutical and nonpharmacological therapies.

In addition to informing the development of interventions, theories and frameworks can also help nurse practitioners to better understand and communicate the underlying principles and rationale for their actions. For example, a nurse practitioner may use a theory of nursing (Peplau 1952) to explain why they are focusing on a particular aspect of care, or why they are using a specific intervention (Smith 2020). This can help to build trust and understanding with patients, as well as foster collaboration with other healthcare professionals.

Theories and frameworks enable study and assessment also (Parse 1987). Nurse practitioners can create research questions and hypotheses based on current information utilizing a well-established theory or framework (Pender et al. 2014). This can help guarantee that study findings are valuable and can inform future practice and decision-making.

This chapter focuses on models and theoretical foundations of care using a biopsychosocial framework. This chapter also introduces the learner to the classifica-

T. Stewart, *Psychiatric-Mental Health Nurse Practitioner Program Companion and Board Certification Exam Review Workbook*,
https://doi.org/10.1007/978-3-031-60894-0_2

tion of psychiatric disorders in the DSM. Developmental and foundational nursing theories that support the nurse practitioner role, along with the importance of the therapeutic relationship, are introduced.

1. ____ are frameworks for organizing and better understanding a body of knowledge. They help PHMNPs take a rational, systematic approach to patient care and decision-making.
2. Match each of the conceptual models in psychiatric care with its description.

Model	Description
_____Psychodynamic	A. Thinking processes including expectations, beliefs, memory, and patterns and how they influence feelings and behavior
_____Behavioral	B. Disease focus including etiology and diagnosis
_____Interpersonal	C. Relationships with significant others and their approval/disapproval shape an individual's self-concept
_____Cognitive	D. Learned behavior, as people are shaped by their environments and the rewards/punishment they receive therein
_____Humanistic	E. Intrapsychic processes, like conflicts, anxiety, defenses, and impulses
_____Biomedical	F. Experiences of the here and now and how humans get meaning from life through choice and responsibility

3. Each stage in Piaget's theory of cognitive development introduces new cognitive skills that help children grasp the environment and think logically. Children's thinking progresses from fundamental physical interactions to complicated, abstract thought processes. Complete the following table using Jean Piaget's cognitive growth stages.

Stage	Age Range	Description
Sensorimotor		
Preoperational		
Concrete operations		
Formal operations		

4. Complete the following chart on Erikson's developmental stages.

Name	Description	Lifespan period
Trust vs. mistrust		

Name	Description	Lifespan period
Autonomy vs. shame and doubt		
Initiative vs. guilt		
Industry vs. inferiority		
Identity vs. role confusion		
Intimacy vs. isolation		
Generativity vs. stagnation		
Ego integrity vs. despair		

5. Label each descriptor as being associated with the Id (I), Ego (E), or Superego (S).

_____Aggression
_____Conscience
_____Defense mechanisms
_____Guilt and shame
_____Hunger
_____Instinct
_____Mediator
_____Morals
_____Pleasure
_____Rational
_____Reality
_____Shaped by authority figures
_____Unconscious

6. According to Pavlov's classical conditioning, a ______________________________ response refers to the pairing of a stimulus with a response. When an individual gains a learned behavioral response, this is called ______________________________. The term ______________________________ is used if the learned response is lost.

7. According to Skinner, positive and negative reinforcers (e.g., patient phone use, off-unit movement) are used to reinforce or discourage a behavior, also known as a(n) ______________________________ behavior. These reinforcers help to change the environment and reduce the likelihood of maladaptive behaviors.

8. Put the following steps of behavior modification therapy into the correct order (1 = first step; 5 = last step).

	Identify replacements to maladaptive behavior
	Identify reinforcers that maintain maladaptive behavior
	Substitute one stimulus for another
	Target maladaptive behavior by defining it
	Identify reinforcers to discourage undesirable, and encourage desirable, behavior

9. Match each of the following treatments used in the behavioral conceptual framework with the best explanation.

Treatment	Explanation
_____Systematic desensitization	A. Practices including deep breathing, progressive muscle relaxation, and meditation alleviate stress and anxiety. These approaches lower heart rate, muscle tension, and calmness, reducing stress's psychological and physiological impacts
_____Flooding	B. A therapy that teaches straightforward, direct, and respectful expression of feelings, wishes, and rights. Teaching passive and aggressive patients how to express their demands and set limits is especially important
_____Aversive therapy	C. A phobia and anxiety treatment. Relaxation and progressive exposure to the fearful object or scenario are used. The patient learns to manage rising anxiety step-by-step, diminishing fear over time
_____Biofeedback	D. A method that eliminates bad habits with unpleasant stimuli. For instance, associating a terrible taste or smell with a harmful action like smoking to deter it
_____Relaxation techniques	E. An intense and immediate exposure therapy for the frightened object or scenario. Exposes the patient to the maximal terror intensity to swiftly eliminate anxiety
_____Assertiveness training	F. Real-time feedback teaches patients to control heart rate, muscle tension, and blood pressure. Patients notice their stress and anxiety responses and utilize relaxation techniques to control them

10. The interpersonal conceptual framework posits that human beings have two basic drives: (1) ______________________________ (e.g., basic needs) and (2) ______________________________ (e.g., culturally defined needs). The health of one's relationships determines the degree of attainment of these two drives.

11. The nurse theorist, ______________________________, developed an interpersonal theory of nursing. She is regarded as "the mother of psychiatric nursing." In order to help patients effectively solve interpersonal difficulties, psychiatric nursing professionals establish a corrective interpersonal relationship with them.

12. According to the cognitive conceptual framework, ____________________ are the automatic thoughts a person uses to evaluate his or her present situation.

13. An individual's conception of why an event is happening, arising from either external or internal to the self, is known as ______________________________.

14. The cognitive framework states that distorted thinking causes disordered behavior.

    TRUE FALSE

15. Describe the basic process of cognitive treatment led by a PMHNP.

16. ______________________________ therapy, as developed by Ellis, helps patients to dispute the underlying irrational beliefs that affect their cognitive processes.

17. Summarize the humanistic view of mental illness.

18. In Rogers' ______________________________ therapy, the therapist makes an effort to develop an empathetic relationship with the patient. Listening to the sufferer, they repeat what they comprehend. Acceptance and understanding help patients acquire self-awareness. Self-awareness brings responsibility and choice.

19. Rogers' three humanistic principles are: (1) ______________________________, (2) ____________________________________, and (3) ______________ ____________________.

20. The idea that everyone possesses the internal resources to solve their problems is at the core of ____, or embracing and assisting another person as they are, without judgment.

21. While psychotherapy has become a part of the biomedical model, ______________________________ remains the most common treatment. Adherence to the treatment regimen can be difficult.

22. In the biopsychosocial framework of care, what does recovery refer to? What are the major dimensions of recovery?

23. The ____is a publication by the American Psychiatric Association (APA) that provides a comprehensive classification and diagnostic criteria for mental disorders. It's used by mental health professionals, researchers, and policymakers across various disciplines as a standard reference for diagnosing and treating mental health conditions.

24. What is a therapeutic relationship/alliance?

25. Name 5 characteristics of a therapeutic relationship.
    1. ____
    2. ____
    3. ____
    4. ____
    5. ____

26. What is the Health Belief Model and why is it important for PMHNPs to understand?

27. List the five stages of the Transtheoretical Model of Change in order. Then, provide behaviors, factors, challenges, or strategies associated with each stage.

Stage	Description and associated elements

28. What is motivational interviewing? What are the four core principles of MI?

29. In the table below, describe each technique of motivational interviewing. Then, provide an example of how each technique may be used with a client in psychiatry-mental health.

Technique/ strategy	Description	Example in psychiatry-mental health
Open-ended questions (O)		
Affirmations (A)		
Reflective listening (R)		
Summarizing (S)		
Addressing ambivalence		
Eliciting change talk		
Dealing with resistance		

Technique/ strategy	Description	Example in psychiatry-mental health
Reflective question		

30. In the table below, compare Motivational Interviewing and traditional therapies across the various listed dimensions.

Feature/aspect	Motivational interviewing	Traditional therapies
Approach and focus		
Role of the therapist		
Goals and outcomes		
Techniques and process		
Collaboration level		
Focus on ambivalence		
Confrontation		
Outcome emphasis		
Session duration		
Technique specificity		

31. Match each of the following nursing theories with the most appropriate description.

Nursing theory	Description of main ideas
_____Hildegard Peplau's interpersonal theory	A. Develops nursing skills and knowledge in five stages. It values experiential learning and clinical judgment and expertise development. This paradigm emphasizes constant learning and adaptation to meet patients' complex needs
_____Jean Watson's theory of human caring	B. Describes the nurse–patient connection as a sequence of phases, stressing the nurse's responsibility in identifying patient needs and difficulties. It emphasizes therapeutic relationship development
_____Dorothea Orem's self-care deficit theory	C. Focuses on patient–environment relationships, emphasizing how the environment affects healing and rehabilitation and how nurses can manipulate it to promote Well-being
_____Betty Neuman's systems model	D. Recognizes that culture affects treatment. Social structure, language, religious and spiritual views, and other elements affecting the patient's worldview are examined. Understanding cultural variations and similarities is crucial to providing comprehensive and tailored care, especially in mental health, where cultural context can greatly affect patient experience and treatment
_____Florence Nightingale's environmental theory	E. Highlights self-care and the nurse's role in supporting it. Patients are educated and encouraged to be independent
_____Patricia Benner's novice to expert theory	F. Nursing is about caring. It lists ten factors to promote mind–body–soul harmony. The theory stresses nursing's humanistic and scientific features
_____Madeleine Leininger's theory of cultural care	G. Based on the idea that each patient needs a customized treatment. Understanding patients' stress responses and using primary, secondary, and tertiary preventative measures to maintain optimal health are its core goals

2.1 Answers and Explanations to Chapter Activities

1. Theoretical models.
2. __E___Psychodynamic.
   __D___Behavioral.
   __C___Interpersonal.
   __A___Cognitive.
   __F___Humanistic.
   __B___Biomedical.
3.

Stage	Age range	Description
Sensorimotor	Birth–2 years	Object permanence: The ability to understand that objects have an existence independent of the child's involvement with them
Preoperational	2–7 years	Extensive use of language and symbolism; engages in magical thinking

Stage	Age range	Description
Concrete operations	7–12 years	Begins to use logic; develops concepts of reversibility and conservation
Formal operations	12 years–adult	Ability to think abstractly, in a formal, logical manner

4.

Name	Description	Lifespan period
Trust vs. mistrust	Basic needs fulfilled; issues of trust development with significant others	Infancy
Autonomy vs. shame and doubt	Initial exploration of separation from significant others; independence; muscle control (toilet training) and self-control	Toddlerhood
Initiative vs. guilt	Examination of love and hate; explores action, sense of purpose	Preschool age
Industry vs. inferiority	Realization of competence and competition; purposeful work; perseverance tested	School age
Identity vs. role confusion	Sense of self; identification of future goals or potentials	Adolescence
Intimacy vs. isolation	Capacity for love and intimacy; commitment to relationships and work	Young adulthood
Generativity vs. stagnation	Concern for others over self; productivity; leaving a mark on society	Middle adulthood
Ego integrity vs. despair	Adjustment to life situations; life review and preparation for death	Late adulthood

5. __I___Aggression.
   __S___Conscience.
   __E___Defense mechanisms.
   __S__Guilt and shame.
   __I___Hunger.
   __I___Instinct.
   __E___Mediator.
   __S___Morals.
   __I___Pleasure.
   __E___Rational.
   __E___Reality.
   __S___Shaped by authority figures.
   __I___Unconscious.
6. Conditioning; acquisition; extinction.
7. Operant.
8.

3	Identify replacements to maladaptive behavior
2	Identify reinforcers that maintain maladaptive behavior
5	Substitute one stimulus for another
1	Target maladaptive behavior by defining it
4	Identify reinforcers to discourage undesirable, and encourage desirable, behavior

9. __C___Systematic Desensitization.
   __E___Flooding.
   __D___Aversive Therapy.
   __F___Biofeedback.
   __A___Relaxation Techniques.
   __B___Assertiveness Training.
10. Satisfaction, security.
11. Hildegaard Peplau.
12. Appraisals.
13. Attributions.
14. TRUE. The cognitive framework states that skewed thinking causes disordered behavior. CBT and other cognitive-based therapies focus on identifying and modifying maladaptive thought processes to enhance emotional control and behavioral responses.
15. PMHNPs record patients' cognition and then help the patient become more aware of their cognitive processes, especially maladaptive ones. The patient should try different ways of thinking to change their cognition. This is cognitive reorganization.
16. Rational-emotive.
17. Humanistic view posits that mental illness inhibits autonomy, accountability, and personal growth by alienating oneself. Lack of self-awareness and unmet needs impact relationships and security. The main human anxiety is death. Recovery includes self-awareness, happiness, love, and growth.
18. Client-centered
19. Unconditional positive regard, empathy, congruence/respect
20. Unconditional positive regard
21. Pharmacotherapy
22. Recovery is achieving a meaningful and satisfying life as defined by the person, not just alleviating symptoms. Even if symptoms persist, recovery is a journey that improves the quality of life and well-being across biological, psychological, and social dimensions. Biological refers to the physical or physiological aspects of health. Psychological pertains to mental health and emotional well-being. Social considers the social and environmental factors that influence one's health.
23. Diagnostic and Statistical Manual of Mental Disorders
24. Therapeutic relationships, also called therapeutic alliances, are professional and collaborative relationships between healthcare providers like therapists, counselors, and nurses and clients or patients. It is essential for treatment in all modalities and healthcare settings. The quality of this relationship greatly affects treatment success and client results.
25. Therapeutic relationships include trust, empathy, respect, genuineness, boundaries, among others.
26. The Health Belief Model (HBM) uses attitudes and beliefs to explain and predict health behaviors. The core components of the HBM include (1) an individual's perceptions of their disease risk and (2) the individual's opinion of a health behavior's benefits, elements that make individuals modify their

behavior, and an individual's belief in their ability to succeed. The HBM is important for PMHNPs to understand so that they can tailor interventions, encourage preventive behaviors, address perceived barriers and benefits, and take into account culture, among others.

27.

Stage	Description and associated elements
1. Precontemplation	Behaviors/factors: Lack of awareness or denial of problem; not considering change Challenges: Overcoming denial and increasing awareness Strategies: Education about the harm and impact of their current behavior; motivational interviewing to elicit self-motivational statements and recognition of the problem
2. Contemplation	Behaviors/factors: Acknowledging the problem; ambivalence about change Challenges: Moving from thinking to action; decisional balance Strategies: Weighing the pros and cons of changing; identifying barriers and facilitators to change; eliciting personal reasons for change; visualization of a healthier future
3. Preparation	Behaviors/factors: Intending to take action; planning for change Challenges: Developing a realistic and effective plan Strategies: Setting goals; creating an action plan; seeking support; arranging the environment to facilitate change
4. Action	Behaviors/factors: Actively engaging in behavior change; making visible modifications Challenges: Sustaining change over time; resisting temptation Strategies: Self-monitoring; seeking feedback; reinforcing success; finding healthy alternatives; using reminders and cues; continuing support and counseling
5. Maintenance	Behaviors/factors: Sustaining the change over time; integrating the behavior into their lifestyle Challenges: Preventing relapse; dealing with setbacks Strategies: Developing coping strategies for potential relapse triggers; reminding oneself of the benefits of change; seeking continued support; rewarding oneself for maintaining the change

28. Motivational Interviewing (MI) is a collaborative, person-centered approach to resolve ambivalence or reluctance to change. The core principles of Motivational Interviewing include showing empathy, developing discrepancies between patient's values and actions, rolling with resistance, promoting, and self-efficacy. Motivational Interviewing works because it respects patients' autonomy and self-direction. It is about inspiring change by aligning with someone's values and aspirations, not forcing them to act. PMHNPs must understand these principles to engage with patients in a way that is compassionate, collaborative, and more likely to result in beneficial outcomes.

29.

Technique/ strategy	Description	Example in psychiatry-mental health
Open-ended questions (O)	Questions that encourage detailed responses and exploration, allowing clients to discuss their thoughts and feelings freely	"What are your thoughts about the changes you want to make in your life?" this invites the client to explore their desires and concerns
Affirmations (A)	Positive statements that recognize a client's strengths and acknowledge behaviors that lead in the direction of positive change	"You've been very consistent in attending these sessions, which shows your commitment to change." this reinforces the client's efforts and boosts their confidence
Reflective listening (R)	A technique where the therapist listens attentively to the client and then reflects back what they hear, often rephrasing or summarizing the client's words	Client: "I'm not sure I can change." therapist: "It sounds like you're unsure about your ability to make this change right now." this shows understanding and encourages further exploration
Summarizing (S)	Providing a concise and coherent recap of what has been discussed during the session, often used to transition or conclude the session	"So today we've discussed how your anxiety affects your daily life and some strategies that might help. Does that sound right to you?" this ensures mutual understanding and sets the stage for future discussions
Addressing ambivalence	Acknowledging and discussing the client's mixed feelings or uncertainties about change to help them resolve their ambivalence and move forward	"On one hand, you feel that smoking relaxes you, but on the other, you're worried about your health. Let's explore these conflicting feelings." this validates the client's feelings and encourages deeper reflection
Eliciting change talk	Encouraging the client to express their desire, ability, reasons, and need for change, which strengthens their motivation and commitment	"What benefits do you think you would gain if you were to make this change?" this question prompts the client to articulate their own motivations for change
Dealing with resistance	Responding to the client's resistance in a nonconfrontational way, using it as an opportunity to understand their perspective and explore their reluctance	When a client objects or denies the need for change, the therapist might say, "it seems like this is a challenging idea for you. Can you tell me more about your concerns?" this approach respects the client's autonomy and encourages open discussion
Reflective question	Asking a question that prompts the client to reflect on their thoughts, feelings, or behaviors, fostering deeper self-awareness and insight	"How do you think your life might be different if you were able to make this change?" this encourages the client to envision a positive future and the impact of change

30.

Feature/aspect	Motivational interviewing	Traditional therapies
Approach and focus	Client-centered, directive, collaborative, and focused on eliciting change talk	Expert-centered, can be prescriptive, variable collaboration, focused on understanding and treating underlying issues
Role of the therapist	Acts as a facilitator, reflective listener, and adopts a nonconfrontational stance	Seen as an authority or guide, often analytical/interpretative, and can be confrontational depending on the therapy type
Goals and outcomes	Immediate behavior change, increasing self-efficacy for change	Broad or long-term psychological change, diverse goals including insight, behavioral change, and emotional processing
Techniques and process	Brief and focused, uses specific techniques like OARS, and focuses on change talk and resolving ambivalence	Varies in duration, uses a wide range of techniques depending on the therapy approach, including cognitive and dynamic tools
Collaboration level	High collaboration with the client guiding the session based on their values and motivations	Collaboration varies; some therapies are more therapist-led with structured interventions
Focus on ambivalence	Specifically addresses and explores ambivalence about change	Ambivalence may be explored but is not the central focus; more focused on diagnosis and treatment planning
Confrontation	Avoids direct confrontation, uses a gentle guiding approach to address resistance	Some traditional therapies use confrontation to challenge beliefs or behaviors directly
Outcome emphasis	Emphasizes immediate and practical changes in specific behaviors	Often addresses deeper or long-term psychological issues, with a broader range of therapeutic outcomes
Session duration	Often brief and time-limited, may require only a few sessions	Duration can vary widely from short-term to long-term treatment
Technique specificity	Uses specific MI techniques (e.g., OARS, eliciting change talk)	Employs a variety of techniques specific to the type of therapy (e.g., CBT techniques, psychodynamic interpretations)

31. Match each of the following nursing theories with the most appropriate description.

- __B___Hildegard Peplau's Interpersonal Theory.
- __F___Jean Watson's Theory of Human Caring.
- __E___Dorothea Orem's Self-Care Deficit Theory.
- __G___Betty Neuman's Systems Model.
- __C___Florence Nightingale's Environmental Theory.
- __A___Patricia Benner's Novice to Expert Theory.
- __D___Madeleine Leininger's Theory of Cultural Care.

References and Resources

American Psychiatric Association. Diagnostic and statistical manual of mental disorders. In: DSM-5-TR. 5th ed. American Psychiatric Association Publishing; 2022.

Cain DJ, Keenan K, Rubin S, editors. Humanistic psychotherapies: handbook of research and practice. 2nd ed. American Psychological Association; 2016. https://doi.org/10.1037/14775-000.

Caughill A. Preserving the art and science of psychotherapy for advanced practice psychiatric mental health nurses. Issues Ment Health Nurs. 2016;37(4):268–72. https://doi.org/10.3109/01612840.2016.1147625.

Fawcett J. Applying Conceptual Models of Nursing: Quality Improvement, Research, and Practice. Springer Publishing Company; 2016.

Haber J. Hildegard E. Peplau: the psychiatric nursing legacy of a legend. J Am Psychiatr Nurses Assoc. 2000;6(2):56–62. https://doi.org/10.1016/S1078-3903(00)90021-1.

Hansen BS, Dysvik E. Expanding the theoretical understanding in advanced practice nursing: framing the future. Nurs Forum. 2022;57:1593–8. https://doi.org/10.1111/nuf.12827.

Johnson K, Vanderhoef D, Magrath N. Psychiatric-mental health nurse practitioner review and resource manual. American Nurses Credentialing Center, American Nurses Association; 2020.

Kim H. The role of theory in clinical nursing practice. Klin Sygepleje. 2012;26:16–29.

Leininger MM. Culture care diversity and universality: a theory of nursing. National League for Nursing; 1991.

McFarland MR, Wehbe-Alamah HB. Leininger's theory of culture care diversity and universality: an overview with a historical retrospective and a view toward the future. J Transcult Nurs. 2019;30(6):540–57. https://doi.org/10.1177/1043659619867134.

Parse RR, Barrett E, Bourgeois M, Dee V, Egan E, Germain C, King I, Koerner J, Neuman B, Newman M, Roy C, Walker L, Watson J, Wolf G. Nursing theory-guided practice: a definition. Nurs Sci Q. 2000;13(2):177. https://doi.org/10.1177/08943180022107474.

Parse RR. Nursing science: major paradigms, theories, and critiques. W.B. Saunders; 1987.

Pender NJ, Murdaugh CL, Parson MA. Health promotion in nursing practice. 7th ed. Pearson; 2014.

Peplau HE. Interpersonal relations in nursing: a conceptual frame of reference for psychodynamic nursing. G.P. Putnam's Sons; 1952.

Prochaska JO, DiClemente CC. Transtheoretical therapy: toward a more integrative model of change. Psychother: Theory, Res Practice. 1982;19(3):276–88. https://doi.org/10.1037/h0088437.

Rogers ME. An introduction to the theoretical basis of nursing. Am J Nurs. 1970;71(10):2026–7.

Smith MC, editor. Nursing theories and nursing practice. 5th ed. Davis: F.A; 2020.

Wedding D, Corsini RJ, editors. Current psychotherapies. 11th ed; 2018. Cengage

Wheeler K. Psychotherapy for the advanced practice psychiatric nurse: a how-to guide for evidence-based practice. 2nd ed. Springer Publishing Company; 2013.

Wortans J, Happell B, Johnstone H. The role of the nurse practitioner in psychiatric/mental health nursing: exploring consumer satisfaction. J Psychiatr Ment Health Nurs. 2006;13:78–84. https://doi.org/10.1111/j.1365-2850.2006.00916.x.

Wilson R, Godfrey CM, Sears K, Medves J, Ross-White A, Lambert N. Exploring conceptual and theoretical frameworks for nurse practitioner education: a scoping review protocol. JBI Database System Rev Implement Rep. 2015;13:146–55. https://doi.org/10.11124/jbisrir-2015-2150.

Zakhari R. The psychiatric-mental health nurse practitioner certification review manual. Springer Publishing Company; 2021.

Notes:

Notes:

3 Ethics and Legal Principles

Test your learning and check your understanding of this book's contents: use the "Springer Nature Flashcards" app to access questions using ▶ https://sn.pub/62J0Ar.

To use the app, please follow the instructions in Chap. 1.

Ethics and legal principles are of central importance for Psychiatric-Mental Health Nurse Practitioners (PMHNPs) as they help to guide decision-making, ensure patient safety, and maintain the integrity of the nursing profession. In order to provide high-quality care, PMHNPs must remain familiar with, and adhere to, both ethical and legal principles.

Ethical principles provide guidance on how to behave in a way that is fair, honest, and respectful toward others. In the healthcare profession, this includes treating patients with dignity and respect, protecting patient confidentiality, and avoiding conflicts of interest. PMHNPs must also be aware of ethical principles related to informed consent, beneficence (doing what is best for the patient), non-maleficence (avoiding harm to the patient), and autonomy (respecting the patient's right to make decisions about their own care) (American Nurses Association 2015; Fry and Veatch 2012; Purtilo and Doherty 2017).

Legal principles, on the other hand, are rules and regulations created by the government to safeguard the public. In the healthcare profession, this includes laws related to the practice of nursing, such as the requirement to obtain a license in order to practice, as well as laws related to patient privacy and confidentiality, such as the Health Insurance Portability and Accountability Act (HIPAA). PMHNPs must be aware of these legal principles in order to practice safely and effectively within the bounds of the law (U.S. Department of Health and Human Services 2021).

PMHNPs must prioritize ethics and law. These values underpin nursing and assist PMHNPs in providing safe, effective, and compassionate care. Understanding

T. Stewart, *Psychiatric-Mental Health Nurse Practitioner Program Companion and Board Certification Exam Review Workbook*,
https://doi.org/10.1007/978-3-031-60894-0_3

these principles will also assist PMHNPs avoid legal and ethical infractions that could potentially harm their patients or their own careers.

This chapter introduces the key areas of ethics as they relate to psychiatric nursing and PMHNP practice. Legal principles and key court cases about duty to warn, involuntary hospitalization, and right to refuse are presented. Lastly, client rights and conflicts of interest are discussed.

3.1 Ethics

1. Match each approach to ethical decision-making with its description.

1. __________Deontological	A. Action based on the action only; no consequences are taken into account
2. __________Teleological	B. Action based on the morality of the individual completing the act or making the decision
3. __________Utilitarianism	C. Action based on the expected outcome; the act itself is not considered
4. __________Virtue ethics	D. Action based on if it will produce the greatest good for the greatest number

2. A(n) ____ refers to a conflict between various courses of action based on their potential positive/negative outcomes.

3. Match each of the following bioethical principles with its key characteristics.

Principle	Characteristics
1. __________Beneficence	A. Distribution of resources/care without regard to individual attributes.
2. __________Autonomy	B. Promote good of client.
3. __________Justice	C. Loyalty and commitment to patient
4. __________Fidelity	D. Doing no wrong to a client
5. __________Veracity	E. Acknowledging rights of a client to make own decisions
6. __________Nonmaleficence	F. Communicating truthfully

4. A(n) ____ develops when the PMHNP's personal circumstances interfere with their ability to make unbiased clinical judgments. These circumstances may include financial, personal, or professional loss or gain.

5. Which of the following is a conflict of interest and should be reported or avoided completely? Mark your answers with an X.

   _____Gift from a patient.

   _____Consultancy with a pharmaceutical company.

   _____Client's public rating of your office's services and professionalism.

   _____Referrals from another PMHNP in the same company.

   _____Establishing a direct referral system with a medical provider between your clients, and then splitting the income between the two offices.

______Former patient of 5 years who moved out of state sent cookies to your office staff.

______Receiving samples of new antidepressants to distribute to clients.

______Acting as therapist for two new clients—a husband and wife, as they go through a divorce. Other providers are available.

______Your next door neighbor receives news at 7 pm on Saturday evening that her parents died in a car accident. Her PCP does not have on-call services on the weekend. You prescribe her clonazepam 0.5 mg #10 to assist with her anxiety. The pharmacy closes at midnight.

______A PMHNP helps a client plan her wedding.

6. How often does a provider need to disclose potential conflicts of interest? To whom?

7. What types of documentation in a medical record evidence objectivity by the PMHNP?

3.2 Legal Principles

8. Name at least five patient's rights.
    1.
    2.
    3.
    4.
    5.

9. The ____ of 1963 deinstitutionalized the mentally ill, shifting care toward community-based options, use of psychotropics, and community integration.

10. What is parity with regard to mental health insurance?

11. If committed involuntarily, a patient loses their ability to make decisions about their healthcare.
    TRUE FALSE

12. What circumstances must be present for a patient to be eligible for involuntary commitment 1to a psychiatric unit?

13. If a patient feels that they have been unlawfully detained and denied due process, they may file a petition called ______________________________ ______________ to a court.

14. Provide a brief explanation of the main takeaways with regard to mental healthcare for each of the following court cases.

Court case	Ruling
Tarasoff v. regents of university of California	
Rennie v. Klein	
Rogers v. Okin (commissioner of the Department of Mental Health)	
Canterbury v. Spence	

Court case	Ruling
Donaldson v. O'Connor	
Durham v. US	
Ford v. wainwright	
Dusky v. US	

15. Define testamentary capacity.

16. Patient confidentiality can never be broken. The closed door of a PMHNP is a sacred space.
    TRUE FALSE

17. The PMHNP has ordered Ativan 1 mg IM q4 hours for a catatonic patient. The patient does not speak when asked if she consents. However, the patient rolls up her sleeve. The patient has provided ____ ________________.

18. Compare and contrast capacity and competency.

Capacity	**Competency**

19. Individuals with a severe mental illness, who would like to specify their wishes about care during acute episodes or disability, may complete a ______________ ______________________________ in some states. This document may identify their preferred treating provider, medical power of attorney, medication preferences or therapies, preferred facilities, and visitation/release of information permissions.

20. Seclusion and restraint orders may be written "as needed" for 24 h at a time.

    TRUE FALSE

21. ______________________________ is professional negligence, a type of unintentional tort. What are the five elements required to prove this type of negligence?
    1.
    2.
    3.
    4.
    5.

22. Upon entry to the geriatric psychiatry inpatient unit, the PMHNP notices that numerous patients in the day area are seated in geri chairs with tray tables

placed in front of them. They are unable to get up on their own. The PMHNP asks the nurses about the setup. The nurses explain that they are short-staffed and these patients are "wanderers." The PMHNP explains to the nurses that what they are doing is considered ____ ______________________.

23. The ____ __ Act aims to protect employees with mental illnesses, and other disabilities, from discrimination due to disclosure to employers. Employers with at least __________ employees must provide reasonable accommodations to applicants and employees self-identifying with a disability.

24. Malpractice insurance will provide financial protection for nurse practitioners who practice outside of their scope of practice.
    TRUE FALSE

25. Label each description with the name of the type of negligence needed to prove malpractice

Type of negligence	Description
	Providing reasonable care to client
	The standard of care was violated while treating the client
	The violation of standard of care and reported injuries are causally linked
	The violation of the standard of care caused negative outcomes to the client

26. ____________________________________ determines that an individual is able to make reasonable judgments and decisions regarding their well-being, including health concerns.

27. ____________________________________ refers to the involuntary admission and evaluation of an individual who is deemed at risk to self or others due to a psychiatric illness and who will receive treatment likely to improve their condition.

28. When an individual is involuntarily admitted to a psychiatric unit, they forfeit all of their civil liberties.
    TRUE FALSE

29. An individual who voluntarily admits themselves for psychiatric care maintains all of their civil liberties
    TRUE FALSE

30. A ____ documents an individual's healthcare preferences regarding medical treatment and end-of-life care should they become unable to make decisions for themselves.

31. An individual who makes healthcare decisions for another person is a _______ ____.

32. ____ are increasingly recommended for clients with severe mental illnesses to designate their preferences for care in the case of relapse. Currently, <30 states offer these plans.

33. What are open note laws? What do they mean for practice as a PMHNP?

34. What federal statute protects a client's right to not have their healthcare information disclosed by their healthcare provider?

35. As long as a psychiatric-mental health nurse practitioner provides written information about confidentiality, they do not have to discuss confidentiality issues with patients.

    TRUE FALSE

36. What are the four patient rights guaranteed under HIPAA?
    1.
    2.
    3.
    4.

37. What is the Health Information Technology for Economic and Clinical Health Act (HITECH) of 2009?

38. Practitioners offering telehealth services must account for the emergency care of their clients.

    TRUE FALSE

39. Name at least five examples of when confidentiality may be broken by the nurse practitioner.
    1.
    2.
    3.
    4.
    5.

40. A provider is guilty of ____________________________ when they practice below the standard of care.

41. What are the four conditions that must be proven by a preponderance of evidence to prove a claim of malpractice?
    1.
    2.
    3.
    4.

42. ____________________________ damages provide the harmed patient with monies to cover medical expenses, lost salary, or physical suffering.

43. Money awarded to the harmed patient in order to punish a provider found guilty of malpractice is called ____________________________ damages.

44. What are exceptions to maintaining confidentiality in a PMHNP-patient relationship?

45. Explain the obligations of the PMHNP under the Tarasoff Rule.

46. What are three situations that do not require informed consent?
    1.
    2.
    3.

47. What are the four elements of informed consent?
    1.
    2.
    3.
    4.

48. It is assumed that informed consent has been obtained with the completion of an intake note by the PMHNP.
    TRUE FALSE

49. Under what conditions are minors considered emancipated?

50. Competence is a clinical term and may be assessed by a physician.
    TRUE FALSE

51. ______________________________ is a legal term, decided only by a judge.

52. To have decisional capacity, a patient must be able to:
    1.
    2.
    3.
    4.

53. When considering the role of guardians and conservators, what is meant by the term "substituted judgment"?

54. Provide three contrasting explanations of voluntary and involuntary admission to psychiatric hospitals.

Voluntary	vs.	Involuntary

55. Involuntary commitment is supported by two legal principles: (1) ____________________________________, or protecting citizens from each other, and (2) ______________________________________, or protecting citizens who can't care for themselves.

56. What is the difference between mental impairment and mental disability? How can a PMHNP determine if an individual with a mental impairment also has mental disability?

57. The legal case ______________________________________ determined that an individual who is not mentally competent cannot stand trial.

58. ______________________________________ differs from Not Guilty by Reason of Insanity in that it does not recognize any criminal insanity defense at all.

59. The ______________________________ is the most stringent test to determine if an individual did not understand what they were doing or its wrongfulness, which a crime is committed.

60. The court case ______________________________________ __ holds that evidence must be generally accepted by the appropriate scientific community.

3.3 Answers and Explanations to Chapter Activities

1. 1/A, 2/C, 3/D, 4/B
2. An ethical dilemma is a decision-making situation involving conflicting morals. In an ethical dilemma, there are no clear solutions; thus, the decision-maker must weigh the pros and drawbacks of each option and evaluate the ethical implications. To address ethical difficulties, decision-makers must assess the advantages and cons of each option and choose the one that best fits their values.
3. 1/B, 2/E, 3/A, 4/C, 5/F, 6/D
4. A conflict of interest develops when a person or organization acts in their personal or relationship interests rather than those of their clients. A PMHNP may have a conflict of interest if they have financial or personal contact with a patient or group that could influence treatment. To avoid conflicts of interest, healthcare providers must declare any financial or personal relationships that may influence their decisions and base clinical decisions on the best evidence and the patient's best interest. This may include disclosing potential conflicts of interest to patients and coworkers, recusing themselves from personal interest decisions, and maintaining ethical and professional standards. Resolving conflicts of interest helps healthcare workers protect patients and public trust.
5. __X___Gift from a patient.
   __X___Consultancy with a pharmaceutical company.
   __X___Establishing a direct referral system with a medical provider between your clients, and then splitting the income between the two offices.
   __X___Acting as a therapist for two new clients—a husband and wife, as they go through a divorce. Other providers are available.
   __X___A PMHNP helps a client plan her wedding.
6. Notify affected parties of potential conflicts of interest when they occur. Otherwise, annual disclosure is normal. This involves alerting patients, coworkers, and other stakeholders affected by the provider's choice.

7. Direct client comments, quotes, and validated instrument/scale data can support the PMHNP's assessment and treatment plan. Direct client statements and quotes disclose patient thoughts, feelings, and impressions. These comments demonstrate that the PMHNP is evaluating the patient's subjective experiences rather than making biased or prejudiced assumptions. Objective data from validated instruments and scales can support the PMHNP's assessment and treatment plan. Since they were developed and tested, these instruments measure specific symptoms or disorders accurately.
8.
    - The right to informed consent.
    - The right to privacy and confidentiality.
    - The right to receive appropriate care and treatment.
    - The right to refuse treatment.
    - The right to access their medical records.
    - Healthy and safe environment.
    - Participation in decision-making.
    - Consent and withdraw it at any time.
    - Access to healthcare.
    - Knowledge of one's health.
    - Insurance/medical aid scheme.
    - Choice of health services.
    - Treated by a named healthcare provider.
    - Confidentiality and privacy.
    - Treatment in the least restrictive environment.
9. The 1963 Community Mental Health Act deinstitutionalized the mentally ill, promoting community-based care, psychotropics, and community integration.
10. Mental health insurance must cover mental health and substance use disorders at the same level as physical health conditions. This law expands mental health treatments. The Affordable Care Act and Paul Wellstone and Pete Domenici Mental Health Parity and Addiction Equity Act are notable.
11. FALSE. Involuntary commitment to a mental health hospital may restrict a patient's independence and autonomy, but it does not necessarily take away their healthcare decisions. Involuntary commitment is usually used to treat and support mentally ill people who may harm themselves or others. Although their freedom may be limited, patients are entitled to obtain information about their condition, participate in treatment decisions as much as they can, and preserve certain healthcare rights. A court may appoint a guardian or conservator to make healthcare decisions for an involuntarily confined person. This is not automatic and requires a legal process to determine guardianship or conservatorship. The rules and regulations of a patient's jurisdiction and their situation will determine their rights and decision-making competence.
12. Involuntary psychiatric unit commitment requires different circumstances based on the jurisdiction and laws and regulations. They may include:

- Grave Disability: The patient must be unable to provide food, shelter, and medical care owing to mental illness.
- Treatment Refusal: The patient must decline or be unable to consent to mental health treatment.
- Imminent Risk of Harm: The patient must be at imminent risk of serious harm to themselves or others without psychiatric care.
- Whenever possible, voluntary treatment is preferred to forced commitment. When the foregoing criteria are met, involuntary commitment may be essential to protect the patient and others.

13. Patients might submit a habeas corpus petition if they believe they were wrongfully held and denied due process. A writ of habeas corpus permits detainees to contest their detention and seek freedom. Many legal systems and constitutions provide it as a fundamental right.
14.

Court case	Ruling
Tarasoff v. Regents of University of California	Mental health professionals have a duty to protect individuals who may be at risk of harm from a patient, even if that requires breaching patient confidentiality. Known as "duty to warn"
Rennie v. Klein	A psychiatrist may be held liable for negligence if they fail to adequately warn potential victims of harm from their patient
Rogers v. Okin (commissioner of the Department of Mental Health)	Individuals involuntarily committed to a mental health facility have the right to receive treatment in the least restrictive environment possible
Canterbury v. Spence	Patients have a right to receive information about the risks and benefits of medical treatment, and healthcare providers have a duty to provide that information in a manner that the patient can understand
Donaldson v. O'Connor	Individuals with mental illnesses have a right to receive treatment in the least restrictive environment possible and to be protected from unnecessary confinement
Durham v. US	The insanity defense may be used if the defendant's crime was the result of a mental disease or defect
Ford v. Wainwright	The execution of individuals with mental illnesses or intellectual disabilities is cruel and unusual punishment and is therefore unconstitutional
Dusky v. US	Defendants must have the mental capacity to understand the charges against them and to assist in their defense in order to stand trial

15. Testamentary capacity is the mental ability to make a valid will. For a will to be legally valid, the testator (the person making the will) must have the mental capacity to understand its nature and effect and to appreciate their property and the people who would normally benefit from it. Wills may be invalidated if the testator lacks testamentary ability. If the testator had a mental illness or dementia when they made the will, testamentary ability may be questioned.

16. FALSE. Patient confidentiality is an important ethical ideal in healthcare, although it might be compromised to protect the patient or others. These conditions may include:

    - Duty to Warn: A PMHNP may have to warn potential victims or take other measures to protect a patient who may hurt herself or others. To prevent harm, confidentiality may need to be broken.
    - Child Abuse or Neglect: PMHNPs must report suspected child abuse or neglect to authorities by law. To safeguard the child, confidentiality may need to be broken.
    - Court Order: A subpoena or other legal procedure may require the release of patient information.
    - PMHNPs should keep patient confidentiality as much as possible and only break it when necessary. Understanding that secrecy is not an absolute right may necessitate balancing it with other ethical values, legal responsibilities, and patient safety and well-being concerns.

17. Implied consent occurs when a patient's behaviors or conduct imply they assent to medical treatment without vocal or written consent. If the patient rolls up her sleeve, she may be willing to undergo the Ativan injection. Verbal or written consent is desirable, however, it may not be practicable or practical in some cases. PMHNPs may utilize clinical judgment to assess if implied consent is appropriate and describe the circumstances in the patient's medical record.
18.

Capacity	Competency
Refers to a person's ability to make decisions about their healthcare and other important aspects of their life.	Refers to a person's ability to participate in legal proceedings, such as a trial or hearing
Usually evaluated on a case-by-case basis and depends on a person's ability to understand the relevant information, weigh the risks and benefits of different options, and communicate their decision in a meaningful way.	Typically evaluated using specific legal standards and procedures and can have significant implications for a person's legal rights and outcomes
Can be affected by a variety of factors, such as mental illness, cognitive impairment, and substance use.	Depends on a person's ability to understand the nature and consequences of the legal proceedings, communicate effectively with their attorney, and make decisions about their defense
Has implications for a person's ability to make informed decisions about their healthcare and other important aspects of their life.	Has implications for a person's legal rights and outcomes in legal proceedings
Ability to make informed decisions	Degree of mental soundness to make decisions or complete tasks
Can change quickly	If incompetent, provide legal guardian to consent and make decisions for the patient
Medical determination	Legal term

19. Patients with serious mental illness can complete a psychiatric advance directive (PAD) to express their care preferences during acute impairment in several states. A psychiatric advance directive helps mentally ill persons say how they want to be treated during acute illness or disability. Their preferred doctor, medical power of attorney, prescription preferences, facilities, and visitation/release of information authorization may be included. Even if they cannot express their views, psychiatric advance directives ensure that mentally ill patients receive treatment that suits them.
20. FALSE. Except for pediatrics, orders are 24 h, however, emergency orders are required. Once unbound, the patient needs a new order.
21. Tort malpractice without intent is professional negligence. Five elements prove malpractice:
    - Patient care was the provider's legal duty.
    - Failure to offer adequate care.
    - Nonperformance hurts the sufferer.
    - Violating duty caused patient damage.
    - A provider's negligence hurt the patient.
22. FALSE incarceration. The PMHNP warns nurses that they are breaching patient rights. Nurses and PMHNP should create non-restraint roaming management.
23. Employee disclosure discrimination against mentally ill and disabled workers is prohibited by the ADA. Employers of 15 or more must accommodate disabled candidates and workers. According to law, a disability is a physical or mental impairment that significantly impairs one or more major life functions, such as walking, talking, hearing, seeing, or learning. Employers must provide reasonable accommodations for disabled applicants and workers without undue hardship under the ADA. Disability-related work schedule, duty, and setting changes may be reasonable accommodations. Disability discrimination in hiring, firing, promotion, and pay is another ADA violation. Medical information must be kept private by employers.
24. FALSE. Nurse practitioners are not covered by malpractice insurance if they practice outside of their scope.
25. Near Cause, Duty, Breach, Damages.
26. Decisional capacity implies making reasonable health and well-being decisions.
    - Health and medical decision-making rely on an individual's capacity. A patient's capacity is usually assessed by their ability to absorb pertinent information, understand potential consequences, and communicate their decision clearly and consistently.
27. Involuntary commitment involves admitting and evaluating a psychiatric patient who is a risk to themselves or others and will receive treatment. Involuntary commitment guidelines normally balance mental illness protection with individual rights and freedoms.
28. FALSE. Involuntarily hospitalized psychiatric patients retain civil liberties. Although the law protects people, involuntary admission may limit freedom

and autonomy, such as hospitalization or medication. Humane and dignified treatment, medical and mental healthcare, and legal knowledge are rights of involuntarily admitted psychiatric patients.

29. TRUE. Civil freedoms are frequently preserved when someone voluntarily receives mental care. They can refuse treatment, make care decisions, and leave the facility at any time (based on evaluation) if they are not a threat to themselves or others. Individuals' individuality and autonomy may be reduced even if they voluntarily enter mental facilities. Staff may restrict guests, phone use, and other activities. Even if they self-admitted, psychiatric crisis patients may be involuntarily admitted and treated if they become a threat.
30. If unable to communicate, a living will documents medical and end-of-life intentions. A person's living will frequently contains medical preferences like mechanical breathing, tube feeding, and CPR. This may include painkillers and other comfort measures.
31. Healthcare decisions are made by a proxy/surrogate or durable power of attorney.
32. Significant mental illness patients are increasingly recommended to have psychiatric advance directives (PADs) to define care preferences in case of relapse.
33. Providers must disclose clinical notes and medical records to patients and their families under open note regulations. These regulations attempt to increase patient–provider communication and empower patients to make healthcare decisions. Each state's laws may allow PMHNPs to share clinical notes and medical information with patients and their families.
34. Healthcare clients' privacy is protected under HIPAA. HIPAA protects medical records and other personal health information nationwide. Under the Privacy Rule, healthcare providers must preserve patients' health information and seek written agreement before using or disclosing it for non-treatment, payment, or operations. People can examine, copy, and request adjustments to their medical records under the Privacy Rule. The Privacy Rule fines or disqualifies healthcare practitioners who violate patients' privacy rights.
35. FALSE. Informed consent in mental health treatment requires written confidentiality information, but it is not enough to guarantee patients understand their rights and confidentiality limits. Professionally and ethically, PMHNPs must discuss confidentiality with patients and address concerns. Keep discussing confidentiality during treatment. When required to report or warn or protect, PMHNPs should tell patients of what information will be kept confidential and when it may be revealed.
36. HIPAA safeguards four patient rights:

    - See and copy sensitive health data. Patients can review and correct medical records.
    - Right to control PHI use and dissemination. Patients can ask their doctors to restrict PHI use and disclosure, such as to certain parties.
    - Secret communication requests. Patients can request paper or phone PHI communication from their doctors.

- Reporting rights violations. HIPAA violations can be reported to HHS by patients.

37. To improve US healthcare quality and efficiency, HITECH pushed EHR and other HIT use. Healthcare providers receive HITECH incentives for EHR and HIT adoption and meaningful usage. Expanded HIPAA enforcement and fines for noncompliance improve health information privacy and security.
38. TRUE. Emergency plans are required for telehealth providers. Telehealth practitioners need emergency management protocols for directing patients to in-person or emergency services and following up. Emergency care and legal compliance can help telehealth providers provide high-quality care and improve patient safety.
39. Law and ethics require healthcare providers to protect patients' privacy. Sometimes confidentiality must be broken to protect patients or others. The nurse practitioner may compromise confidentiality:

    - Healthcare providers must report suspected child, elder, or self-harm in many countries.
    - Healthcare practitioners may need to warn clients of potential violence or injury.
    - Court orders or subpoenas: Doctors may have to reveal patient data.
    - Insurance and other third-party payers may require healthcare providers to share information for billing and reimbursement.
    - Collaboration and treatment: Clinicians may need to share confidential patient information or collaborate to provide coordinated care. Patient care providers, consultants, and specialists may receive information.

40. Malpractice happens when a provider falls below the standard of care, which is reasonable and careful practice.
41. Evidence must predominate for four malpractice situations. There are four conditions:

    - Medical professionals have a legal and ethical duty to treat patients.
    - Healthcare providers breached duty when they fell short of professional standards. Evidence from experts and others sets the standard of treatment.
    - Healthcare provider negligence hurt the patient. An action or inaction by the provider must cause injury.
    - Damages: Duty violation hurt the patient. Damages may be physical, emotional, financial, or other.

42. Compensatory damages cover medical expenditures, lost wages, and pain and suffering.
43. Punitive damages deter healthcare providers from acts of extreme or irresponsibility. Instead of compensating patients, punitive damages benefit society. All malpractice claims don't award punitive damages. They are frequently imposed on flagrant or malicious healthcare providers. Punitive damages may be limited or commensurate to patient harm in some jurisdictions.

44. PMHNPs must maintain confidentiality, although they may compromise it to protect patients or others. Examples of PMHNP-patient confidentiality exceptions:

- Healthcare providers must report suspected child, elder, or self-harm in many countries.
- Healthcare practitioners may need to warn clients of potential violence or injury.
- Court orders or subpoenas: Doctors may have to reveal patient data.
- Insurance and other third-party payers may require healthcare providers to share information for billing and reimbursement.
- Collaboration and treatment: Clinicians may need to share confidential patient information or collaborate to provide coordinated care. Patient care providers, consultants, and specialists may receive information.
- When a patient is in imminent danger, a PMHNP may need to release confidential patient information to authorities or take other measures to protect the patient and others.

45. Healthcare practitioners, including PMHNPs, must warn or take other reasonable efforts to protect patients under the Tarasoff rule. This may involve:

- A PMHNP must notify and protect potential victims if they believe a patient is a significant hazard.
- When a patient poses a significant risk to self or others, a PMHNP may call the police.
- Hospitalization: A PMHNP may hospitalize a dangerous patient.

46. Healthcare providers may provide emergency care without informed permission.

- If informed consent could hurt a patient, doctors may withhold information or treatment. In clinical trials or research studies where informed consent is impossible, patients may waive their rights.

47. Four components of informed consent:

- Healthcare decisions must be made by patients. Understanding the information and choice consequences is crucial.
- Information: The patient must know the therapy's risks, benefits, alternatives, and side effects.
- Understand: The patient must demonstrate understanding of the topic and choice consequences. Clarification from their doctor may assist.
- Voluntary consent: The patient must consent independently. Healthcare autonomy is needed.
- Any medical practice needs these four elements for informed patient consent. Professionals must provide clear and complete information about healthcare options so patients can make educated decisions. Informed consent helps doctors empower patients to make smart decisions.

48. FALSE. Providers must regularly advise patients about their treatment options, including risks, benefits, and alternatives. After discussing informed consent, the patient can ask questions and clarify healthcare issues. Written documents or other resources from healthcare providers may assist patients decide.

Discussions, written materials, and other informed consent resources should be in the patient's medical record. Patients can understand their healthcare options and protect healthcare personnel in court with this paperwork.

49. A juvenile can become emancipated before 18 if they married, living independently and managing their own affairs, have children, in military service, or directly by courts.
50. FALSE. To determine competence, courts assess cognitive and functional ability. But clinically, capacity means a patient's ability to make life or healthcare decisions. Informed decision-making and information comprehension are assessed by healthcare providers.
51. Only judges may assess competence.
52. Patients must decide:

    - The patient must understand their medical condition, treatment risks and benefits, and choice outcomes.
    - The patient must comprehend their medical condition and how their choices affect their health.
    - Reason: Patients must rationally assess facts and make decisions.
    - Express: Patients must articulate their choices.
    - Clinicians evaluate patients' healthcare decision-making. This assessment helps patients make best-interest decisions. For incompetent patients, doctors may appoint a legal guardian or surrogate.

53. "Substituted judgment" occurs when a court appoints a guardian or conservator to make decisions for an incapable member. In these situations, the guardian or conservator must make decisions that benefit the person they represent and reflect their beliefs, preferences, and perspectives. The person empowered to make decisions for an incapacitated individual may not share their values or preferences. Family, friends, and healthcare providers who know the person's intentions and values may help the guardian or conservator review written instructions or advance directives.
54.

	Voluntary admission	Involuntary admission
1.	Patient voluntarily seeks treatment and agrees to be admitted to a psychiatric facility	Patient is admitted to a psychiatric hospital against their will
2.	Patient has the right to make decisions about their treatment and can choose to leave the facility at any time	Patient may be required to remain in the facility and undergo treatment until they are deemed to be no longer a danger to themselves or others
3.	Patient retains control over their treatment and can refuse or consent to specific treatments, medications, or therapies	Patient may be required to undergo treatment, medication, or therapy without their consent, if it is deemed necessary to address their condition and ensure their safety
4.	May be a less restrictive option as the patient maintains some degree of control over their treatment	May be more restrictive as the patient may be required to remain in the facility and undergo treatment until they are deemed to be no longer a danger to themselves or others

55. Police power protects citizens from each other and harm. Parens patriae permits the government to interfere if a mental disease prevents self-care.
56. The phrases "mental impairment" and "mental disability" are typically interchangeable, but their meanings vary by context. A mental impairment is any condition that impairs mental functioning, such as a mental disease, developmental issue, or cognitive impairment. However, a mental disability is usually a more severe and long-term impairment that severely affects daily activities and social participation. Mentally impaired people must be assessed for mental disability by PMHNPs. A thorough evaluation of the patient's medical history, symptoms, and functional abilities can do this. Standardized tests may be used by the PMHNP to examine cognitive, social, and adaptive skills. The PMHNP must consider the severity of the impairment, the individual's age and developmental stage, and the impact of the impairment on daily life and independence to determine if an individual with a mental impairment has a mental disability. The PMHNP may also include the person's social and cultural background and any other physical or medical issues that may be affecting their disability.
57. Dusky v. United States established that mentally incompetent defendants cannot stand trial. This 1960 Supreme Court case set the criterion for assessing a person's ability to stand trial in federal court. The court found that a defendant must have "sufficient present ability to consult with his lawyer with a reasonable degree of rational understanding" and a "rational as well as factual understanding of the proceedings against him." Many US state and federal courts apply this test to determine competency to stand trial.
58. Unlike "not guilty by reason of insanity" (NGRI), "guilty but mentally ill" (GBMI) does not recognize any criminal insanity defense. A defendant with a GBMI plea may be judged guilty yet have a mental condition or defect that contributed to their offense. GBMI permits the offender to obtain psychiatric therapy while serving their sentence, but they are still liable for their acts and must complete their term. In contrast, the NGRI plea permits a defendant to claim mental illness or defect absolves them of guilt. Instead of prison, the defendant may be confined to a mental health hospital if the plea is accepted. The GBMI plea is not accepted in all states and its use varies. Both GBMI and NGRI pleas are contentious because some believe they allow dangerous offenders to avoid accountability.
59. The M'Naghten rule is the strictest criteria for whether a criminal did not grasp their actions or their wrongfulness. In 1843, Daniel M'Naghten attempted to assassinate the British Prime Minister but was acquitted due to insanity. The M'Naghten rule requires that the defendant did not recognize the nature and quality of their actions or that they were wrong at the time of the offense to establish insanity. Many US and international jurisdictions use the M'Naghten rule.
60. Frye v. United States established that scientific evidence must be broadly recognized. The 1923 United States Court of Appeals for the District of Columbia Circuit case established the "Frye standard" for scientific evidence admissibility. Scientific evidence must be generally acknowledged by the scientific

community to be admissible in court under the Frye standard. Scientific methodology, procedures, and concepts utilized to generate evidence must be widely accepted in the relevant scientific community. Many US state and federal courts employ the Frye criterion to determine scientific evidence admissibility. In Daubert v. Merrell Dow Pharmaceuticals, the US Supreme Court replaced the Frye standard in 1993. For court admissibility, scientific evidence must be relevant and credible under the Daubert standard. Judges must also evaluate scientific evidence and determine admissibility under the standard.

References and Resources

American Nurses Association. Code of ethics for nurses with interpretive statements. 2nd ed. American Nurses Association; 2015.

American Psychiatric Association, editor. Diagnostic and statistical manual of mental disorders. DSM-5-TR (Fifth edition, text revision) ed. American Psychiatric Association Publishing; 2022.

Balestra ML. Liability risks for psychiatric mental health nurse practitioners. J Nurse Pract. 2018;14(9):671–6. https://doi.org/10.1016/j.nurpra.2018.08.005.

Dunne JP, Blackwell EK, Ursini E, Milliken A. Ethical issues in psychiatric and mental health care. In: Grace P, Milliken A, editors. *Clinical ethics handbook for nurses* (the international library of bioethics, vol 93). Springer; 2022. https://doi.org/10.1007/978-94-024-2155-2_9.

Fry ST, Veatch RM. Case studies in nursing ethics. 4th ed. Jones & Bartlett Publishers; 2012.

Johnson K, Vanderhoef D, Magrath N. Psychiatric-mental health nurse practitioner review and resource manual. American Nurses Association: American Nurses Credentialing Center; 2020.

Limandri BJ. Ethical reasoning in prescribing and monitoring psychotropic medications. J Psychosoc Nurs Ment Health Serv. 2019;57(1):7–10. https://doi.org/10.3928/02793695-20181212-03.

Manderius C, Clintståhl K, Sjöström K, et al. The psychiatric mental health nurse's ethical considerations regarding the use of coercive measures—a qualitative interview study. BMC Nurs. 2023;22:23. https://doi.org/10.1186/s12912-023-01186-z.

Purtilo RB, Doherty R. Ethical dimensions in the health professions. 6th ed. Jones and Bartlett Learning; 2017.

Sadock BJ, Sadock VA, Ruiz P. Synopsis of psychiatry: behavioral sciences clinical psychiatry. 11th ed. Wolters Kluwer; 2015.

U.S. Department of Health and Human Services. (2021). Health insurance portability and accountability act (HIPAA). https://www.hhs.gov/hipaa/index.html.

Ventura CAA, Austin W, Carrara BS, de Brito ES. Nursing care in mental health: human rights and ethical issues. Nurs Ethics. 2021;28(4):463–80. https://doi.org/10.1177/0969733020952102.

Zakhari R. The psychiatric-mental health nurse practitioner certification review manual. Springer Publishing Company; 2021.

Zheng C, Li S, Chen Y, Ye J, Xiao A, Xia Z, Liao Y, Xu Y, Zhang Y, Yu L, Wang C, Lin J. Ethical consideration on use of seclusion in mental health services. Int J Nurs Sci. 2020;7(1):116–20. https://doi.org/10.1016/j.ijnss.2019.10.001.

Notes:

Notes:

Anatomy and Physiology of the Brain and Nervous System

4

Test your learning and check your understanding of this book's contents: use the "Springer Nature Flashcards" app to access questions using ▶ https://sn.pub/62J0Ar.

To use the app, please follow the instructions in Chap. 1.

Knowledge of the anatomy and physiology of the brain and nervous system is paramount for psychiatric-mental health nurse practitioners (PMHNPs) in order to be able to assess, diagnose, and treat patients with a variety of mental health conditions. After all, the brain is the control center of the body and is responsible for the majority of functions that keep the body functioning properly. While there is still much research to be done on the specific brain structures and functions that are involved in mental illnesses, the physiology of numerous brain structures has already been implicated in various mental illnesses.

- The amygdala is hyperactive in people with anxiety disorders and depression (McEwen and Morrison 2013; Sheline et al. 1999).
- The prefrontal cortex is less active in people with depression and schizophrenia (Akbarian et al. 1995; Kolb and Whishaw 2015; Mayberg et al. 1999).
- The hippocampus is smaller in people with depression and post-traumatic stress disorder (PTSD) (Bremner et al. 1995; McEwen and Morrison 2013; Sheline et al. 1999).
- The thalamus is abnormal in people with schizophrenia (Akbarian et al. 1995; Purves et al. 2017).
- The insula is hyperactive in people with anxiety disorders (Etkin et al. 2015) and depression (Siegle et al. 2007).
- The cingulate cortex is hyperactive in people with depression (Mayberg et al. 1999) and schizophrenia (Carter et al. 2001).

T. Stewart, *Psychiatric-Mental Health Nurse Practitioner Program Companion and Board Certification Exam Review Workbook*,
https://doi.org/10.1007/978-3-031-60894-0_4

- The striatum is abnormal in people with addiction (Goldstein and Volkow 2011) and obsessive-compulsive disorder (OCD).
- The ventral tegmental area (VTA) is hyperactive in people with addiction (Goldstein and Volkow 2011).

The nervous system is a complex network of cells and tissues that is responsible for transmitting and processing information throughout the body. The nervous system consists of two main parts: the central nervous system (CNS) and the peripheral nervous system (PNS). The CNS is made up of the brain and the spinal cord and is responsible for processing and integrating information from the body. The PNS consists of nerves that extend from the CNS to the rest of the body and are responsible for transmitting information to and from the CNS.

In addition to its clinical applications, knowledge of the anatomy and physiology of the brain and nervous system is also important for PMHNPs to be able to educate patients about their conditions and treatment options. By having a strong understanding of the underlying physiological processes involved, PMHNPs can provide patients with clear and accurate information about their conditions and help them make informed decisions about their care.

This chapter reviews the anatomy and physiology of the brain and the central nervous system. Particular attention is placed on neurotransmitters and their pathways and connections to mental illnesses. Neuroimaging assessment and diagnostic procedures are included.

4.1 Foundations and Brain Anatomy

1. What is the main purpose of the nervous system?

2. Complete the table with the divisions and secondary systems of the nervous system. Under each label, provide 1–2 functions of the system parts.

Division	Secondary system	Function(s)
Central nervous system (CNS)	Brain	
		Receives sensory input from the body and sends motor signals to muscles and organs. It also contains reflex pathways that allow for rapid, automatic responses to certain stimuli
	Cerebrospinal fluid (CSF)	

Division	Secondary system	Function(s)
Peripheral nervous system (PNS)		Controls voluntary movements of the skeletal muscles, and receives and processes sensory information from the body's surface and joints. The sensory subsystem detects changes in the environment and sends information to the CNS, while the motor subsystem sends signals from the CNS to the muscles to initiate movement
	Autonomic nervous system (ANS)	
		Controls the functions of the gastrointestinal tract, including motility, secretion, and blood flow. It can operate independently of the CNS but is also influenced by it

3. White and gray matter in the brain and spinal cord are vital to the neurological system. The following table compares white and gray matter. Explain their composition, function, location, similarities, and differences.

	White	Gray
Composition		
Function		
Location		
Similarities		

	White	Gray
Differences		

4. Why does the human brain have numerous folds, grooves, and dips?

5. ______________________ are shallow grooves on the brain. _______________ are deep grooves.

6. Areas of raised tissue on the cortex, or outer surface of the brain, are called _________________.

7. The left and right hemispheres of the brain make up the ______________________.

8. Which hemisphere of the brain is dominant in most people?

9. The ________________________________ connects the two cerebral hemispheres. Composed of _________________________, this structure supports interhemispheric sensorimotor signals.

10. Label the brain structures in the image below (Fig. 4.1).

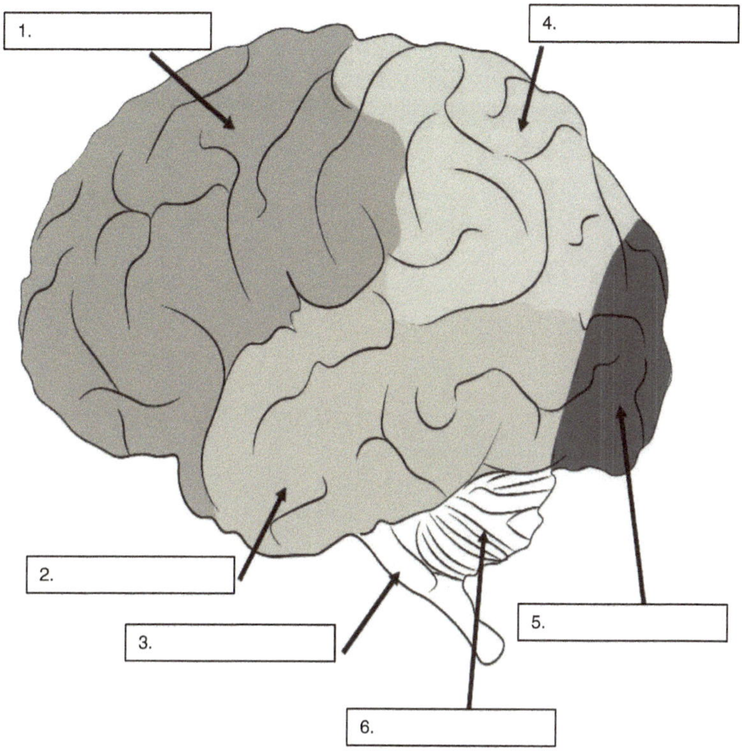

Fig. 4.1 Sagittal view of the brain, external (With permission from: Farnsworth von Cederwald, B. (2020). Brain Basics in Neuroergonomics. In: Nam, C. (eds) Neuroergonomics. Cognitive Science and Technology. Springer, Cham. https://doi.org/10.1007/978-3-030-34784-0_2)

11. Complete the table by listing the major functions of each lobe of the brain.

Lobe	Major functions
Frontal	
Temporal	
Parietal	
Occipital	

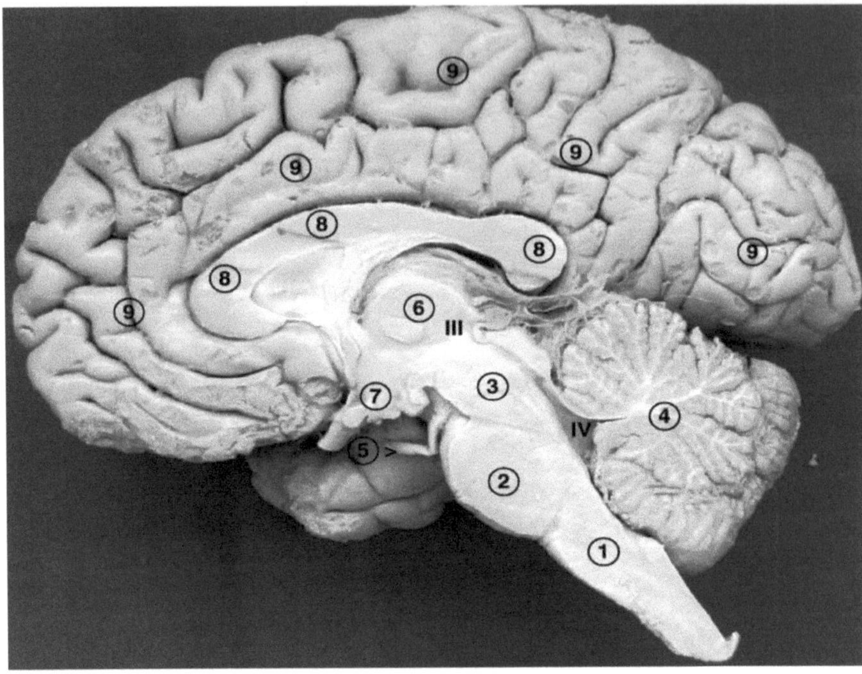

Fig. 4.2 Sagittal view of the brain, internal (With permission from: Schröder, H. et al. (2023). General Considerations. In: The Human Brainstem. Springer, Cham. https://doi.org/10.1007/978-3-030-89980-6_1)

12. Below is a median section of the brain. Label each of the following anatomical parts: mesencephalon, medulla oblongata, cerebellum, thalamus, hypothalamus, pons, corpus callosum, and telencephalon (Fig. 4.2).
    1. ______________________________
    2. ______________________________
    3. ______________________________
    4. ______________________________
    5. Oculomotor nerve CNIII.
    6. ______________________________
    7. ______________________________
    8. ______________________________
    9. ______________________________.

13. The limbic system is a set of structures in the brain that deal with emotions, memories, arousal, and autonomic functions. Place an X next to the following brain structures which are part of the limbic system. This list is not exhaustive.
    ______Amygdala
    ______Basal Ganglia
    ______Cerebellum
    ______Cerebral Cortex
    ______Cingulate Cortex
    ______Corpus Callosum

_____Fornix
_____Hippocampus
_____Hypothalamus
_____Medulla Oblongata
_____Midbrain
_____Olfactory Bulb
_____Pons
_____Thalamus
_____Ventral Tegmental Area

14. Match each of the following brain structures with its function.

_________1. Amygdala	A. Motor signals from CNS to skeletal muscles, movement, automatic actions
_________2. Basal ganglia	B. Sensory relay except for smell, strong emotion regulator, memory
_________3. Hippocampus	C. Hunger, thirst, circadian rhythms, libido, body temperature, overall homeostasis
_________4. Hypothalamus	D. Smell, mood, powerful emotions
_________5. Thalamus	E. Short-term to long-term memory, learning
_________6. Cingulate gyrus	F. Emotion, behavior, motor regulation
_________7. Cerebellum	G. Dopamine
_________8. Medulla oblongata	H. Reflexes, vital signs, involuntary muscle movement, respiration
_________9. Midbrain	I. Balance, gross motor movement, cognition, impulse control
_________10. Pons	J. Regulate body functions
_________11. Reticular formation	K. Norepinephrine

15. Below is a list of the most applicable imaging techniques to the work of PMHNPs. Match each test with the best explanation on the right.

Category	Test	Explanation
Structural	_____X-ray	A. EEG complement
	_____Computed tomography (CT)	B. Visualizes cerebral blood flow, expensive
	_____Magnetic resonance imaging (MRI)	C. 3-D, structures, differences in density, inexpensive, cannot view deep into the brain, no differentiation of white/gray matter, limited points of view
Functional	_____Electroencephalogram (EEG)	D. Specialized brain images from radionuclei and electron interaction, expensive
	_____Magnetoencephalography (MEG)	E. 2-D, deep brain images, differentiate white/gray matter, high resolution, expensive, not for patients with metal implants or claustrophobia
	_____Single photon emission computed tomography (SPECT)	F. 2-D using electromagnetic waves, blocked by dense objects like bone, tumors, and metal materials, contrast dyes may be used to highlight certain areas (white), air-filled structures appear black, inexpensive, limited use
	_____Positron emission tomography (PET)	G. Electrical functioning of CNS, inexpensive

16. It is important for PMHNP to complete a neurological examination on clients. Complete the following table on the cranial nerves and their potential association with mental health disorders.

CN	Name	Connection to mental health disorders
CN I		
CN II		
CN III		
CN IV		
CN V		
CN VI		
CN VII		
CN VIII		
CN IX		

CN	Name	Connection to mental health disorders
CN X		
CN XI		
CN XII		

17. ______________________________ refers to the brain's continuous development and alteration throughout one's life as influenced by the interactions between genetics and life experiences.

18. The brain's efficacy is focused by the removal of inactive and irrelevant synapses. Adolescence is a key period for this refinement. This activity is known as ______________________________.

4.2 Neuron and Action Potentials

19. The basic cell of the nervous system is called the ______________. It is composed of three principal parts: ______________, ______________, ______________.

20. To assist impulse conduction along axons, ______________ form a protective sheath called ______________, which gives the axons their white color.

21. Name three structures or proteins that are contained in the neuronal cell body's cell membrane.
    1. ______________________________
    2. ______________________________
    3. ______________________________.

22. Label the following on the neuron: receptor, dendrite, axon, synapse, soma, oligodendrocyte, myelin sheath, vesicle, and node of Ranvier (Fig. 4.3).

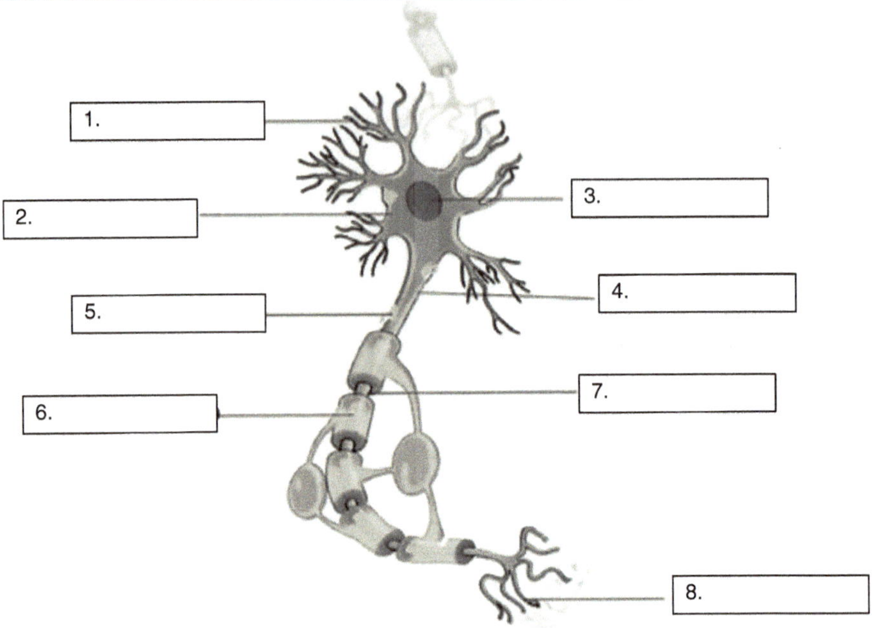

Fig. 4.3 Neuron (With permission from: Gautam, A. (2017). Nerve Cells. In: Vonk, J., Shackelford, T. (eds) Encyclopedia of Animal Cognition and Behavior. Springer, Cham. https://doi.org/10.1007/978-3-319-47829-6_1282-1)

23. ________________ collect signals coming into the neuron. The ________________ transmit signals away from the soma.

24. Reuptake pumps are located on the ________________________ terminal of the neuron.

25. An action potential is a brief electrical signal that travels along the axon of a neuron, leading to the release of neurotransmitters at the synapse. Number the order of the steps in an action potential and neurotransmitter release. Then, provide a short explanation of what happens at each step.

Order	Step	Explanation
	Action potential	
	Depolarization	

Order	Step	Explanation
	Hyperpolarization	
	Neurotransmitter release	
	Repolarization	
	Resting potential	

26. During depolarization, ________ and ________ions flow ________ the cell, causing an excitatory response.

27. During repolarization, ________ ions flow into the cell and ________ ions exit the cell, resulting in an inhibitory response.

28. A postsynaptic neuron being activated too often can reduce its number of receptors via ______________________________. In contrast, a neuron making itself more sensitive to stimulation by increasing its number of neurons is called ______________________________.

4.3 Neurotransmitters

29. ____________________________________ are chemical messengers released from a neuron and then bind to a receptor on another neuron or cell, transmitting signals between neurons and cells in the nervous system. These chemicals are synthesized from dietary substrates, like amino acids, fatty acids, and nucleotides.

30. In addition to receptor linkage, name three other ways in which neurotransmitters in a synapse go away so the synapse can "reset."
    1. ______________________________
    ______
    2. ______________________________
    ______
    3. ______________________________
    ______.

31. Where in the brain would we find the cells that produce each of the following neurotransmitters?

Neurotransmitter	Production location(s)
Dopamine	
Serotonin	
Norepinephrine	
Acetylcholine	
Histamine	
GABA	
Glutamate	

32. The abbreviation 5-HT for serotonin stands for ______________________________.

33. What are the pharmacological functions/uses of serotonin?

34. While 5-HT is produced in the ____________________ in the brain, 90% of the neurotransmitter is located in the ____________________.

35. What is serotonin syndrome? Name 5–7 symptoms associated with serotonin syndrome.
    1. ______________________________
    2. ______________________________
    3. ______________________________
    4. ______________________________
    5. ______________________________
    6. ______________________________
    7. ______________________________.

36. The reward function of dopamine is produced in what area of the brain?

37. What are the effects/functions of dopamine?

38. The ________________ dopamine receptor is implicated in the pharmacology of antipsychotics.

39. Which three neurotransmitters are catecholamines?
    1. ____
    2. ____
    3. ____.

40. Which catecholamine most strongly mediates the sympathetic nervous system?

41. Match the following drug effect terms with their definition.

Drug effect term	Definition
__________Full agonist	A. A drug that binds to and activates a receptor, producing a maximal response. These can elicit the same response as an endogenous ligand for that receptor
__________ Partial agonist	B. A drug that binds to the same receptor as an agonist but produces the opposite effect, decreasing the basal activity of the receptor. These can have therapeutic applications in diseases where the receptor is constitutively active
__________ Antagonist	C. A drug that binds to and activates a receptor, but produces a submaximal response. These have lower intrinsic activity than full agonists and can block the activity of full agonists at the same receptor
__________ Inverse agonist	D. A drug that binds to a receptor but does not activate it, and prevents the binding of endogenous ligands or other agonists. These can block the effects of agonists at the same receptor

42. Norepinephrine, a key neurotransmitter and hormone in the body, primarily acts on adrenergic receptors to regulate various physiological responses. For each receptor, explain its effect and an example medication.

Adrenergic receptor	Effect	Example medication
α1		
α2		

Adrenergic receptor	Effect	Example medication
β1		
β2		

43. Acetylcholine acts on ______________________ and ____________________ receptors in the ________________________ nervous system and central nervous system, respectively.

44. Acetylcholine's effects on the parasympathetic nervous system will result in what symptoms?

45. Acetylcholine acting at nicotinic receptors affects skeletal muscles and learning, memory, and attention. In the latter cases, it is implicated in ___________ ________________________________.

46. Damage to the ____ in the brain is linked to Alzheimer's dementia because this area is rich in acetylcholine.

47. In addition to helping lessen allergies, antihistamines are also used for _______________________ and _________________________.

48. Newer antihistamines do not cause drowsiness because they only act on the _______________________ nervous system.

49. Label each medication as H1 or H2 medication.

	Diphenhydramine
	Doxylamine
	Cimetidine
	Hydroxyzine
	Ranitidine
	Cetirizine
	Famotidine
	Loratadine
	Fexofenadine

50. _______________ neurotransmitter blockers cause sedation. _______________ neurotransmitter blockers work mostly on gastric mucosa to help reduce acid reflux.

51. Endorphins and enkephalins are endogenous ______________________.

52. ________ is the primary opioid receptor subtype bound to create an analgesic effect.

53. ______________________ is the brain's inhibitory neurotransmitter, slowing neuronal transmission.

54. The brain's excitatory neurotransmitter is ____________________, as it amplifies neuronal signals.

55. Glutamate binds to ______________________________________ and _____________________________________ receptors to affect learning, memory, and thought processing.

56. Identify each of the following neurotransmitters as an amino acid (AA), cholinergic (C), monoamine (M), or neuropeptide (N).
    _____Acetylcholine
    _____Aspartate
    _____Dopamine
    _____Dynorphins
    _____Endorphins
    _____Enkephalins
    _____Epinephrine
    _____Gamma-aminobutyric acid
    _____Glutamate
    _____Glycine
    _____Norepinephrine
    _____Serotonin
    _____Somatostatin
    _____Substance P.

57. All of the monoamines are classified as a catecholamine, except for ______________________.

58. The precursor to dopamine is ______________________.

59. The precursor to norepinephrine is ______________________.

60. The precursor to serotonin is ____________________________.

61. ____________________________ and ____________________________ are both precursors to acetylcholine.

62. Monoamine oxidase (MAO) enzyme removes an excess of which neurotransmitters from the synaptic cleft?

63. How are excess norepinephrine and serotonin removed from the synaptic cleft?

64. Complete the table with information about each neurotransmitter.

Neurotransmitter	Receptors	Function	High levels	Associated disorders	Low levels	Associated disorders
Dopamine	D1-like D2-like		Mild: Improved creativity Improved ability for Abstract thinking Improved Executive Functioning Improved spatiality Severe: Disorganized Thinking Loose association Tics Stereotypic Behavior			Substance abuse Anhedonia Parkinsonian symptoms
Norepinephrine		Alertness Focused attention Orientation Primes "fight or Flight" Learning Memory				
	5HT1a 5HT1d 5HT2 5HT2a 5HT3 5HT4		Sedation Increased Aggression Hallucinations (rare)			Depression OCD Anxiety Schizophrenia

Neurotransmitter	Receptors	Function	High levels	Associated disorders	Low levels	Associated disorders
Glutamate		Memory Sustained Automatic Functions		Seizure disorder Bipolar disorder Psychosis		
γ-Aminobutyric acid (GABA)	GABAa GABAb		Reduced cellular Excitability Sedation Impaired memory			Anxiety
	Nicotinic Muscarinic	Attention Memory Thirst Mood regulation REM sleep Sexual behavior Muscle tone		Parkinsonian symptoms	Lack of inhibition Decreased Memory Euphoria Antisocial action Speech decrease Dry mouth, blurred Vision, constipation	
	μ (mu) k (kappa) ε (epsilon) δ (delta) σ (sigma)		Insensitivity to pain Catatonic-like Movement Disturbance Auditory Hallucinations Decreased Memory		Decreased Pleasure sensation Dysphoria	Substance abuse

65. What is the function of catechol-O-methyltransferase (COMT)?

66. What is kindling? What neurotransmitter is involved in this process?

67. ______________________________ and glutamate both work as excitatory neurotransmitters.

68. __________________________ and GABA are both inhibitory neurotransmitters.

69. Name the four dopamine pathways. Then, provide key characteristics about each pathway, including any notable symptoms or disorders.

Pathway	Characteristics

70. ______ and ______ dopamine receptors stimulate adenyl cyclase. _______, _______, and _______ inhibit cAMP formation.

71. Antipsychotics block ____________________ neurotransmitter receptors in the mesolimbic pathway. These medications also block dopamine in the nigrostriatal pathway which can lead to ____________________________________ ____________________.

72. ______________________________ is a second-generation antipsychotic that blocks the tuberoinfundibular pathway. Noted side effects from this medication include ______________________________ and _____________________ ___________.

73. ______________________________ affects the amygdala causing anxiety.

74. Amphetamine salts increase ______________________________ and ______________________________ neurotransmitters in the brain.

75. In order to have sufficient melatonin, one must have sufficient ______________________________ neurotransmitter levels.

76. Why is GI distress a common side effect of medications that result in increased serotonin levels?

77. Buspirone is a _________________________ to 5-HT1A.

78. Mirtazapine (Remeron) antagonizes 5-HT2 and 5-HT3 receptors causing increased energy.

TRUE FALSE

79. Individuals with migraines already taking serotonergic medications should be warned of increased risks for serotonin syndrome if prescribed a ___________ ________________________ for their migraines.

80. Sedation and weight gain are associated with some psychiatric medications which antagonize the ________________ receptor.

81. ___________________ is a precursor to GABA.

82. ____ is the key receptor for glutamate. When blocked, symptoms associated with schizophrenia may result.

83. ______________________ is a controversial treatment for treatment-resistant depression and is a noncompetitive antagonist for the NMDA receptor, paradoxically causing an increase in glutamate.

84. Name 3–5 types of medications or substances that bind to GABA receptors.
   1. ______________________
   2. ______________________
   3. ______________________
   4. ______________________
   5. ______________________.

85. Donepezil is a ______________________ which prevents the breakdown of acetylcholine. It is used as a drug to slow cognitive loss in Alzheimer's dementia.

4.4 (Dys-)Function

86. What are five examples of executive functions?
   1. ______________________
   2. ______________________
   3. ______________________
   4. ______________________
   5. ______________________.

87. Expressive speech is located in ______________________area in the ______________ lobe. Receptive speech is located in ______________ area in the ______________ lobe.

88. Match the lobe with the potential symptoms from damage.

________	1. Frontal	A. Field defects, blindness, and visual hallucinations.
________	2. Temporal	B. Personality changes, emotional, and intellectual changes.
________	3. Parietal	C. Visual or auditory hallucinations, aphasia, and amnesia.
________	4. Occipital	D. Sensory–perceptual disturbances and agnosia.

89. An individual who develops promiscuous behaviors and poor judgment after a car accident may have damaged the ______________ lobe of the brain.

90. A patient with increasing difficulty recognizing familiar objects and decreasing sense of proprioception may have a lesion on the ______________ lobe of the brain.

91. New onset of auditory hallucinations with no other signs or symptoms may warrant radiological imaging of the ______________ lobe of the brain.

92. The ______________ is considered the "relay station" for sensory information in the brain.

93. What does the term "contralateral" mean in regard to the functioning of the cerebral cortex?

94. Dementia may be attributable in part to damage or dysfunction in the ______ ______________________________, part of the limbic system.

95. Irritability and aggression seen in some patients with schizophrenia and autism spectrum disorder may be linked to the ______________________________, in the emotional center of the brain.

96. Anorexia nervosa may have roots in the brain's ________________________ ______________, which is associated with appetite and metabolism.

97. Another name for the basal ganglia is the ______________________________.

98. Extrapyramidal side effects from psychotropic medications are caused by motor nerve irritation in the ____________________________________.

99. What two structures are located in the basal ganglia and associated with motor control?

100. Emotions and memory are regulated in the ____________________________ __________.

101. Autism spectrum disorder and ADHD may be attributed to dysfunction in which part of the brainstem?

102. Do cerebellar hemispheres have ipsilateral or contralateral control of the body?

103. If cerebellar dysfunction is suspected, the PMHNP should conduct the ________________________ test.

104. Complete the following table with the appropriate term, definition, or associated disorder/medication.

Term	Definition	Associated disorder or medication
	Restlessness or an inability to remain still; a common side effect of antipsychotic medication	Schizophrenia; antipsychotic medication
Akinesia		Parkinson's disease; parkinsonian medication
Agnosia	Inability to recognize or identify familiar objects or people	
	Abnormal physical weakness or lack of energy	Depression; anxiety
Dyskinesia		Parkinson's disease; antipsychotic medication
Dyspraxia	Difficulty with motor planning or coordination	
	Repeating or mimicking the words or movements of others	
Neologism	Inventing new words or phrases that have no recognizable meaning	
Perseveration		Obsessive-compulsive disorder; traumatic brain injury
	Speech that is unrelated to the topic at hand, often including loose associations	Schizophrenia; bipolar disorder
Word salad		Schizophrenia; mania
	Loss or impairment of the ability to communicate through language	

Term	Definition	Associated disorder or medication
Amnesia		
	Involuntary muscle contractions that cause repetitive or twisting movements	Parkinson's disease; antipsychotic medication
Ataxia		Multiple sclerosis; alcohol use disorder
	Inability to swallow or difficulty swallowing	

4.5 Answers and Explanations to Chapter Activities

1. The nervous system functions to regulate the body's reaction to internal and external stimuli. It processes sensory data from the environment and responds appropriately. Our nervous system also regulates and maintains homeostasis, the balance of physiological processes that keep us healthy. The nervous system controls movement, sensation, perception, thinking, memory, and emotion. It transmits information and impulses across the body.
2.

Division	Secondary System	Function(s)
Central nervous system (CNS)	Brain	Controls physiological functions, interprets sensory data, initiates voluntary and involuntary motor responses, stores memories, and permits emotions and higher cognitive functions
	Spinal cord	Receiving bodily sensory input and sending motor signals to muscles and organs. It has reflex pathways for quick, automatic responses to stimuli
	Cerebrospinal fluid (CSF)	Cushions and protects the brain and spinal cord, delivers nourishment and waste removal, and stabilizes the nervous system
Peripheral nervous system (PNS)	Somatic nervous system (SNS)	Receives and analyzes sensory input from the body's surface and joints and controls voluntary skeletal muscle movements. The sensory subsystem registers environmental changes and conveys them to the CNS, whereas the motor subsystem instructs muscles to move
	Autonomic nervous system (ANS)	Controls heart rate, digestion, respiration, and blood pressure. The sympathetic and parasympathetic nerve systems affect these processes oppositely. The sympathetic subsystem increases heart rate, dilates pupils, and decreases digestive function to prepare the body for "fight or flight" responses, while the parasympathetic subsystem decreases heart rate, constricts pupils, and increases digestive function to promote "rest and digest" responses

Division	Secondary System	Function(s)
	Enteric nervous system (ENS)	Regulates gastrointestinal motility, secretion, and blood flow. It can function independently but is impacted by the CNS

3.

	White	Gray
Composition	Made up of myelinated axons. Myelination gives white matter its characteristic pale color. It also contains some glial cells, which support and protect the neurons	Composed primarily of neuronal cell bodies, dendrites, and unmyelinated axons, along with neuroglia and capillaries. It appears gray due to the lack of myelin
Function	Its main function is to transmit signals between gray matter areas and between the gray matter and the rest of the body. The myelinated fibers enhance the speed and efficiency of information transmission	The primary role is to process and regulate information. It is where most of the brain's synaptic activity occurs, leading to the processing of information. Functions include muscle control, sensory perception such as seeing and hearing, memory, emotions, and speech
Location	Found beneath the gray matter cortex, making up the bulk of the deeper parts of the brain. It forms connections between the various gray matter areas and between these areas and the spinal cord. Encircles the gray matter and extends throughout the spinal cord	Located in the outer layer of the brain, known as the cerebral cortex, and also found in regions called the basal ganglia and brainstem. It forms the cortex of the cerebellum as well. Located in the core of the spinal cord, it is shaped like a butterfly or the letter "H" in cross-section
Similarities	Both are integral parts of the nervous system and are necessary for transmitting and processing information Both contain some amount of glial cells, which support and maintain the neurons	Both are integral parts of the nervous system and are necessary for transmitting and processing information Both contain some amount of glial cells, which support and maintain the neurons
Differences	White due to myelin Primarily involved in signal transmission On the inside of the brain but outside of the spinal cord	Gray due to neuron cell bodies and lack of myelin Processes information On the outside of the brain but inside the spinal cord

4. The numerous folds, grooves, and dips in the human brain, also called convolutions, increase the surface area of the brain and allow for a greater number of neurons to be packed into a smaller space.
5. Sulci are shallow grooves on the brain, while fissures are deep grooves.
6. Areas of raised tissue on the cortex are called gyri.
7. The left and right hemispheres of the brain make up the cerebrum.

8. Most people's left hemisphere dominates linguistic and analytical processing, whereas the right dominates visual-spatial processing and creativity. Most people are left-hemisphere dominant.
9. Brain hemispheres are connected by the corpus callosum. By communicating and coordinating brain functions, this white matter structure promotes inter-hemispheric sensorimotor impulses.
10.
    - Frontal lobe.
    - Temporal lobe.
    - Brain stem.
    - Parietal lobe.
    - Occipital lobe.
    - Cerebellum.

11.

Lobe	Major functions
Frontal	– Voluntary motor movement and coordination of muscles – Memory and decision-making through sensory input – Executive functions (planning, reasoning, problem-solving, decision-making) – Expressive speech (Broca's area) – Personality and social behavior
Temporal	– Receptive speech, including comprehension (Wernicke's area) – Auditory senses – Memory (especially declarative memory) – Emotion (limbic system)
Parietal	– Senses (touch, temperature, pressure, pain) – Spatial awareness and perception – Perception and integration of sensory information from multiple sources – Reading and writing (left parietal lobe)
Occipital	– Vision integration and processing (primary visual cortex)

12.
    1. Medulla oblongata.
    2. Pons.
    3. Mesencephalon (Midbrain).
    4. Cerebellum.
    5. Oculomotor nerve CNIII.
    6. Thalamus.
    7. Hypothalamus.
    8. Corpus callosum.
    9. Telencephalon (Neocortex).

13. _____X___Amygdala
_____Basal Ganglia.
_____Cerebellum.
_____Cerebral Cortex.
_____X___Cingulate Cortex.
_____Corpus Callosum.

_____X___Fornix.
_____X___Hippocampus.
_____X___Hypothalamus.
_____Medulla Oblongata.
_____Midbrain.
_____Olfactory Bulb.
_____Pons.
_____Thalamus.
_____Ventral Tegmental Area

14. ____D______1. Amygdala
____A______2. Basal ganglia.
____E______3. Hippocampus.
____C_____4. Hypothalamus.
____B_____5. Thalamus.
____F_____6. Cingulate gyrus.
____I______7. Cerebellum.
____J______8. Medulla oblongata.
____G_____9. Midbrain.
____K______10. Pons.
____H_____11. Reticular formation

15. ____F___X-ray
____C__Computed tomography (CT).
____E___Magnetic Resonance Imaging (MRI).
____G___Electroencephalogram (EEG).
____A___Magnetoencephalography (MEG).
____B___Single photon emission computed tomography (SPECT).
____D___Positron emission tomography (PET).

16.

CN	Name	Connection to mental health disorders
CN I	Olfactory	Anosmia (loss of smell) can be associated with depressive symptoms. Changes in smell can also be early signs of neurodegenerative disorders like Parkinson's or Alzheimer's. Some medications, particularly antipsychotics and mood stabilizers, can lead to anosmia or altered smell, which can affect taste and appetite
CN II	Optic	Visual impairments can lead to anxiety and depression. Visual hallucinations can be a sign of neurological issues affecting mental health, like in some cases of schizophrenia. Certain antipsychotics and antidepressants can cause blurred vision or changes in vision due to their anticholinergic effects
CN III	Oculomotor	Abnormal eye movements or pupillary response can indicate a neurological disorder that may have psychiatric symptoms. Antipsychotics can sometimes cause an oculogyric crisis, leading to involuntary upward eye movement. Other medications may cause blurred vision or changes in pupil size
CN IV	Trochlear	Double vision (diplopia) can cause disorientation, anxiety, and challenges with spatial navigation. Most psychotropic drug effects on eye movement are related to the oculomotor nerve

CN	Name	Connection to mental health disorders
CN V	Trigeminal	Trigeminal neuralgia can cause chronic pain, leading to depression or anxiety. Sensory disturbances may also affect mental health. Tegretol, a mood stabilizer, is actually used to treat trigeminal neuralgia
CN VI	Abducens	Psychotropic medications rarely affect the abducens nerve directly, but blurred vision or difficulty focusing can be side effects of many psychotropic drugs
CN VII	Facial	Facial paralysis (e.g., Bell's palsy) can affect emotional expression and social interaction, potentially leading to anxiety or depression. Taste disturbances can affect appetite and mood. Some antipsychotics can cause tardive dyskinesia, which may include facial twitching or grimacing
CN VIII	Vestibulocochlear	Hearing loss or tinnitus can lead to social withdrawal, depression, and anxiety. Balance issues can also lead to fear of falling and related anxiety. Some antidepressants and antipsychotics can cause dizziness or unsteadiness
CN IX	Glossopharyngeal	Swallowing difficulties can lead to fear of eating and social anxiety, while taste disturbances can affect appetite and mood. Some medications can cause dry mouth, which can indirectly affect taste and swallowing. Rarely, they may contribute to swallowing difficulties
CN X	Vagus	The vagus nerve is a direct link between the gut and brain; issues can lead to or exacerbate conditions like anxiety and depression. It is also involved in calming responses. Many psychotropic medications can cause tachycardia or palpitations. Some, particularly SSRIs, can lead to gastrointestinal side effects, potentially affecting the vagus nerve
CN XI	Accessory	Impaired movement can lead to physical discomfort and restrictions, affecting mental health due to decreased mobility and independence. Chronic use of antipsychotics can lead to tardive dyskinesia, which might include unusual movements affecting the neck and shoulders
CN XII	Hypoglossal	Difficulties in speech can lead to social withdrawal and frustration, potentially affecting mental health. Antipsychotic medications can sometimes cause tongue protrusion or unusual movements as part of tardive dyskinesia

17. Neuroplasticity.
18. Synaptic pruning.
19. Neurons are nervous system cells composed of three main parts:
    - Cell body (soma): This core of the neuron contains the nucleus and other metabolic components.
    - Dendrites: These branched extensions of the neuron receive signals from neighboring neurons and sense receptors.
    - Axon: This long, thin fiber sends impulses from the cell body to other neurons, muscles, and glands. Axons are sheathed in myelin to facilitate signal transmission.
20. Glial cells—oligodendrocytes in the central nervous system and Schwann cells in the peripheral nervous system—form myelin, which gives axons their

white appearance, to aid impulse conduction. Myelin insulates the axon and prevents electrical signals from being lost.

21. The neuronal cell body's membrane is a lipid bilayer with proteins and channels. The neuronal cell body's ability to communicate with other neurons and transfer electrical signals depends on these proteins and channels, which govern molecule flow. Neuronal cell membrane proteins include:

    - Ion channels: These proteins let sodium, potassium, and calcium ions enter and exit the cell. This helps neurons create and transmit electrical signals.
    - Neurotransmitter receptors: These cell membrane proteins bind to neurotransmitters to start a signaling cascade.
    - Enzymes: Cell membrane-bound enzymes catalyze chemical processes.
    - Transporters: These proteins move neurotransmitters and ions inside and outside the cell.

22. The numbers on the neuron structure graphic refer to these parts:

    1. Dendrites receive neuron or sensory receptor impulses.
    2. Nuclear and organelle-containing cell body/soma.
    3. Cell genetic material is in the nucleus.
    4. Axon hillock: axon origin.
    5. Long fiber that transmits electrical impulses away from cell body: axon.
    6. Myelin sheath: a fatty coating that insulates and speeds up axon signaling.
    7. Nodes of Ranvier: myelin sheath gaps for action potentials Terminal buttons/synaptic knobs: smaller structures at axon ends that release neurotransmitters for communication with other neurons or muscle cells.
    8. Synapse: the space between two neurons' terminal buttons and dendrites or cell bodies.

23. Dendrites receive impulses from the soma, whereas axons send them out.
24. Presynaptic terminal.
25.

Order	Step	Explanation
1	Resting potential	The neuron is at rest, negative inside and positive outside. Potassium (K+) is inside the cell and sodium (Na+) outside
2	Depolarization	Neuron membrane sodium channels open when stimulated. The inside of the neuron becomes more positive than the outside when sodium ions enter
3	Action potential	After the action potential peaks, membrane potential rapidly returns to resting. K+ ions leave the cell through potassium channels, repolarizing it
4	Repolarization	After the peak of the action potential, the membrane potential rapidly returns to its resting state. Potassium channels open, allowing K+ ions to flow out of the cell, leading to repolarization
5	Hyperpolarization	The movement of K+ ions continues past the resting potential, causing a brief period of hyperpolarization where the membrane potential becomes more negative than the resting potential

Order	Step	Explanation
6	Neurotransmitter release	The action potential opens voltage-gated calcium channels at the axon terminal. Ca^{2+} ions enter the axon terminal and fuse neurotransmitter-containing vesicles with the presynaptic membrane neurotransmitters enter the synaptic cleft and attach to postsynaptic membrane receptors, signaling the next cell

26. During depolarization, sodium (Na+) and calcium (Ca^{2+}) ions flow into the cell, causing an excitatory response.
27. During repolarization, chloride (Cl-) ions flow into the cell and potassium (K+) ions exit the cell, resulting in an inhibitory response.
28. Downregulation; Upregulation.
29. Neurotransmitters.
30. In addition to receptor linkage, three other ways neurotransmitters can vanish to "reset" a synapse are:

    - Neurotransmitters produced in the synaptic cleft can diffuse away and be absorbed by extracellular fluid. Neurotransmitters are removed from the synaptic cleft.
    - Enzyme breakdown: Monoamine oxidase (MAO) degrades dopamine and serotonin in the synaptic cleft. This method quickly ceases synaptic cleft neurotransmitter activities.
    - The presynaptic neuron receives several neurotransmitters from transporters. The synaptic cleft is cleared and neurotransmitters recycled. Transporters reuptake dopamine.
31.

Neurotransmitter	Production location(s)
Dopamine	Substantia nigra, ventral tegmental area (VTA)
Serotonin	Raphe nuclei in the brainstem
Norepinephrine	Locus coeruleus in the pons
Acetylcholine	Basal forebrain (nucleus basalis, medial septal area), brainstem (pedunculopontine nucleus, laterodorsal tegmental nucleus)
Histamine	Tuberomammillary nucleus of the hypothalamus
GABA	Cerebral cortex, basal ganglia, hippocampus, thalamus
Glutamate	Widespread throughout the cerebral cortex

32. 5-Hydroxytryptamine
33. DOMAINS: depression, obsessions, mood, anxiety, impulsivity, nausea, sleep.
34. Raphe nuclei; intestines.
35. Serotonin syndrome due to increased central nervous system's serotonin activity can be fatal. Serotonin-boosting medications are usually to blame. These include SSRIs, SNRIs, MAOIs, and others, especially when used concurrently or with other serotonin-affecting drugs. Symptoms range from moderate to severe and include:

- Restlessness/agitation.
- Confused or lost.
- Fast heartbeat, high BP.
- Muscle stiffness and pupil dilation.
- Diarrhea, nausea, vomiting.
- High fever.
- Shivering and sweating.
- Headache, tremors.
- Lack of coordination and muscular twitching.
- In severe situations, seizures and unconsciousness.

36. The ventral tegmental area (VTA) neurons in the midbrain regulate motivation, reinforcement, addiction, and the reward system. Dopamine from the VTA travels to the nucleus accumbens, prefrontal cortex, and amygdala. Other VTA functions include learning, memory, mood modulation, and stress response. Addiction, depression, and Parkinson's disease have been linked to VTA and dopaminergic pathway dysfunction.
37. Drug addiction, psychosis, prolactin inhibition, attention, motivation, involuntary movements, nausea, energy (DOPAMINE).
38. D2.
39. Dopamine, epinephrine (adrenaline), norepinephrine (noradrenaline).
40. Norepinephrine.
41. ____A______Full agonist
    ____C______Partial agonist.
    ____D______Antagonist.
    ____B______Inverse agonist.
42.

Adrenergic Receptor	Effect	Example medication
α1	Widespread vasoconstriction, sweat, glucose	Prazosin, doxazosin, terazosin
α2	Blocks sympathetic nervous system	Clonidine, methyldopa, Guanfacine
β1	Increases cardiac output	Propranolol, metoprolol, atenolol
β2	Lungs, relax smooth muscle	Albuterol, Salmeterol, Formoterol

43. Muscarinic; nicotinic; parasympathetic.
44. SLUDGEM: salivation, lacrimation, urination, diaphoresis, GI effects, emesis, miosis.
45. Alzheimer's dementia.
46. Nucleus basalis of Meynert.
47. Insomnia; acid reflux.
48. Peripheral.
49. H1 blockers, often called H1 antihistamines, alleviate allergic reactions such as itching, sneezing, and runny noses. H2 blockers or antagonists inhibit stomach acid production. GERD, peptic ulcers, and gastritis are often treated

with them. They reduce stomach acid by inhibiting H2 receptors on stomach cells.

H1	Diphenhydramine
H1	Doxylamine
H2	Cimetidine
H1	Hydroxyzine
H2	Ranitidine
H1	Cetirizine
H2	Famotidine
H1	Loratadine
H1	Fexofenadine

50. H1; H2.
51. Opioids.
52. Mu.
53. GABA.
54. Glutamate.
55. Glutamate binds to NMDA (N-methyl-D-aspartate) and AMPA (alpha-amino-3-hydroxy-5-methyl-4-isoxazolepropionic acid) receptors to affect learning, memory, and thought processing.
56. ___C__Acetylcholine
    ___AA___Aspartate.
    ___M___Dopamine.
    ___N___Dynorphins.
    ___N___Endorphins.
    ___N___Enkephalins.
    ___M___Epinephrine.
    ___AA___Gamma-aminobutyric acid.
    ___AA___Glutamate.
    ___AA___Glycine.
    ___M__Norepinephrine.
    ___M___Serotonin.
    ___N___Somatostatin.
    ___N___Substance P
57. All of the monoamines are classified as a catecholamine, except for serotonin, which is an indolamine.
58. Tyrosine.
59. Dopamine.
60. Tryptophan.
61. Acetyl Coenzyme A (CoA), choline.
62. Monoamine oxidase (MAO) enzyme eliminates excess dopamine, norepinephrine, and serotonin from the synaptic cleft.
63. Presynaptic neuron reuptake pumps remove excess norepinephrine and serotonin from the synaptic cleft. These pumps return excess neurotransmitters to the presynaptic neuron for metabolization or vesicle storage. Monoamine oxidases (MAOs) in the synaptic cleft break down norepinephrine and serotonin to remove excess neurotransmitters.

64.

Neurotransmitter	Receptors	Function	High levels	Associated disorders	Low levels	Associated disorders
Dopamine	D1-like D2-like	Thinking Decision-making Reward-seeking Behavior Fine muscle action Integrated Cognition	Mild: Improved creativity Improved ability for Abstract thinking Improved Executive Functioning Improved spatiality Severe: Disorganized Thinking Loose association Tics Stereotypic Behavior	Schizophrenia Psychosis	Mild: Poor impulse Control Poor spatiality Lack of abstractive Thought Severe: Parkinson's disease Endocrine Alterations Movement Disorders	Substance abuse Anhedonia Parkinsonian symptoms
Norepinephrine	α1 α2	Alertness Focused attention Orientation Primes "fight or Flight" Learning Memory	Anxiety Hyperalertness Increased startle Paranoia Decreased Appetite	Anxiety	Dullness Low energy Depressive affect	Depression
Serotonin	5HT1a 5HT1d 5HT2 5HT2a 5HT3 5HT4	Regulation of sleep Pain perception Mood states Temperature Regulation of Aggression Libido Precursor for Melatonin	Sedation Increased Aggression Hallucinations (rare)		Irritability Hostility Depression Sleep Dysregulation Loss of appetite Loss of libido	Depression OCD Anxiety Schizophrenia
Glutamate	AMPA MNDA	Memory Sustained Automatic Functions	Kindling Seizures Anxiety or panic	Seizure disorder Bipolar disorder Psychosis	Poor memory Low energy Distractible	Mood disorders Memory Negative Sx of schizophrenia

Neurotransmitter	Receptors	Function	High levels	Associated disorders	Low levels	Associated disorders
γ-Aminobutyric acid (GABA)	GABAa GABAb	Reduces arousal Reduces Aggression Reduces anxiety Reduces excitation	Reduced cellular Excitability Sedation Impaired memory		Irritability Hostility Tension and worry Anxiety Seizure activity	Anxiety
Acetylcholine	Nicotinic Muscarinic	Attention Memory Thirst Mood regulation REM sleep Sexual behavior Muscle tone	Over-inhibition Anxiety Depression Somatic Complaints Self-consciousness Drooling Extrapyramidal Movements	Parkinsonian symptoms	Lack of inhibition Decreased Memory Euphoria Antisocial action Speech decrease Dry mouth, blurred Vision, constipation	Alzheimer's Memory
Neuropeptides	μ (mu) k (kappa) ε (epsilon) δ (delta) σ (sigma)	Modulate Emotions Reward-center Function Consolidation of Memory Modulate reactions To stress	Insensitivity to pain Catatonic-like Movement Disturbance Auditory Hallucinations Decreased Memory		Hypersensitivity to Pain and stress Decreased Pleasure sensation Dysphoria	Substance abuse

65. Catechol-O-methyltransferase (COMT) degrades dopamine, norepinephrine, and epinephrine in the brain and other organs. It turns neurotransmitters into urine-excreted metabolites. Some drugs for schizophrenia and Parkinson's disease target COMT, which regulates brain neurotransmitter levels.
66. Neuroscience uses kindling, a phenomenon in which repeated, subthreshold stimulations lead to a stronger, longer-lasting response, to research seizures and epilepsy. After repeated brain electrical stimulations, which were too weak to trigger a seizure at first, animal models developed full-blown seizures. This effect was long-lasting and could cause spontaneous seizures, imitating human epilepsy. Important igniting features:

    - Progressive sensitization: Each subthreshold stimulation increases brain sensitivity and reaction, causing overactivity and seizures.
    - Kindling alters neuronal circuits and synapses throughout time. Once ignited, the brain may permanently be seizure-prone.
    - Application: It is used to mimic epilepsy development, seizure processes, and antiepileptic medication effects.
    - Glutamate is the main igniting neurotransmitter. Glutamate, the brain's principal excitatory neurotransmitter, increases neuronal excitability. Changes in glutamate receptors (such as NMDA receptors) and glutamatergic transmission during kindling cause and intensify seizures. Kindling increases glutamate-sensitive neuronal response, causing hyperexcitability. Kindling also involves GABA, the brain's principal inhibitory neurotransmitter. Kindling's excitability may be heightened by GABAergic system changes that diminish inhibition. Kindling is important for understanding and treating epilepsy and other brain hyperexcitability disorders. It helps explain how repeated small neural injuries might cause substantial brain function alterations.

67. Aspartate.
68. Glycine.
69.

Pathway	Characteristics
Mesolimbic	Reward feedback loop, drug abuse, positive (+) symptoms of schizophrenia due to excessive DA in this pathway
Nigrostriatal	Movements; parkinsonian symptoms associated with deficient DA in this pathway
Mesocortical	Planning, behavior, cognition; associated with frontal lobe disorders; deficient DA in this pathway associated with negative (−) symptoms of schizophrenia
Tuberoinfundibular	Pituitary gland affecting prolactin levels

70. D1 and D5 dopamine receptors stimulate adenyl cyclase. D2, D3, and D4 dopamine receptors inhibit cAMP formation.
71. Antipsychotics block D2 receptors in the mesolimbic pathway. These medications also block dopamine in the nigrostriatal pathway which can lead to extrapyramidal side effects.

72. TRisperidone can cause increased levels of prolactin and result in side effects such as galactorrhea and sexual dysfunction.
73. Norepinephrine.
74. Dopamine and norepinephrine.
75. In order to have sufficient melatonin, one must have sufficient serotonin.
76. Because serotonin regulates gastrointestinal function, medicines that raise serotonin levels can cause GI distress. Nausea, vomiting, diarrhea, and abdominal pain can result from serotonin-induced gastrointestinal motility and secretion. Increased serotonin levels can also cause gut pain hypersensitivity.
77. Partial agonist.
78. FALSE. Mirtazapine (Remeron) is actually an antagonist at 5-HT2A and 5-HT3 receptors, and a potent antagonist of histamine H1 receptors, leading to sedation and weight gain as common side effects.
79. Triptan: 5-HT1B/1D agonists.
80. H1, histamine 1, which affects wakefulness, appetite, and feeding behaviors.
81. Glutamate.
82. The key receptor for glutamate is the N-methyl-D-aspartate (NMDA) receptor.
83. 83. Ketamine
84. Benzodiazepines, barbiturates, some sleep meds (e.g., zolpidem, zopiclone), some anticonvulsants (e.g., topiramate), gabapentinoids (e.g., pregabalin), ethanol.
85. Acetylcholinesterase inhibitor.
86. Working memory, reasoning, planning, prioritizing, sequencing behavior, insight, flexibility, judgment, impulse control, behavioral cueing, intelligence, abstraction.
87. Expressive speech is located in Broca's area in the frontal lobe. Receptive speech is located in Wernicke's area in the temporal lobe.
88. ____B______ 1. Frontal
    ____C______ 2. Temporal.
    ____D______ 3. Parietal.
    ____A______ 4. Occipital
89. Frontal.
90. Parietal.
91. Temporal.
92. Thalamus.
93. The term "contralateral" alludes to the cerebral cortex's left and right hemispheres, which govern the body's sides. Nerves from one side of the brain cross the spinal cord to the other.
94. Dementia, especially Alzheimer's, can impair the limbic system's hippocampus. Dementia symptoms include memory loss and spatial navigation issues caused by hippocampal dysfunction or injury.
95. The limbic system's amygdala regulates fear and anger. Amygdala dysregulation may cause irritability and hostility in schizophrenia and autism spectrum disorder individuals.

96. The hypothalamus may cause anorexia nervosa, an eating condition characterized by a skewed body image and a fear of weight increase. The hypothalamus regulates hunger and metabolism, and anorexia nervosa patients have anomalies in this region.
97. Basal ganglia are called "corpus striatum." Caudate, putamen, and accumbens nuclei make up the striatum, the biggest basal ganglia component.
98. Basal ganglia motor nerve stimulation causes psychotropic drug extrapyramidal side effects. These side effects may be caused by basal ganglia dopamine receptor blockage, which increases acetylcholine activity and causes tremors, rigidity, and akathisia.
99. The substantia nigra and striatum (caudate nucleus and putamen) are basal ganglia components that control motor function.
100. Limbic system.
101. Brainstem reticular activating system (RAS) impairment is linked to autism spectrum disorder and ADHD. Arousal, attentiveness, and other functions are regulated by the RAS.
102. The cerebellum controls the body ipsilaterally. The cerebellum's hemispheres mostly control the same side of the body. The right cerebellar hemisphere coordinates right arm and leg motions, while the left does the same for the left. The cerebellum is remarkable in its ipsilateral organization, while most other brain regions, including the cerebral cortex, have contralateral control, where each hemisphere affects the opposing side. The cerebellum receives input from the spinal cord and cerebral cortex regarding desired movements and present location and transmits corrective feedback to coordinate smooth, precise, and accurate movements. The fact that it operates ipsilaterally helps diagnose cerebellar diseases.
103. Cerebellar function is often assessed with the Romberg test. The test requires the patient to stand with feet together and eyes closed. Losing balance or swaying excessively indicates a positive Romberg test.
104.

Term	Definition	Associated disorder or medication
Akathisia	Restlessness or an inability to remain still; a common side effect of antipsychotic medication	Schizophrenia; antipsychotic medication
Akinesia	Loss or impairment of the ability to initiate voluntary movement	Parkinson's disease; parkinsonian medication
Agnosia	Inability to recognize or identify familiar objects or people	Alzheimer's; stroke
Asthenia	Abnormal physical weakness or lack of energy	Depression; anxiety
Dyskinesia	Involuntary muscle movements, often caused by medication side effects	Parkinson's disease; antipsychotic medication
Dyspraxia	Difficulty with motor planning or coordination	Autism spectrum disorder; developmental coordination disorder

Term	Definition	Associated disorder or medication
Echolalia: Echopraxia	Repeating or mimicking the words or movements of others	Autism spectrum disorder; schizophrenia
Neologism	Inventing new words or phrases that have no recognizable meaning	Schizophrenia; mania
Perseveration	Persistent repetition of a response, idea, or activity	Obsessive-compulsive disorder; traumatic brain injury
Tangential speech	Speech that is unrelated to the topic at hand, often including loose associations	Schizophrenia; bipolar disorder
Word salad	Incoherent and disconnected speech that makes no sense	Schizophrenia; mania
Aphasia	Loss or impairment of the ability to communicate through language	Stroke; traumatic brain injury
Amnesia	Loss of memory or inability to recall past events	Dementia; alcohol use disorder
Dystonia	Involuntary muscle contractions that cause repetitive or twisting movements	Parkinson's disease; antipsychotic medication
Ataxia	Loss of coordination or unsteady movements	Multiple sclerosis; alcohol use disorder
Aphagia	Inability to swallow or difficulty swallowing	Stroke; Parkinson's disease

References and Resources

Akbarian S, Kim JJ, Potkin SG, Hetrick WP, Bunney WE Jr, Jones EG. Gene expression for glutamic acid decarboxylase is reduced without loss of neurons in the prefrontal cortex of schizophrenics. Arch Gen Psychiatry. 1995;52(2):258–66. https://doi.org/10.1001/archpsyc.1995.03950160008002.

American Psychiatric Association (Ed.). (2022). Diagnostic and statistical manual of mental disorders: DSM-5-TR (5th edition). American Psychiatric Association Publishing.

Bear MF, Connors BW, Paradiso MA. Neuroscience: exploring the brain. 4th ed. Lippincott Williams & Wilkins; 2015.

Bishir M, Bhat A, Essa MM, Ekpo O, Ihunwo AO, Veeraraghavan VP, Mohan SK, Mahalakshmi AM, Ray B, Tuladhar S, Chang S, Chidambaram SB, Sakharkar MK, Guillemin GJ, Qoronfleh MW, Ojcius DM. Sleep deprivation and neurological disorders. Biomed Res Int. 2020;2020:5764017. https://doi.org/10.1155/2020/5764017.

Bremner JD, Randall P, Scott TM, Bronen RA, Seibyl JP, Southwick SM, Charney DS. MRI-based measurement of hippocampal volume in patients with combat-related posttraumatic stress disorder. Am J Psychiatry. 1995;152(7):973–81. https://doi.org/10.1176/ajp.152.7.973.

Carter CS, MacDonald AW, Ross LL, Stenger VA, Bench CJ. Anterior cingulate cortex activity and impaired self-monitoring of performance in patients with schizophrenia: an event-related fMRI study. Am J Psychiatry. 2001;158(8):1423–8. https://doi.org/10.1176/appi.ajp.158.9.1423.

Etkin A, Büchel C, Gross JJ. The neural bases of emotion regulation. Nat Rev Neurosci. 2015;16(11):693–700. https://doi.org/10.1038/nrn4044. PMID: 26481098.

Goldstein RZ, Volkow ND. Dysfunction of the prefrontal cortex in addiction: neuroimaging findings and clinical implications. Nat Rev Neurosci. 2011;12(11):652–69. https://doi.org/10.1038/nrn3119.

Ho TC, Connolly CG, Henje Blom E, LeWinn KZ, Strigo IA, Paulus MP, Frank G, Max JE, Wu J, Chan M, Tapert SF, Simmons AN, Yang TT. Emotion-dependent functional connectivity of the default mode network in adolescent depression. Biol Psychiatry. 2015;78(9):635–46. https://doi.org/10.1016/j.biopsych.2014.09.002.

Johnson K, Vanderhoef D, Magrath N. Psychiatric-mental health nurse practitioner review and resource manual. American Nurses Association: American Nurses Credentialing Center; 2020.

Kneisl CR, Trigoboff E. Contemporary psychiatric mental health nursing. 3rd ed. Pearson; 2012.

Kolb B, Whishaw IQ. Fundamentals of human neuropsychology. Worth Publishers; 2015.

Mayberg HS, Liotti M, Brannan SK, McGinnis S, Mahurin RK, Jerabek PA, Tekell JL. Reciprocal limbic-cortical function and negative mood: converging PET findings in depression and normal sadness. Am J Psychiatry. 1999;156(5):675–82. https://doi.org/10.1176/ajp.156.5.675.

McEwen BS, Morrison JH. Brain on stress: vulnerability and plasticity of the prefrontal cortex over the life course. Neuron. 2013;79(1):16–29. https://doi.org/10.1016/j.neuron.2013.06.028.

Purves D, Augustine GJ, Fitzpatrick D, Katz LC, LaMantia A-S, McNamara JO, Williams SM, (Eds.). Neuroscience. 6th ed. Oxford University Press; 2017.

Sheline YI, Sanghavi M, Mintun MA, Gado MH. Depression duration but not age predicts hippocampal volume loss in medically healthy women with recurrent major depression. J Neurosci. 1999;19(12):5034–43. https://doi.org/10.1523/JNEUROSCI.19-12-05034.1999.

Siegle GJ, Thompson W, Carter CS, Steinhauer SR, Thase ME. Increased amygdala and decreased dorsolateral prefrontal BOLD responses in unipolar depression: related and independent features. Biol Psychiatry. 2007;61(2):198–209. https://doi.org/10.1016/j.biopsych.2006.05.048.

Zakhari R. The psychiatric-mental health nurse practitioner certification review manual. Springer Publishing Company; 2021.

Notes:

Notes:

Assessment and Diagnosis Fundamentals

5

Test your learning and check your understanding of this book's contents: use the "Springer Nature Flashcards" app to access questions using ▶ https://sn.pub/62J0Ar.

To use the app, please follow the instructions in Chap. 1.

Before advancing to the role of a nurse practitioner, one must first become a registered nurse. This prerequisite is grounded in the fundamental importance of maintaining the nurse identity, not only as a philosophical commitment to holistic care but also as a repository of essential nursing science knowledge that accompanies practitioners in their new roles as healthcare providers. Even Psychiatric-Mental Health Nurse Practitioners (PMHNPs) must rule out thyroid problems, malignancies, and nutritional deficiencies before diagnosing a mental illness.

To comprehend patients' health and mental health therapy, PMHNPs obtain a complete medical and psychiatric history. Data on current symptoms, medical problems, medications, and mental health family history are collected. PMHNPs check for mental illness and physical health issues throughout the physical exam. This may involve vital signs, neurological evaluation, and bodily inspection for injuries or illness. A screening history and physical exam enable the PMHNP to rule out psychiatric-causing medical conditions.

The mental status exam is key to the PMHNP evaluation. This test evaluates appearance, behavior, emotion, affect, thought processes, and cognition. PMHNPs can assess mental health by asking and observing. They may assess mood, energy, concentration, communication, mental processes, and judgment. To examine mental health, PMHNPs may use standardized tests like the MMSE or PHQ-9. These methods standardize and objectively evaluate depression and cognitive function.

PMHNPs diagnose mental health issues using several signs. PMHNPs evaluate symptoms' severity, duration, and impact on life. Medical and psychiatric history,

T. Stewart, *Psychiatric-Mental Health Nurse Practitioner Program Companion and Board Certification Exam Review Workbook*,
https://doi.org/10.1007/978-3-031-60894-0_5

including previous therapy and physical or environmental factors that may be producing symptoms, is also assessed.

PMHNPs can diagnose mental illness using the DSM or ICD-10. These tools help providers standardize mental health diagnoses. The most widely used US mental health diagnostic manual is the DSM. Detailed descriptions and diagnostic criteria are provided for mood, anxiety, psychotic, personality, and substance use disorders. Many nations diagnose and classify mental illness using the World Health Organization's ICD-10. It detects various mental and physical illnesses and injuries.

This chapter reviews important fundamental information from general nursing that will continue to be necessary as a psychiatric-mental health nurse practitioner. This information will include important laboratory values and their meanings, such as hypo- vs. hyperthyroidism, renal and liver function tests, and electrolyte levels. This chapter also discusses nurse practitioners' assessment and diagnosis.

5.1 Foundations

1. What are some differences between a sign and a symptom?

Sign	Symptom

2. In the table below are ten common signs and symptoms seen in psychiatry. Label each as a sign (S) or a symptom (Sx).

S/Sx	Sign/Symptom
	Flat affect (reduced emotional expression)
	Auditory hallucinations (hearing voices)
	Delusions (false beliefs)
	Suicidal ideation (thoughts of suicide)
	Disorganized speech (incoherence)
	Agitation or restlessness
	Anxiety (feelings of worry, nervousness)
	Depressed mood (feeling sad or empty)
	Catatonia (abnormal motor behaviors)
	Insomnia (difficulty sleeping)

3. What are the differences between a side effect and an adverse effect?

Side effect	Adverse effect

4. In the table below are ten common side effects and adverse effects seen with psychiatric medications. Label each as a side effect (SE) or adverse effect (AE).

SE/AE	Effect
	Agranulocytosis (a severe drop in white blood cells) from clozapine
	Dry mouth from anticholinergic medications (e.g., TCAs)
	Sedation or drowsiness from benzodiazepines or antipsychotics
	Serotonin syndrome from SSRIs (when taken in high doses or with other serotonergic drugs)
	Weight gain from atypical antipsychotics or mood stabilizers
	Suicidal thoughts, particularly in young people starting antidepressants
	Extrapyramidal symptoms (EPS) like tremors or rigidity from typical antipsychotics
	Sexual dysfunction from SSRIs and other antidepressants
	Tardive dyskinesia from long-term use of antipsychotics
	Stevens-Johnson syndrome (a severe skin reaction) from certain medications like lamotrigine

5. Write the range of normal results for each lab test. Exact matches to the answers are not necessary as the ranges differ by laboratory.

	Attempt #1	Attempt #2	Attempt #3
Sodium (Na)			
Potassium (K)			
Calcium (ca)			
Magnesium (mg)			
Phosphorus (PO)			
Glucose (fasting)			
pH			
Pa CO_2			

	Attempt #1	Attempt #2	Attempt #3
Pa O_2			
HCO_3 (bicarb)			
Cl (chloride)			
RBC's males			
RBC's females			
HGB			
HCT			
WBC's			
Erythrocyte sedimentation rate			
Total serum cholesterol			
LDL			
HDL			
Triglycerides			
Therapeutic INR			
PT			
PTT			
INR			
Albumin			
Ammonia			
Total bilirubin			
Total protein			
Urine specific gravity			
Urine pH			
Glucose, RBCs, WBCs, albumin in urine			
Bacteria in urine			
Serum creatinine			
BUN			
GFR			
Digoxin level			
Lithium level			
Magnesium sulfate			
Phenobarbital			
Theophylline			
Hb A1C			
Platelets			
CVP			
AST/ALT			
Lactic acid			
Troponin			
Creatine kinase (rhabdo marker, ALS)			
Brain natriuretic peptide (heart failure marker)			
Uric acid			
Acceptable Lead level			

6. For each thyroid hormone, provide the normal accepted range and signs and symptoms of its dysfunction.

Hormone	Normal range	Signs and symptoms of low levels	Signs and symptoms of high levels
Triiodothyronine (T3)			
Thyroxine (T4)			
Thyroid-stimulating hormone (TSH)			

7. Label each of the following test results as euthyroid, hypothyroid, or hyperthyroid.

	TSH = 84 mU/L, free T4 = 3 nmol/L
	TSH = 0.15 mU/L, free T4 = 79 nmol/L
	TSH = 8.9 mU/L, free T4 = 15 nmol/L
	TSH = 2.2 mU/L, free T4 = 82 nmol/L
	TSH = 24 mU/L, free T4 = 3 nmol/L
	TSH = 1.9 mU/L, free T4 = 22 nmol/L

8. What are the five psychiatric symptoms that may be caused by a disordered thyroid?

   1.____
   2.____
   3.____
   4.____
   5.____.

9. A patient takes Depakote for their mood disorder. What laboratory tests will be important for the PMHNP to monitor?

10. The therapeutic range for Valproate is ________—________ mcg/mL.

11. A PMHNP might be expected to see an elevated ____ lab value in a patient who abuses alcohol.

12. The lab test for ______________________________ is the most sensitive and specific indicator for kidney disease. ______________________________ lab test is best to monitor overall kidney function.

13. For a patient on lithium therapy, which lab tests will be key to monitor, in addition to lithium blood levels?

14. The therapeutic range for lithium is ________—________ mmol/L.

15. For each patient scenario, would we expect their lithium level to be normal, high, or low?

	Patient is dehydrated
	Patient's sodium levels are elevated
	Patient's sodium intake is reduced
	Patient is taking ACEIs, diuretics, and metronidazole

16. To initiate clozapine therapy, a patient's ANC must be at least _______________ mm^3.

17. For each of the following laboratory findings, provide a diagnosis and an example of how this abnormality may present in mental health.

Laboratory finding	Potential diagnosis	Psychiatric example
Hemoglobin 10.2 g/dL		
Hemoglobin 10.2 g/dL and MCV 77 fL		
Hemoglobin 10.2 g/dL and MCV 105 fL		
PLT 70,000/mm^3		

18. For each of the following high and low electrolyte levels, provide potential signs and symptoms and causes.

Imbalance	Lab value	Signs and symptoms	Potential causes
↓Na^+	<135		
↑Na^+	>145		

Imbalance	Lab value	Signs and symptoms	Potential causes
↓ Mg+	<1.3 mg/dL		
↑Mg+	>2.7 mg/dL		
↓K+	<3.5 mEq/L		
↑K+	>5.0 mEq/L		
↓Ca+	<8.5 mg/dL		
↑Ca+	>10.5 mg/dL		

19. A normal hemoglobin A1C level would be < ______%. A normal fasting glucose level would be < _______ mg/dL.

20. For hypoglycemia and hyperglycemia, provide the serum glucose level for diagnosis and common signs and symptoms.

Hypoglycemia		
Hyperglycemia		

21. For patients on second-generation antipsychotics, which laboratory tests should be ordered to monitor for dyslipidemia?

22. Label each of the following as most characteristic of Diabetes mellitus Type 1, Type 2, or normal.

	Autoimmune
	Insulin resistance
	Acute onset, weight loss, ketonuria
	Few symptoms
	Often diagnosed through routine screening/blood work
	Beta cell destruction
	Polydipsia, polyphagia, polyuria

23. What is anemia?

24. Cushing's syndrome is characterized by an excess of cortisol, a hormone that plays a crucial role in stress response, metabolism, and immune function. What are some potential mental health effects of this syndrome?

25. ________________________________ is characterized by insufficient production of cortisol and often aldosterone. This deficiency can significantly affect the body's ability to respond to stress and maintain homeostasis. What are three potential mental health sequelae associated with this disease?

    1.________________________________
    2.________________________________
    3.________________________________.

26. Epilepsy is a neurological disorder characterized by recurrent seizures. In individuals with epilepsy, certain psychiatric medications and treatments can lower the seizure threshold, making seizures more likely to occur. Name three psychiatric medications that may lower the seizure threshold and two procedures that should be avoided in clients with epilepsy or a history of seizures.

    Medications:

    1.________________________________
    2.________________________________
    3.________________________________

    Procedures:

    1.________________________________
    2.________________________________.

27. How might epilepsy affect mental health?

28. The connection between infections and mental health is an area of increasing interest and research, highlighting the intricate interplay between the immune system, the brain, and psychological well-being. Various infections can influence mental health in both acute and chronic phases, and the impact can range from mild mood disturbances to severe psychiatric conditions. Name five ways in which infections can be connected to mental health.

    1.______________________________
    2.______________________________
    3.______________________________
    4.______________________________
    5.______________________________.

29. Complete the following table on commonly ordered lab tests in psychiatry.

Lab test	What is included	Purpose/Common use
Complete blood count (CBC)		
Comprehensive metabolic panel (CMP)		
Thyroid function tests		
Lipid profile		
Vitamin levels		

Lab test	What is included	Purpose/Common use
Drug screening		
Liver function tests (LFTs)		
Electrolyte panel		
Renal function tests		
Fasting blood glucose		
Hemoglobin A1c (HbA1c)		
Prolactin level		

30. If the PMHNP completes a physical examination of a new client, then the client does not need to continue seeing their primary healthcare provider.
TRUE FALSE

31. Name three to five reasons why a PMHNP should be familiar with how to conduct and review findings from a physical exam.

1.
2.
3.
4.
5.

32. Give three examples of assessments or procedures that are often included in a physical examination that a PMHNP is not qualified to complete, or is deferred by a PMHNP. Then, explain why.

1.
2.
3.

33. What are the three to five goals of the initial assessment or intake interview?

1.
2.
3.
4.
5.

34. For each statement, identify its best descriptor. Each descriptor is only used once.

_____Empathic Statement	A. What brings you in today?
_____Fact finding question	B. Describe your initial reaction to me
_____Open-ended question	C. You seem sad when you talk about her
_____Clarifying question	D. Sounds very lonely
_____Gentle command	E. General summary of what has been said
_____Feelings question	F. Can you tell me more about that?
_____Reflective statement	G. How did that make you feel?
_____Paraphrasing	H. What medication are you taking?

35. PMHNPs should be skilled at checking a client's reflexes. What mental illnesses or side effects to which medications may present as abnormal reflexes?

36. What is the Babinski reflex? What is a positive Babinski sign in adults? What does this mean?

37. For each cranial nerve, write its name, whether it is sensory (S), motor (M), or both (B), and how to test its function.

CN #	Name	Function	Assessment
I			
II			
III			
IV			

CN #	Name	Function	Assessment
V			
VI			
VII			
VIII			
IX			
X			
XI			
XII			

38. To check a patient's equilibrium, the PMHNP can conduct a ______________________________ test. What directions would the PMHNP give the patient? Abnormal findings would suggest what possible dysfunctions?

39. ____ refers to an individual's ability to rapidly alternate their movements without pausing or breaking the rhythm. It is particularly useful in identifying cerebellar dysfunction.

40. In the table below, explain how a PMHNP would test each of the sensory functions.

Graphesthesia	

Pain	
Stereognosis	
Superficial touch	
Temperature	
Two-point discrimination	

41. Part of the physical examination requires testing muscle mass, tone, and strength. What abnormal findings might be of particular interest to a PMHNP?

42. Cranial nerve II and a patient's vision is tested using the __________________ chart.

43. Nystagmus and blurry vision may be caused by psychotropic medications.

TRUE FALSE

44. ______________________ is a common second-generation antipsychotic that is linked to cataract formation.

45. A patient is taking lithium for Bipolar Disorder I, so the PMHNP should visually inspect and palpate the ______________________ gland.

46. Patients taking ______________________ should be asked about breast growth, tenderness, and milk production.

47. Why should a PMHNP check for peripheral edema on a client taking lithium?

48. What elements should be included in a suicide risk assessment?

49. What should be included in a safety plan for clients with suicidal ideation?

50. The ______________________________ is a questionnaire used for suicide assessment developed to systematically assess the severity of a person's suicidal ideation and behavior.

51. List the core components of a mental status exam. Then, provide five descriptive words that could be used to describe normal and abnormal findings for each component.

Component	Description of component	Normal findings	Abnormal findings

52. What signs might evidence tardive dyskinesia? The ____________________ ____________________________ Scale is the most widely used tool to objectively assess for tardive dyskinesia.

53. For each area of physical health, list three to five topics about which you could ask the client during the medical review of systems.

Area	Topics
General/constitutional	
HEENT (head, eyes, ears, nose, throat)	
Pulmonary	
Cardiovascular	
Gastrointestinal	
Urogenital	
Hematological	
Female sexual/reproductive health	

Area	Topics
Male sexual/reproductive health	
Neurological	
Endocrine	
Musculoskeletal	
Dermatological	

54. Complete the crossword puzzle using different thought process terminology.

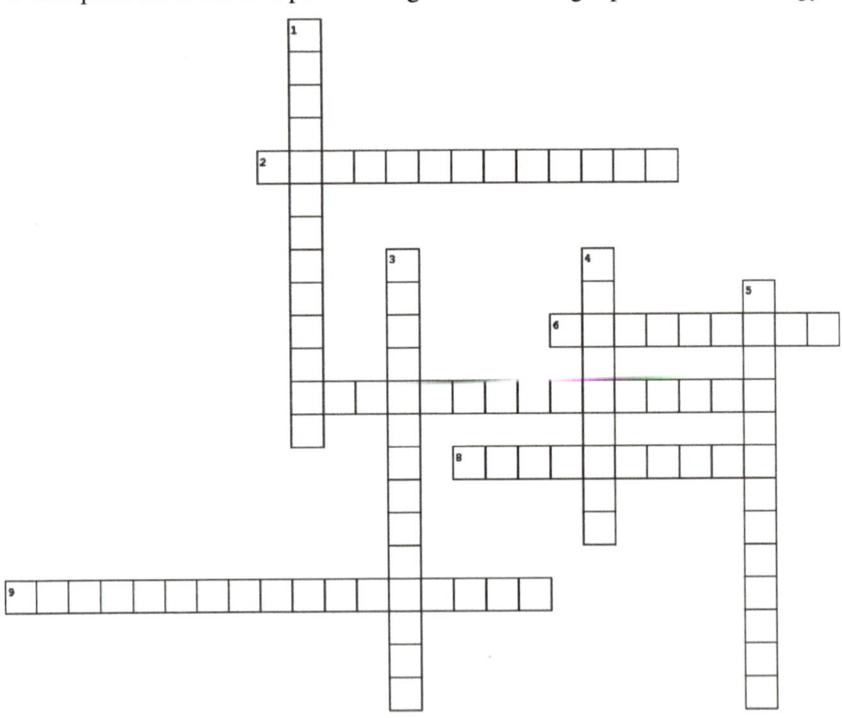

Across	Down
2. Repetition of words, phrases, or concepts taken out of context	1. Answering a question with a statement that is pertinent to the overall subject without actually responding to the initial question
6. Severe illogical or unclear links between ideas	3. Excessive inclusion of unimportant or irrelevant elements that make it difficult to understand the point
Interruption of the mental process before an idea has fully developed, and may accompany a lack of recall	4. Creation of novel words or phrases or the unconventional use of common ones
8. Disruption in the logical flow of thoughts, or loose associations, making sentences illogical	5. Series of varied connections that give the impression that ideas are changing suddenly from one to the next; frequently represented through hurried, strained speech
9. Sounds of words, like rhyming, are associated with thought meanings	

5.2 Answers and Explanations to Chapter Activities

1. Signs and symptoms differ in observation and reporting.

Sign	Symptom
Objective discovery that can be witnessed and measured by someone other than the patient clinician or spectator can see, hear, measure, or feel it factual Examples: A clinician or other person notices weight loss or gain, not just the patient A clinician notices trembling hands or profuse sweating during a consultation A PMHNP sees chaotic speech or behavior during an assessment, or a patient speaks to oneself as if to someone elsewhere	Patient-reported Patient views as abnormal, which others may not notice Patients report feelings, sensations, and impressions of normal functioning alterations as symptoms Subjective Examples: The patient feels hopeless or melancholy, which is different from their usual mood The patient worries about many things, feels out of control, or feels doomed The patient hears voices or believes delusions that are not shared by others in their culture

2.

S/Sx	Sign/Symptom
S	Flat affect (reduced emotional expression)
Sx	Auditory hallucinations (hearing voices)
Sx	Delusions (false beliefs)
Sx	Suicidal ideation (thoughts of suicide)
S	Disorganized speech (incoherence)
S	Agitation or restlessness
Sx	Anxiety (feelings of worry, nervousness)

S/Sx	Sign/Symptom
Sx	Depressed mood (feeling sad or empty)
S	Catatonia (abnormal motor behaviors)
Sx	Insomnia (difficulty sleeping)

3. In medication and treatment, "side effect" and "adverse effect" refer to unwanted outcomes, but they range in intensity and meaning. In psychiatric-mental health, side and unfavorable effects must be distinguished for medication management and patient safety. To ensure therapy benefits outweigh concerns, clinicians must evaluate both types of outcomes and change treatment regimens as needed. Patients should know what to expect and when to seek care for concerns.

Side effect	Adverse effect
Unpleasant but are usually minimal and predictable may be beneficial, but they are not the medication's main goal Examples: Nausea or dry mouth may occur initially starting the medicine, but it usually goes away Weight gain or sleepiness, which can be managed with dose modifications or lifestyle changes Drowsiness or minor cognitive impairment which are usually harmless but may impact daily activities	Pharmaceutical or treatment's more severe, damaging, or unanticipated impact can cause harm, health hazards, or extra treatment might be unpredictable and cause medication discontinuation Examples: High doses or combination of SSRIs with other serotonergic medicines can produce serotonin syndrome, a potentially fatal brain disorder Tardive dyskinesia, a dangerous, sometimes permanent movement disease marked by repeated, involuntary lower facial motions Dependence and withdrawal syndrome might be severe and necessitate medical attention

4.

SE/AE	Effect
AE	Agranulocytosis (a severe drop in white blood cells) from clozapine
SE	Dry mouth from anticholinergic medications (e.g., TCAs)
SE	Sedation or drowsiness from benzodiazepines or antipsychotics
AE	Serotonin syndrome from SSRIs (when taken in high doses or with other serotonergic drugs)
SE	Weight gain from atypical antipsychotics or mood stabilizers
AE	Suicidal thoughts, particularly in young people starting antidepressants
AE	Extrapyramidal symptoms (EPS) like tremors or rigidity from typical antipsychotics
SE	Sexual dysfunction from SSRIs and other antidepressants
AE	Tardive dyskinesia from long-term use of antipsychotics
AE	Stevens-Johnson syndrome (a severe skin reaction) from certain medications like lamotrigine

5.

Sodium (Na)	135–145 meq
Potassium (K)	3.5–5 meq
Calcium (ca)	9.0–10 mg/dL
Magnesium (mg)	1.3–2.1 mg/dL
Phosphorus (PO)	3.0–4.5
Glucose (fasting)	70–105
pH	7.35–7.45, over 90 years 7.25–7.45
Pa CO_2	35–45 mmHg

Pa O_2	>80–100 mm hg
HCO_3 (bicarb)	21–26 meq
Cl (chloride)	98–106 meq
RBC's males	4.7–6.1 million
RBC's females	4.2–5.4 million
HGB	Males: 14–18 Females: 12–16
HCT	Males: 42–52% (50%) Females: 37–47% (45%)
WBC's	5000–10,000 mm^3
Erythrocyte sedimentation rate	<20 mm/h
Total serum cholesterol	Desirable less than 200 mg/dL, less than 150 mg/dL is the target range for therapy to reduce the risk of CV
LDL	Less than 100 mg/dL
HDL	Greater than 40 for men Greater than 50 for women
Triglycerides	Less than 150
Therapeutic INR	2.0–3.0
PT	11–14 s. Therapeutic range for anticoag therapy is 1.5–2 X normal range
PTT	16–40 range, remain <40 s. Therapeutic range for anticoag therapy is 1.5–2.5 X the normal value
INR	Normal 0.9–1.2 If a client needs anti-coagulation, the desired value is 2–3
Albumin	3.8–5
Ammonia	35–65
Total bilirubin	0.0–1.5
Total protein	6–8
Urine specific gravity	1.005–1.030
Urine pH	Average 6.0, range 4.6–8.0
Glucose, RBCs, WBCs, albumin in urine	Negative
Bacteria in urine	< 10,000 colonies/mL
Serum creatinine	Males: 0.6–1.2 Females: 0.5–1.1
BUN	10–20
GFR	90–120 mL/min
Digoxin level	0.8–2.0 ng/mL
Lithium level	0.5–1.2 meQ/L
Magnesium sulfate	4–8
Phenobarbital	10–30
Theophylline	10–20
Hb A1C	5–7
Platelets	150–400,000
CVP	2–8 mmHg
AST/ALT	10–40 μ/L
Lactic acid	5–20 mg/dL
Troponin	<0.5 ng/mL
Creatine kinase (rhabdo marker, ALS)	<200 μ/L
Brain natriuretic peptide (heart failure marker)	<100 pg/mL
Uric acid	5–6
Acceptable lead level	<10 mcg/dL

6.

Hormone	Normal range	Signs and symptoms of low levels	Signs and symptoms of high levels
Triiodothyronine (T3)	Total T3: 80–200 ng/dL Free T3: 2.0-4.4 pg/mL	– Fatigue and sluggishness – Unintentional weight gain – Cold intolerance–dry skin and hair–depression – Constipation – Slow heart rate – Muscle weakness	– Nervousness and irritability – Unintentional weight loss – Heat intolerance–sweating – Palpitations – Diarrhea – Muscle weakness – Insomnia
Thyroxine (T4)	Total T4: 5.0–12.0 μg/dL Free T4: 0.9–1.7 ng/dL	– Fatigue and sluggishness – Unintentional weight gain – Cold intolerance – Dry skin – Hair loss – Depression – Constipation – Slow heart rate - memory problems	– Rapid heartbeat – Hand tremors – Nervousness – Excessive sweating – Heat intolerance – Frequent bowel movements – Weight loss – Sleep disturbances
Thyroid-stimulating hormone (TSH)	0.5–5.0 mIU/L (varies slightly by lab)	– Often detected by elevated TSH levels as it is a response to low T4/T3. – Symptoms are generally reflective of low T3 and T4	– Often detected by low TSH levels as it is a response to high T4/T3. – Symptoms are generally reflective of high T3 and T4

7.

Hypothyroid	TSH = 84 mU/L, Free T4 = 3 nmol/L
Hyperthyroid	TSH = 0.15 mU/L, free T4 = 79 nmol/L
Hypothyroid	TSH = 8.9 mU/L, free T4 = 15 nmol/L
Euthyroid	TSH = 2.2 mU/L, free T4 = 82 nmol/L
Hypothyroid	TSH = 24 mU/L, free T4 = 3 nmol/L
Euthyroid	TSH = 1.9 mU/L, free T4 = 22 nmol/L

8. Depression: Underactive thyroid glands can cause depression. Patients may suffer depression, weariness, loss of interest in activities, and malaise.

    1. Hyperthyroidism can cause anxiety and panic attacks. They include anxiety, restlessness, high heart rate, tremors, and panic attacks.
    2. Both hypo- and hyperthyroidism can cause mood swings and irritability. Rapid mood shifts, impatience, and increased emotional responses can result.
    3. Cognitive impairment: Hypothyroidism can induce memory impairments, sluggish thinking, and concentration issues, similar to dementia and depression.
    4. Fatigue and sleep issues: Thyroid abnormalities can cause insomnia or excessive sleepiness. Despite appropriate sleep, hypothyroidism causes chronic fatigue.

5. Psychosis: Myxedema madness, an uncommon form of severe hypothyroidism, can cause hallucinations and delusions.
6. Thyroid diseases can cause significant personality or behavior changes, but this is rare.

9. ALT, AST, ALP liver function tests.
10. 50–120 mcg/mL
11. Gamma-glutamyl transferase (GGT).
12. Creatinine; GFR.
13. Creatinine, BUN, GFR kidney function tests, thyroid TSH, electrolytes.
14. 0.6–1.2 mmol/L
15.

High	Patient is dehydrated
High	Patient's sodium levels are elevated
Low	Patient's sodium intake is reduced
High	Patient is taking ACEIs, diuretics, and metronidazole

16. 1500 mm^3
17.

Laboratory finding	Potential diagnosis	Psychiatric example
Hemoglobin 10.2 g/dL	Mild anemia	A patient with anemia might present with symptoms like fatigue and low mood, which can exacerbate depressive symptoms
Hemoglobin 10.2 g/dL and MCV 77 fL	Microcytic anemia (e.g., iron deficiency anemia, heavy menstruation)	Iron deficiency anemia can lead to impaired cognitive function and concentration, potentially affecting anxiety and mood disorders
Hemoglobin 10.2 g/dL and MCV 105 fL	Macrocytic anemia (e.g., vitamin B12 or folate deficiency)	Deficiencies in B12 or folate can cause neurological changes, leading to symptoms like memory loss or mood disturbances
PLT 70,000/mm^3	Thrombocytopenia	A patient with thrombocytopenia may experience increased anxiety about health or bleeding, impacting their overall mental Well-being

18.

Imbalance	Lab value	Signs and symptoms	Potential causes
↓Na+	<135	Anorexia, N/V, HA, lethargy, dizziness, confusion, muscle cramps/weakness, seizures, papilledema, dry skin, increased pulse, hypotension, weight gain, edema	Polydipsia, fluid loss, renal disease, adrenal insufficiency, SIADH, head trauma, hyperglycemia, heart failure, meds (diuretics, oxytocin)
↑Na+	>145	Thirst, hyperthermia, lethargy, hypertension, tachycardia, restless, weak, swollen tongue	Dehydration, DI, heatstroke, sea water, burns, hyperventilation, diarrhea, meds (corticosteroids, sodium)

Imbalance	Lab value	Signs and symptoms	Potential causes
↓ Mg+	<1.3 mg/dL	Neuromuscular irritability, + trousseau, + Chvostek, insomnia, mood changes, anorexia, N/V, hyperreflexivity, hypertension, EKG changes (PVCs, inverted T waves, ↓ST, prolonged PR, widened QRS)	Alcoholism, diarrhea, ↓K+ and ↓ca+, hyperparathyroidism, hyperaldosteronism, renal or heart failure, DKA, referring syndrome, MI, meds (gentamicin, cisplatin, cyclosporine, laxative)
↑Mg+	>2.7 mg/dL	Flushed skin, thirst, hypotension, muscle weakness, fatigue, N/V, hyporeflexivity, ↓respirations, dizziness, cardiac arrest, coma, diaphoresis, EKG changes (bradycardia, prolonged PR interval, QRS, peaked T waves, arrhythmias, palpitations)	Renal failure, ↓adrenal fx (Addison's dz), DKA, hypothyroidism, mg + administration (IV or parenteral for pregnant women with pre-eclampsia)
↓K+	<3.5 mEq/L	Fatigue, anorexia, N/V, polyuria, decreased bowel motility, ventricular systole or fibrillation, paresthesias, leg cramps, postural hypotension, coma, ileum, hyporeflexivity, EKG (flat T waves, prominent U waves, decreased ST, prolonged PR)	Diarrhea, vomiting, gastric suction, hyperaldosteronism, bulimia, diuresis, alkalosis, starvation, meds (corticosteroids, carbenicillin, amphotericin B, diuretics, digoxin)
↑K+	>5.0 mEq/L	Muscle weaknesses, dysrhythmias, flaccid paralysis, paresthesias, hyperactive GI, cramps, abdominal distention, irritability, anxiety EKG (tented T waves, prolonged PR intervals and QRS, absent P waves, decreased ST)	Pseudohyperkalemia, renal failure, metabolic acidosis, Addison's, crush injury, burns, blood transfusions, meds (ACE inhibitors, NSAIDs, cyclosporine, K+ sparing diuretics)
↓Ca+	<8.5 mg/dL	Anxiety, irritability, mouth twitching, convulsions, finger numbness, diarrhea, muscle cramps, arrhythmias, hypotension, + trousseau, + Chvostek, seizures, increased deep tendon reflexes, decreased clotting and prothrombin, EKG (prolonged QT, lengthened ST)	Low albumin, renal failure, hyperthyroidism, hypermagnesmia, pancreatitis, Crohn's dz., hypoparathyroidism, alkalosis, low Vit D, peritonitis, diarrhea, burns, fistulas
↑Ca+	>10.5 mg/dL	Weakness, fatigue, anorexia, N/V, constipation, polyuria, polydipsia, renal stones, HTN, fractures, tingling lips, muscle cramps, confusion, hypoactive bowels, EKG (shortened ST segments and QT intervals, bradycardia, heart blocks)	Hyperparathyroidism, renal failure, immobilization, metabolic acidosis, meds (thiazides, ca+, corticosteroids, digoxin, Vit D, lithium)

19. 6%, 100 mg/dL
20.

Hypoglycemia	<55 mg/dL	– Shakiness, nervousness, or anxiety – Sweating, chills, and clamminess – Irritability or impatience – Confusion, including delirium – Rapid/fast heartbeat – Lightheadedness or dizziness – Hunger and nausea–sleepiness – Blurred/impaired vision – Tingling or numbness in the lips or tongue–headaches–weakness or fatigue – Anger, stubbornness, or sadness – Lack of coordination – Seizures or loss of consciousness (in severe cases)
Hyperglycemia	>350 mg/dL	– Frequent urination – Increased thirst – High levels of sugar in the urine – Headaches – Difficulty concentrating – Blurred vision – Fatigue (weak, tired feeling) – Weight loss – Blood sugar of more than 180 mg/dL – Nausea, vomiting, shortness of breath (in severe cases) – A very dry mouth and skin – A rapid heartbeat – Ketones in the urine (especially for type 1 diabetics in case of diabetic ketoacidosis)

21. Total cholesterol, LDL, HDL, triglycerides.
22.

Type 1	Autoimmune
Type 2	Insulin resistance
Type 1	Acute onset, weight loss, ketonuria
Type 2	Few symptoms
Type 2	Often diagnosed through routine screening/blood work
Type 1	Beta cell destruction
Type 1	Polydipsia, polyphagia, polyuria

23. Anemia, a hemoglobin shortage, can cause physical and mental health difficulties. Anemia commonly causes weariness and lethargy. Fatigue can cause melancholy, lethargy, and low motivation, hurting quality of life and mental health.
24. Cushing's Syndrome can affect mental health. Cushing's elevated cortisol levels can cause mood issues. Patients may feel hopeless, depressed, or prone to panic attacks and anxiety. People may be irritable and have trouble controlling their emotions. Memory, focus, and decision-making can suffer like chronic stress. Trouble sleeping might worsen mental health difficulties. Rarely, elevated cortisol levels might cause hallucinations or delusions. Weight gain, acne, and stretch marks can lower self-esteem and cause sadness and social anxiety.
25. Addison's Disease can affect mental health.

- Apathy and depression: Addison's disease's lethargy and low energy can worsen depression. Patients may lose interest in hobbies or activities they used to like.
- Cognitive fog: Patients often experience concentration and memory issues, called "brain fog."
- Stress Intolerance: Reduced stress response can increase anxiety and make stressful situations harder to handle.
- Some people may be irritable or moody.
- Fatigue, physical weakness, and weight loss might impair everyday activities, mood, and quality of life.

26.

- Tricyclic antidepressants (TCAs): Higher doses can lower the seizure threshold. Example: amitriptyline with clomipramine.
- Bupropion (Wellbutrin): At larger doses or in people with a history of seizures, this antidepressant may lower the seizure threshold.
- Certain antipsychotics: Chlorpromazine, thioridazine, and clozapine can lower the seizure threshold, even though newer ones are safer.
- Stimulants: ADHD and narcolepsy medications like amphetamine and methylphenidate may increase seizure risk.
  Avoid these treatments:
- Electroconvulsive therapy (ECT): ECT creates a controlled seizure but can treat severe depression and other mental health issues. It can be utilized in epilepsy patients, but a neurologist must coordinate it and alter antiepileptic drugs.
- Transcranial magnetic stimulation (TMS): Safe, however susceptible people may have seizures.

27. Epilepsy increases the likelihood of these diseases. These mental health concerns might be caused by chronic disease management stress, seizure fear, and social stigma. Epilepsy can cause mood disorders like bipolar disorder in addition to despair and anxiety. Epilepsy can impair memory, attention, and executive functioning depending on the kind and location of seizures. Cognitive problems can cause dissatisfaction, low self-esteem, and loneliness. Rarely, epilepsy patients with temporal lobe seizures may experience psychosis. Epilepsy can alter behavior and personality. If epilepsy affects certain brain areas, people may be irritable, aggressive, or otherwise behave poorly.
28. Diseases that directly damage the brain, such as encephalitis or meningitis, can cause mental health issues like confusion, delirium, and long-term cognitive impairments. Viruses like HSV and bacteria like *Neisseria meningitidis* cause similar consequences. The immune system can alter brain function even if an infection does not reach the CNS. Cytokines, immune system proteins released during infection, can affect brain chemistry and cause weariness, depression, and cognitive fog.

    Infections' indirect mental health effects:

- Chronic illness and stress: Chronic infectious diseases including HIV, hepatitis, and Lyme disease can cause stress, which increases the risk of mental health disorders like depression and anxiety.
- Psychosocial impact: Stigma, solitude, and life changes might influence mental health after infections. Social stigma and discrimination can cause anxiety and sadness in HIV patients.

Mental Health Disorders and Specific Infections:

- PANDAS: Pediatric Autoimmune Neuropsychiatric Disorders Associated with Streptococcal Infections A strep infection that causes brain inflammation due to a misdirected immune response. This can cause sudden obsessive-compulsive behaviors, tics, and mood changes in youngsters.
- Toxoplasmosis: The parasite Toxoplasma gondii has been linked to schizophrenia and bipolar disorder. Parasites can change brain neurotransmitters.
- Severe flu can cause neurological symptoms and, in rare circumstances, long-term neuropsychiatric consequences.

29.

Lab test	What is included	Purpose/common use
Complete blood count (CBC)	White blood cells, red blood cells, hemoglobin, hematocrit, and platelets	Used to check for anemia, infection, and other conditions that can cause fatigue, weakness, or psychiatric symptoms
Comprehensive metabolic panel (CMP)	Glucose, calcium, proteins, electrolytes, kidney, and liver function tests (BUN, creatinine, ALT, AST, bilirubin)	Used to assess general health status, liver and kidney function, and electrolyte balance; important for medication management
Thyroid function tests	Thyroid stimulating hormone (TSH), free T4, sometimes free T3	Used to assess for hypo- or hyperthyroidism, which can mimic or exacerbate psychiatric conditions
Lipid profile	Total cholesterol, LDL, HDL, triglycerides	Often ordered for patients on antipsychotics or other medications that can affect lipid metabolism
Vitamin levels	Commonly vitamin D, vitamin B12, and folate levels	Deficiencies can contribute to depression and cognitive issues
Drug screening	Tests for the presence of various drugs and substances	Used to detect substance use which can contribute to or mimic psychiatric conditions
Liver function tests (LFTs)	Alanine transaminase (ALT), aspartate transaminase (AST), alkaline phosphatase (ALP), bilirubin	Ordered to monitor the effects of medications that can impact liver function
Electrolyte panel	Sodium, potassium, chloride, bicarbonate (or total CO_2)	Electrolyte imbalances can affect mental status and are important to monitor with certain medications
Renal function tests	GFR, blood urea nitrogen (BUN), creatinine	Important for dosing and monitoring the side effects of certain psychiatric medications

Lab test	What is included	Purpose/common use
Fasting blood glucose	Blood glucose levels	Ordered to monitor for diabetes or prediabetes, especially important for patients on antipsychotics that can increase glucose levels
Hemoglobin A1c (HbA1c)	Measures average blood glucose over the past 3 months	Used to monitor blood sugar control, particularly in patients on medications that affect glucose metabolism
Prolactin level	Prolactin hormone levels	Often ordered to check for hyperprolactinemia, especially in patients taking antipsychotics known to increase prolactin

30. FALSE. A new client should still see their primary healthcare provider. PMHNPs specialize in mental care, while the primary healthcare provider manages the patient's physical health and medical conditions. Regular visits to a primary care practitioner ensure complete care and management of nonpsychiatric health concerns.
31. A Psychiatric-Mental Health Nurse Practitioner (PMHNP) must know how to conduct and review physical exams for numerous important reasons:

    - Holistic Care: Mental and physical health are intertwined. PMHNPs can diagnose and treat psychiatric problems holistically by being familiar with physical tests.
    - Identifying Physical Health Disorders: Many psychiatric drugs have physical adverse effects, and some physical disorders can worsen psychiatric symptoms. Physical examination skills enable PMHNPs to spot these concerns early and intervene.
    - Comprehensive Assessment: A complete physical exam can reveal the patient's health and well-being. Understanding these clues helps PMHNPs choose therapy programs that meet each patient's needs.
    - Collaborative Care: PMHNPs frequent multidisciplinary teams. Being able to perform and interpret physical exams helps them communicate with other healthcare practitioners and provide coordinated patient care.
    - Patient Education: PMHNPs who understand how physical health affects mental health can better educate patients about physical health, drug side effects, and when to seek medical assistance.
    - Early detection and prevention: Regular physical checkups can discover diseases that would otherwise go unnoticed. PMHNPs who know these examinations can help avoid disease.

32. Breast, Urology, Gynecology Complex Imaging Interpretation, Surgery: These require urological anatomy, intervention, and procedure complications training. It maintains trust, balances power dynamics, and preserves the therapeutic relationship, making the patient feel supported and valued throughout their care journey.

33. Answers will vary, but may include: Developing a therapeutic relationship with the patient, establishing a compassionate understanding of the patient, decreasing the anxiety of the patient, instilling hope about receiving help, and ensuring that the patient will return.
34. __D___Empathic Statement
    __H___Fact finding Question.
    __A___Open-Ended Question.
    __F___Clarifying Question.
    __B___Gentle Command.
    __G___Feelings Question.
    __C___Reflective Statement.
    __E___Paraphrasing
35. PMHNPs should be adept at examining clients' reflexes during a neurological exam. Mental diseases and drug side effects might cause abnormal responses. Some examples:

    - Neurodegenerative Diseases: Abnormal reflexes can accompany psychological symptoms such depression, anxiety, and cognitive impairments in Huntington's and Parkinson's diseases. The "cogwheel rigidity" and limited arm swing of Parkinson's disease are examples.
    - TBI: These diseases may include irritability, mood fluctuations, cognitive impairment, and aberrant reflex responses.
    - Medication and Substances Side Effects:
    - Haloperidol and risperidone, used to treat schizophrenia, can cause extrapyramidal side effects. EPS can cause tardive dyskinesia, uncontrollable movements. Neuroleptic malignant syndrome (NMS), an uncommon but life-threatening event, can cause mental confusion and muscle rigidity.
    - Selective Serotonin Reuptake Inhibitors (SSRIs): Although rare, SSRIs used for depression and anxiety can cause Serotonin Syndrome, which can cause hyperreflexia, agitation, tremors, and confusion.
    - Bipolar disorder medication with lithium can cause tremors and abnormal muscle responses.
    - Delirium tremens and severe alcohol withdrawal can cause autonomic hyperactivity, including tremors and hyperactive reflexes.
    - Muscle discomfort and uncontrollable leg motions might result from opioid withdrawal.

36. The Babinski reflex is a neurological test used during a physical exam to evaluate the corticospinal tract, which travels from the brain to the spinal cord. This tract controls voluntary movement and coordination. The exam involves stroking the lateral sole of the foot with a blunt item from heel to toe. Adults and children over 2 curl their toes downward (plantar flexion). Positive results frequently indicate neurological issues in adults and children over 2 years old.

37.

CN #	Name	Function	Assessment
I	Olfactory	S	Test the sense of smell by having the patient identify different smells with each nostril separately
II	Optic	S	Test visual acuity using a Snellen chart, assess visual fields by confrontation, and examine the optic disc with an ophthalmoscope
III	Oculomotor	M	Test pupillary reaction to light and accommodation, assess extraocular movements, and test for ptosis
IV	Trochlear	M	Test extraocular movements and the patient's ability to look downward and inward
V	Trigeminal	B	Test sensation in the face by touching different areas with a cotton swab, and test motor function by assessing the strength of jaw clenching
VI	Abducens	M	Test extraocular movements and the patient's ability to look outward
VII	Facial	B	Test the patient's ability to make different facial expressions, assess taste on the anterior two-thirds of the tongue, and test the corneal reflex
VIII	Vestibulocochlear	S	Test hearing using a tuning fork or audiometry, and test balance and coordination
IX	Glossopharyngeal	B	Test the gag reflex, assess taste on the posterior one-third of the tongue, and test the patient's ability to swallow
X	Vagus	B	Test the patient's ability to speak and swallow, assess the palate and uvula for symmetry, and listen to the patient's voice for hoarseness or weakness
XI	Accessory	M	Test the patient's ability to shrug the shoulders and turn the head against resistance
XII	Hypoglossal	M	Test the patient's ability to stick out the tongue and move it from side to side

38. The PMHNP can perform a "Romberg Test." to assess patient balance and proprioception—the awareness of one's body's relative location and movement effort. The PMHNP instructs the patient to stand up straight with feet together. "Close your eyes and hold your arms out to the side or in front of you." "Remain in this position for about 20–30 s." The patient should be told to stay still. To ensure patient safety, the PMHNP or another person should be there to catch them if they fall. A positive Romberg sign is when the patient sways or loses balance with their eyes closed but not open. Abnormalities may indicate sensory ataxia, peripheral neuropathy, vestibular dysfunction, and cerebellar ataxia. If the patient sways with their eyes open, they may have cerebellar or central nervous system disorders causing significant balance impairment.
39. Diadochokinesia.

40.

Graphesthesia	The PMHNP asks the patient to close their eyes. Using a blunt object, the PMHNP "draws" a number or letter on the patient's hand
Pain	The PMHNP lightly pricks different areas of the patient's skin with a sharp object and asks the patient to identify the sensation as "sharp" or "dull"
Stereognosis	With their eyes closed, the patient is given a common object to hold and asked to identify it
Superficial touch	Using a piece of cotton or a brush, the PMHNP lightly touches different areas of the patient's skin and asks them to indicate when they feel the sensation
Temperature	The PMHNP uses objects at different temperatures to touch the patient's skin and asks them to report whether they feel warm or cold and to identify the location of the sensation
Two-point discrimination	Using a caliper or two points of a compass, the PMHNP gently presses on the skin, gradually increasing the distance between points, and asks if the patient feels one point or two

41. A Psychiatric-Mental Health Nurse Practitioner (PMHNP) must examine muscle mass, tone, and strength during a physical exam to identify neurological or physical problems that may impair mental health. PMHNPs may be interested in these abnormalities:

- Muscle atrophy: Possible Implications. Muscle atrophy can suggest psychological problems such severe depression, which can cause inactivity. It can potentially indicate nerve damage or ALS.
- Possible Implications: Increased Muscle Tone (Spasticity or Rigidity) Central nervous system disorders might cause muscular tone increase. Rigidity may indicate Parkinson's disease, while spasticity may indicate MS. Mental illness can accompany both illnesses.
- Possible Implications: Decreased Muscle Tone (Hypotonia) Hypotonia can occur in peripheral nerve diseases and cerebellar ataxia. Long-term inactivity owing to serious psychiatric disorders might also cause it.
- Implications of Muscle Weakness May Include: Generalized muscle weakness in Myasthenia Gravis can cause weariness that may mimic or worsen depression. Localized weakness may suggest a neurological disorder.
- Tremors, tics, or chorea may be adverse effects of psychiatric drugs, such as tardive dyskinesia after long-term antipsychotic usage. They may also signal neurological diseases like Parkinson's or Huntington's disease.
- Possible Implications of Abnormal Gait: Neurological diseases including Parkinson's and cerebellar ataxia can cause abnormal gait. Musculoskeletal difficulties or drug side effects may cause it.
- Possible Implications of Muscle Strength or Tone Asymmetry: Asymmetry may signal a stroke or damage. It may also indicate an illness that affects one side of the body more than the other, like Multiple Sclerosis.
- Fasciculations: Usually harmless, these involuntary muscle twitches may indicate neurological diseases like ALS or electrolyte imbalances.

42. Snellen Chart.
43. TRUE. Psychotropic medicines can cause nystagmus and hazy vision. These side effects are common with lithium, antiepileptics, and some antipsychotics. Healthcare practitioners must monitor and manage these adverse effects.
44. Quetiapine.
45. Thyroid.
46. Antipsychotics.
47. Lithium affects renal function. It affects kidney sodium and water processing, causing fluid retention. Lower extremity edema can result from fluid retention.

    - Lithium can influence thyroid function, causing hypothyroidism. Fluid retention and edema can result from reduced metabolism and interstitial mucopolysaccharides in hypothyroidism. There is some evidence that lithium may directly damage blood arteries, causing them to leak fluid into the surrounding tissue and cause edema.
    - Lithium can cause weight gain, which increases edema risk.

48. A complete suicide risk assessment should include:

    - Current and Past Suicide:

      - Asking about suicide thoughts, plans, behaviors, and intent.
      - Suicide attempt history, including frequency, methods, severity, and context.
      - Ideation: Suicidal thoughts' frequency, intensity, and duration.
      - Specific timing, place, and method planned.
      - Access to suicide weapons and drugs.
      - Intent and lethality: The patient's wish for suicide's fatal outcome.
      - Lethality of the approach.

    - Possible Risks:

      - Mental illness, especially depression, bipolar disorder, schizophrenia, PTSD, and substance misuse.
      - Bereavement, divorce, or other major life changes.
      - Past trauma or abuse.
      - Chronic pain, incapacity, or sickness.
      - Mental illness or suicide in family.
      - Lack of assistance or socialization.
      - Impulsiveness or aggression.
      - Factors for protection include effective therapeutic care for mental, physical, and substance addiction illnesses.
      - Strong familial and friend bonds.
      - Coping and problem-solving.
      - Culture or religion that discourages suicide.

    - Warning Signs:

      - Wishing to die or commit suicide.

- Substance misuse rises.
- Leave friends, family, and society.
- Agitation, insomnia, or perpetual sleep.
- Dramatic mood swings.
- Expressing pessimism, trappedness, or no purpose in life.
- Patients' Perspective and Response to Sickness: Understanding the sickness and its impact on life.
- Treatment attitudes and aid perception.
- Safety Planning: Create a documented plan with warning signals, coping skills, social settings, distractions, family/friends, professionals/agency contacts, and safe surroundings.

- Documentation:

  - The patient's statements, your observations, risk factors, protective factors, and the strategy are recorded.
    Plan for follow-up care, including hospitalization if necessary or referral to mental health providers for continued treatment and monitoring.
  - A suicide risk assessment should be repeated often, especially if the patient's circumstances change. Healthcare practitioners must be sensitive and empathetic during assessments to make patients feel heard and supported.

49. A suicidal client's safety plan is a prioritized written list of coping methods and support sources prepared with the healthcare professional. It helps people notice crisis indicators and respond correctly to lessen suicide risk. Include these essentials:

    - Triggers are warning signs.

      - Identifying personal crisis signs such thoughts, pictures, mood, situation, or conduct.
      - Internal coping strategies are self-help methods that can help individuals resist self-harm tendencies. Relaxation, exercise, and mental distractions are examples.

    - Distraction-causing people and places:

      - List of friends, family, and social settings that can help and divert from the problem.
      - Identifying persons who can assist during a crisis and are aware of the person's suicidal ideas. This list should include names and contact info.

    - Professionals or Agencies for Help:

      Mental health, crisis, and emergency contact information. This must include reliable and accessible materials.

- To ensure environmental safety, strategies should be implemented to secure or remove harmful means from the area. This may involve a trusted person keeping medications or firearms or making home safety measures.
- Reasons for Living: Individual motivations for survival. These might remind them of their life's significance and influence.

- Plan Usage:
  - This safety plan's use and timing should be clearly explained, emphasizing that it is a tool for warning indicators.
  - A statement stating the individual's commitment to implementing the safety plan and not acting on self-harm thoughts impulsively.
- Update and review:
  - Review and update the strategy as warning signals, coping mechanisms, and support networks change.
  - The safety plan should always be available so the person may refer to it when they see warning signs. Collaborating on the strategy makes the client feel invested and more inclined to use it in a crisis. A safety plan is not a contract or promise, but a tool to help people detect and act in emergencies. The plan must be reviewed and updated during treatment to be effective.

50. Healthcare professionals, researchers, communities, and schools use the Columbia Suicide Severity Rating Scale (C-SSRS) to assess suicide risk and determine support and intervention needs. The C-SSRS is simple, easy to use, and encourages suicide and suicidal thought discussions. It is multilingual and proven for diverse age groups and contexts. Clinical, educational, community, and research contexts can use the measure to detect suicide risk and establish intervention levels. The C-SSRS can estimate risk, but it should be used in conjunction with professional judgment.
51.

Component	Description of component	Normal findings	Abnormal findings
Appearance	Observations of the client's physical appearance including clothing, grooming, and visible physical abnormalities	Neat, appropriate, clean, orderly, composed	Disheveled, inappropriate, neglected, bizarre, unkempt
Behavior	The client's actions, level of eye contact, and any motor activity observed during the interview	Calm, cooperative, still, engaged, attentive	Agitated, hostile, restless, withdrawn, catatonic
Speech	Assessing the rate, volume, amount, and articulation of speech	Clear, coherent, fluent, moderate, articulate	Slurred, rapid, mute, pressured, incoherent
Mood	The client's self-reported emotional state	Content, stable, positive, calm, euthymic	Sad, euphoric, irritable, labile, depressed

Component	Description of component	Normal findings	Abnormal findings
Affect	The observed emotional state, often described in terms of range, intensity, and appropriateness	Congruent, appropriate, broad, stable, reactive	Blunted, flat, incongruent, restricted, labile
Thought process	The way the client thinks, as inferred from speech patterns and associations	Logical, goal-directed, coherent, linear, organized	Circumstantial, loosened, tangential, illogical, disorganized
Thought content	What the client is actually thinking about, including the presence of delusions, obsessions, or preoccupations	Reality-based, relevant, consistent, rational, focused	Delusional, obsessive, paranoid, phobic, suicidal
Perception	Assessing for hallucinations or distortions, including auditory, visual, or other sensory experiences	Accurate, clear, realistic, grounded, normal	Hallucinations, illusions, derealization, depersonalization, distorted
Cognition	Evaluation of memory, concentration, and ability to think and calculate	Alert, oriented, focused, intact, sharp	Confused, disoriented, impaired, distracted, forgetful
Insight	The client's awareness and understanding of their current situation and condition	Aware, realistic, insightful, understanding, perceptive	Denial, impaired, unaware, limited, poor
Judgment	The client's ability to make sound, reasonable, and responsible decisions	Good, sound, safe, responsible, rational	Poor, impulsive, unsafe, irresponsible, impaired

52. Tardive dyskinesia (TD) is an adverse effect of long-term use of neuroleptic (antipsychotic) drugs, characterized by involuntary, repetitive body movements. The Abnormal Involuntary Movement Scale (AIMS) is the most widely used tool to assess for tardive dyskinesia. Here are some signs that might evidence tardive dyskinesia:

- Facial Movements:
  - Grimacing or twisting of the face.
  - Puckering, pursing or smacking of lips.
  - Rapid blinking or eye movements.
- Limb Movements:
  - Rapid, involuntary movements of the fingers.
  - Movements of the arms, legs, or torso such as swaying, rocking, or jerking.
- Oral Movements:
  - Tongue protrusion or darting in and out of the mouth.
  - Chewing or biting movements.

- Respiratory Irregularities:
  - Irregular breathing patterns or grunting sounds.
- Other:
  - Difficulty with fine motor movements and tasks.
  - Impaired gait or walking pattern.

53. This table offers a set of topics that a PMHNP or other healthcare professional might cover during a medical review of systems to get a holistic view of the patient's health. The PMHNP should tailor the questions to the individual's specific history and presenting concerns.

Area	Topics
General/constitutional	1. Recent weight gain or loss 2. Fatigue or lethargy 3. Fever or chills 4. Night sweats 5. General sense of health
HEENT (head, eyes, ears, nose, throat)	1. Headaches or head injuries 2. Changes in vision or eye pain 3. Hearing changes or ear pain 4. Sinus problems or nasal congestion 5. Throat soreness or difficulty swallowing
Pulmonary	1. Shortness of breath 2. Cough 3. Wheezing or asthma 4. History of bronchitis or pneumonia 5. Chest pain with breathing
Cardiovascular	1. Chest pain or discomfort 2. Palpitations or irregular heartbeat 3. High or low blood pressure 4. Swelling of legs or feet 5. History of heart disease or stroke
Gastrointestinal	1. Nausea or vomiting 2. Diarrhea or constipation 3. Abdominal pain or discomfort 4. Changes in appetite or eating habits 5. History of liver or kidney disease
Urogenital	1. Frequency of urination 2. Pain or burning during urination 3. Blood in urine 4. Sexual dysfunction 5. History of urinary tract infections
Hematological	1. Easy bruising or bleeding 2. History of anemia or blood disorders 3. Transfusion history 4. Swollen lymph nodes 5. Fatigue or weakness
Female sexual/reproductive health	1. Menstrual history and irregularities 2. Pregnancy history and complications 3. Menopause symptoms 4. Breast changes or discharge 5. History of gynecological disorders or surgeries

Area	Topics
Male sexual/reproductive health	1. Erectile function or sexual issues 2. Testicular pain or masses 3. Prostate issues 4. Urinary symptoms 5. History of reproductive health disorders or surgeries
Neurological	1. Seizures or convulsions 2. Tremors or involuntary movements 3. Weakness or paralysis 4. Sensory changes or numbness 5. Headaches or migraines
Endocrine	1. Heat or cold intolerance 2. Thyroid problems 3. Diabetes symptoms or management 4. Changes in hair or skin 5. Unexplained weight changes
Musculoskeletal	1. Joint pain or stiffness 2. Muscle pain or weakness 3. History of arthritis or fractures 4. Limitations in movement or activities 5. Back pain
Dermatological	1. Rashes or itching 2. Changes in moles or skin color 3. Wounds that do not heal 4. Hair or nail changes 5. History of skin diseases

54.

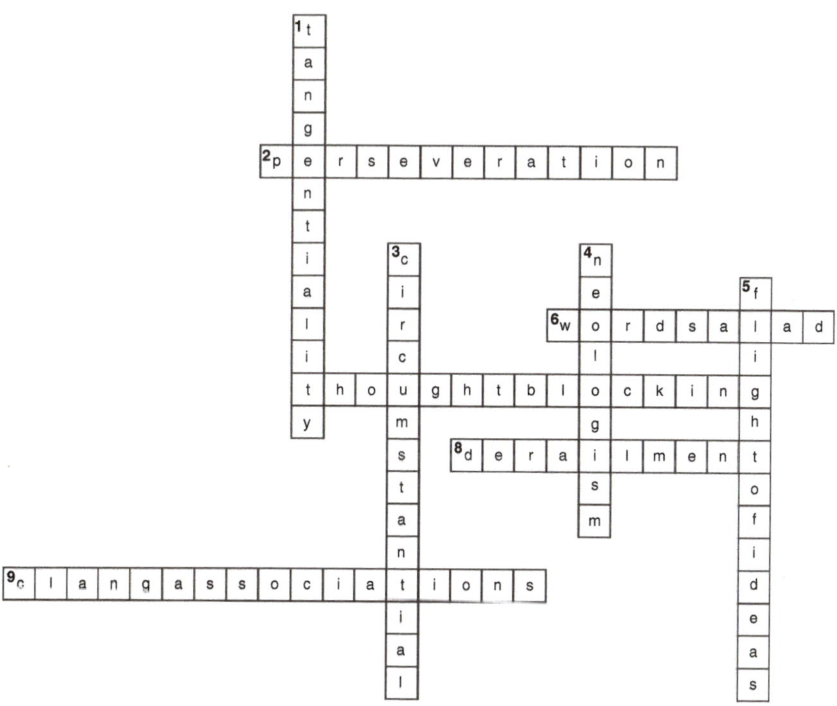
1 tangentiality
2 perseveration
3 circumstantial
4 neologism
5 flightofideas
6 wordsalad
thoughtblocking
8 derailment
9 clangassociations

References and Resources

American Psychiatric Association, editor. Diagnostic and statistical manual of mental disorders: DSM-5-TR. 5th ed. American Psychiatric Association Publishing; 2022.

Bekhet AK, Zauszniewski JA, Matel-Anderson DM, Suresky MJ, Stonehouse M. "evidence for psychiatric and mental health nursing interventions: an update (2011 through 2015)" *OJIN: the*. Online J Issues Nurs. 2018;23(2):1–28.

Bernstein KS, Kaplan R. Psychiatric mental health assessment and diagnosis of adults for advanced practice mental health nurses. 1st ed. Routledge; 2022. https://doi.org/10.4324/9781003137597.

Carlat DJ. The psychiatric interview. 4th ed. Lippincott Williams and Wilkins; 2016.

Ennis G, Happell B, Broadbent M, Reid-Searl K. The importance of communication for clinical leaders in mental health nursing: the perspective of nurses working in mental health. Issues Ment Health Nurs. 2013;34(11):814–9. https://doi.org/10.3109/01612840.2013.829539.

Johnson K, Vanderhoef D, Magrath N. Psychiatric-mental health nurse practitioner review and resource manual. American Nurses Credentialing Center, American Nurses Association; 2020.

Kumar A, Kearney A, Hoskins K, Iyengar A. The role of psychiatric mental health nurse practitioners in improving mental and behavioral health care delivery for children and adolescents in multiple settings. Arch Psychiatr Nurs. 2020;34(5):275–80. https://doi.org/10.1016/j.apnu.2020.07.022.

McInerney J, Lasater K, editors. Advanced practice nursing: an integrative approach. 5th ed. Elsevier; 2014.

McMillan SS, Stewart V, Wheeler AJ, Kelly F, Stapleton H. Medication management in the context of mental illness: an exploratory study of young people living in Australia. BMC Public Health. 2020;20(1):1188. https://doi.org/10.1186/s12889-020-09237-9.

Institute of Medicine (US) Committee on the Robert Wood Johnson Foundation Initiative on the Future of Nursing, at the Institute of Medicine. The future of nursing: leading change, advancing health. National Academies Press (US); 2011.

Shea SC. Psychiatric interviewing: the art of understanding. 3rd ed. Elsevier; 2017.

Zakhari R. The psychiatric-mental health nurse practitioner certification review manual. Springer Publishing Company; 2021.

Notes:

Notes:

Psychopharmacology 6

Test your learning and check your understanding of this book's contents: use the "Springer Nature Flashcards" app to access questions using ▶ https://sn.pub/62J0Ar.

To use the app, please follow the instructions in Chap. 1.

Psychopharmacology is the study of the effects of medications on the mind and behavior. It is a vital aspect of psychiatric-mental health nursing, as medication is often used to manage and treat mental health conditions. The use of medication in the treatment of mental health conditions has been shown to be effective in reducing symptoms and improving quality of life.

One of the key responsibilities of Psychiatric-Mental Health Nurse Practitioners (PMHNPs) is to assess and diagnose mental health conditions. This includes determining the appropriate treatment plan for each patient, which may involve the use of medication. PMHNPs must be able to evaluate the potential benefits and risks of using medication, as well as determine the appropriate dosage and frequency of administration (American Nurses Association 2015).

In addition to prescribing medication, PMHNPs also play a crucial role in monitoring their patients' response to treatment. This involves regularly evaluating the effectiveness of the medication, as well as monitoring for any adverse effects or interactions with other medications the patient may be taking (American Nurses Association 2015). PMHNPs must have a thorough understanding of the pharmacokinetics and pharmacodynamics of the medications they prescribe in order to properly monitor their patients and make adjustments to treatment as needed.

PMHNPs also play a key role in patient education and support. This includes educating patients about their medications, including how to take them properly and any potential side effects or interactions (American Nurses Association 2015). PMHNPs may also work with patients to develop strategies for managing side effects or to identify alternative treatments if necessary.

T. Stewart, *Psychiatric-Mental Health Nurse Practitioner Program Companion and Board Certification Exam Review Workbook*,
https://doi.org/10.1007/978-3-031-60894-0_6

There are a wide variety of psychiatric medications available, each with its specific mechanisms of action and potential side effects. PMHNPs must have a broad knowledge of these medications and their indications in order to make informed treatment decisions for their patients. They must also stay up-to-date on the latest research and developments in the field of psychopharmacology in order to provide the best possible care for their patients.

This chapter presents key concepts in pharmacology that will be useful when reviewing medications for each mental illness. Principles of pharmacology such as pharmacodynamics, pharmacokinetics, half-life, and therapeutic range are covered.

6.1 Foundations

1. ______________________________ refers to a drug's action on the body and how it achieves these responses based on dose.
2. ______________________________ is how the body acts on the drug once it's introduced to the system.
3. Match each step of pharmacokinetics with the appropriate description.

_____1. Absorption	A. How the body gets rid of the drug or its metabolites.
_____2. Distribution	B. How the drug is moved around the body, from systemic to cellular receptor levels.
_____3. Metabolism	C. How the drug is taken up into the blood.
_____4. Excretion	D. How the drug is transformed for use.

4. Which helps us decide on the most effective route, dosage, and schedule of drugs—pharmacodynamics or pharmacokinetics?
5. A small dose of a drug is required for it to be efficacious. This drug has a high ________________________.
6. ______________________________ is a relative measure of the safety of a drug by providing a ratio between toxic and median effective doses.
7. The wider the difference between the therapeutic and toxic doses of a drug means it is ______________________________ safe because it has a __________________________ therapeutic index.

8. A patient taking a Z drug for insomnia for several years complains that their sleep over the past 2 months is not as restful as it used to be. The PMHNP might need to increase the dose of the drug due to ______________________.
If the lack of response occurred quickly, over two to three nights, then the patient may be experiencing ______________________.

9. ______________________ provides a genetic explanation of why some people and ethnic groups may react differently to certain drugs. For example, individuals of Asian descent with the ______________________ allele are at increased risk for Stevens–Johnson Syndrome when taking the anti-convulsant, ______________________.

10. The most active site of drug metabolism in the human body is the ______________________.

11. ______________________ drugs mimic neurotransmitters. They bind to receptor sites and stimulate an action just as natural chemicals would.

12. ______________________ drugs block receptor sites, disallowing the body's neurotransmitters from attaching. No action results.

13. A drug that binds to a receptor, but causes the opposite effect, is called a(n) ______________________.

14. ______________________ do not completely activate receptors to which they bind.

15. What is the best way to avoid the first-pass effect?

16. Define metabolism.

17. Which class of enzymes is charged with first-pass metabolism? In what two body organs does this occur?

18. Oral medications are normally absorbed in the ______________________________.

19. Most medications used in psychiatry are hydrophilic.

    TRUE FALSE

20. Most medications used in psychiatry are highly protein-bound, and thus not active.

    TRUE FALSE

21. How might underweight vs. overweight individuals experience the same dose of psychotropic medication differently?

22. It takes ________ half-lives to eliminate a drug from the body. It takes the same number of half-lives to reach a steady state.

23. A drug's half-life (t1/2) is helpful when determining how often we should dose a medication.

    TRUE FALSE

24. When the amount of drug eliminated equals the amount of drug administered is referred to as ___________________________.

25. Children have faster first-pass metabolism thanks to over-active CYP450 enzymes ________, ________, ________, ________, and ________.

26. Explain how inducers and inhibitors affect the metabolism of other medications. What adverse effects can each lead to?

27. If a patient has liver disease, their medication dose may need to be ___________________________.

28. What changes in the body's composition make older adults more susceptible to drug toxicity?

29. Identify if each of the following characteristics is typical of an inducer (D) or an inhibitor (H).

______Can decrease drug efficacy
______Can decrease safety or increase the toxicity of other drugs
______Can decrease safety or increase the toxicity of other drugs
______Can increase drug efficacy
______Decreases the activity of drug-metabolizing enzymes
______Decreases the effectiveness of other medications
______Examples: cimetidine, fluconazole, and grapefruit juice
______Examples: rifampin, phenytoin, and carbamazepine

______Increases the activity of drug-metabolizing enzymes
______Increases the effectiveness and toxicity of other medications
______Increases the risk of adverse effects or toxicity
______Increases the risk of treatment failure or therapeutic resistance
______Leads to decreased metabolism and clearance of other drugs
______Leads to increased metabolism and clearance of other drugs.

30. In the following table, list as many CYP450 inhibitors and inducers as possible.

Inhibitors	Inducers

31. Ion channels undergoing an excitatory response allow ________ and ________ ions to enter a cell, causing a(n) ______________________________.

32. ______________________________ takes place when there is an inhibitory response in ion channels. __________ ions enter the cell; __________ exits the cell.

33. Reuptake pumps are found on the ____________________________ part of the neuron.

34. For each of the following descriptions, identify if it pertains to a Schedule I, II, III, IV, or V drug. Some descriptions may apply to more than one scheduled drug.

	High abuse and dependency
	No refills
	5 refill limit
	Testosterone, suboxone
	Research use only
	Wake-promoting drugs
	Lowest abuse potential
	Benzodiazepines, Z drugs
	Can telephone order, but follow with a written prescription
	Written prescription only
	Opioids, stimulants
	Heroin, marijuana
	Cough syrups with codeine
	Prescription renewal 6 months

35. Identify which of the following medications may induce depression (D), mania (M), or both (B).

_____steroids
_____antidepressants
_____beta blockers
_____progesterone
_____benzodiazepines
_____disulfiram
_____interferon
_____antineoplastics
_____isoniazid
_____retrovirals
_____isotreretinoin.

36. For each drug listed, identify if it can give a false positive for amphetamines (A), Alcohol (E), Benzodiazepines (B), Cocaine (C), Heroin/morphine (H), or Methadone/PCP (M).

_____Amoxicillin
_____Antibiotics
_____Bupropion
_____Codeine
_____Dextromethrophan
_____Fluoxetine
_____Nasal decongestants
_____Nefazodone
_____NSAIDs
_____Poppy seeds
_____Pseudoephedrine
_____Quinolones
_____Ranitidine
_____Rifampin
_____Sertraline
_____Stimulants
_____Trazodone
_____Valium.

37. A reduced ______________________________ in the kidneys may lead to the increased serum concentration of some drugs, putting the patient at risk of toxicity.

38. What are two reasons why drug doses may need to be adjusted during pregnancy?

39. What is the difference between side effects and adverse effects?

40. ______________________________ refers to inability to stop or control symptoms with medication.

41. Natural substances, like vitamins or herbs, do not have potential negative effects, and should be offered to patients prior to prescription medication.
    TRUE FALSE

42. In order to experience a toxic effect from a drug, patients must be on a suprath- erapeutic dose.
    TRUE FALSE

43. All adverse effects are reversible with the proper psychopharmacological intervention.
    TRUE FALSE

44. An individual whose serum drug levels show the achievement of a steady state in 5 half-lives evidence that the individual is a ______________________________ metabolizer.

45. Why should the PMHNP monitor sodium levels in patients on antidepressants?

46. In addition to cancer and other respiratory ailments, why should the PMHNP ask patients who smoke if they would like assistance in smoking cessation?

47. Provide a definition of each term.

Titration	
Taper	

48. The goal of _________________________ is to address a patient's signs and symptoms on the least effective dose of medication.

49. Medications with ________________________ half-lives are easier from which to wean patients.

50. One side effect of SSRIs can be hyperhidrosis. ________________________________ or ______________________________ may be prescribed to help address this issue.

51. Complete the following table.

Side effect	Signs/symptoms	Causes
Neuroleptic malignant syndrome (NMS)		
Tardive dyskinesia (TD)		
Hyperprolactinemia		
Extrapyramidal side effects (EPS)		
Hypertensive crisis		
Serotonin syndrome		
HAM (antihistamine, antiadrenergic, and antimuscarinic)		

52. ______________________________ medications worsen neurocognitive disorders, like dementia.

6.2 Antidepressants and Mood Stabilizers

53. Patients should trial an antidepressant for at least __________ weeks at a therapeutic dose before the PMHNP changes medications.

54. What symptoms may an individual experience when withdrawing from antidepressants?

55. What are five considerations that a PMHNP should take into account when choosing an antidepressant for a patient?

    1.______________________________
    2.______________________________
    3.______________________________
    4.______________________________
    5.______________________________.

56. Patients on anti-clotting agents should be monitored if started on an SSRI, particularly fluoxetine, because they may be at (increased/decreased) risk for bleeding.

57. Match the following antidepressants with information on the right.

Antidepressant	Information
_____Fluoxetine	A. Can increase blood pressure, used for major depression and anxiety disorders
_____Sertraline	B. Weekly dosing form, safe in pregnancy and with pediatric populations
_____Paroxetine	C. Also used for pain syndromes, can affect liver function
_____ Fluvoxamine	D. Highly protein bound so potential for drug drug interactions, short half-life increases withdrawal phenomena if missed dose
_____(Es) citalopram	E. Atypical antidepressant, can be stimulating, lowers the seizure threshold
_____Venlafaxine	F. QTc prolongation risks, low drug–drug interactions
_____Duloxetine	G. Atypical, can cause sedation and weight gain, minimal sexual side effects
_____Vortioxetine	H. Derivative of venlafaxine, a similar uses and side effect profile
_____ Desvenlafaxine	I. FDA-approved for OCD, inhibits CYP
_____Bupropion	J. Increased GI disturbances
_____Mirtazapine	K may improve cognitive symptoms in depression, low sexual side effects

58. SSRIs are relatively safer in overdose than other antidepressants because they act selectively on serotonin and not on ______________________________ ___, ______________________________, or ______________________________ ______________ receptors.

59. (Des)Venlafaxine and duloxetine are ______________________________ ______________________________ reuptake inhibitors. They are often used for depression, anxiety, and concurrent pain.

60. Why should bupropion be used with caution in patients with eating disorders?

61. Bupropion may be useful as an adjunct to SSRIs if patients are experiencing what side effects?

62. Although acting on serotonin receptors, trazodone is not used for depression. It is prescribed for insomnia. Men should be warned that trazodone may cause ______________________________, which requires immediate care.

63. Mirtazapine is a ______________________________ receptor antagonist. It is used to treat major depression, insomnia, and weight loss, often in the elderly.

64. TCAs inhibit the reuptake of both ______________________________ and ______________________________ by presynaptic receptors.

65. TCA overdose may be treated with IV ______________________________ ______________________.

66. Match the following heterocyclic antidepressants (tricyclic and tetracyclic) with the appropriate description on the right.

Antidepressant	Description
_____amitriptyline	A. Useful in chronic pain, migraines, and insomnia
_____imipramine	B. Chronic pain, least orthostatic hypotension
_____clomipramine	C. Chronic pain, sleep aid
_____doxepin	D. Activating, least anticholinergic
_____nortriptyline	E. Metabolite of antipsychotic with similar side-effect profile, EPS risk
_____desipramine	F. Enuresis and panic disorder
_____amoxapine	G. OCD

67. A client may overdose on a TCA by taking _______ week(s) worth of the medication.

68. Using a 3Cs mnemonic, what are the three major complications of TCAs?

1.____
2.____
3.____.

69. Label each possible side effect of TCAs as antihistamine (H), antiadrenergic (A), or antimuscarinic/anticholinergic (M).

__________Arrhythmias
__________Blurred vision
__________Constipation
__________Dizziness
__________Dry mouth
__________Glaucoma exacerbation
__________Orthostatic hypotension
__________Sedation
__________Urinary retention
__________Weight gain
__________Widening of QRS, QT and PR intervals.

70. Tyramine is an intermediate between tyrosine and the neurotransmitter ____________________________________.

71. Which three MAOIs are used for refractory depression and anxiety disorders?

1.____
2.____
3.____.

72. ________________________________ is an MAOI that does not require dietary modification when used at low doses. But, other serotonergic drugs should still be avoided.

73. ________________________________ is a serotonin antagonist that can be used to treat serotonin syndrome.

74. How long of a "wash out" period between an SSRI and MAOI is recommended?

75. Name five symptoms of hypertensive crisis.

1.____
2.____
3.____
4.____
5.____

76. For each of the disorders below, identify which antidepressants may be used as a treatment. Place an X in the box.

	SSRI	SNRI	TCA	MAOI	Other
Obsessive-compulsive disorder					
Panic disorder					
Eating disorder					
Dysthymia (persistent depressive disorder)					
Social anxiety disorder					
Generalized anxiety disorder					
Posttraumatic stress disorder					
Irritable bowel syndrome					
Enuresis					
Neuropathic pain					
Chronic pain					
Fibromyalgia					
Migraines					
Smoking cessation					
Premenstrual dysphoric disorder					
Insomnia					

77. ____ may be used to augment antidepressants and antipsychotics in patients with major depressive disorder and schizophrenia.

78. The gold standard treatment for acute mania is the medication ____________ ________________________. It is also useful in depressive disorders.

79. Which tests should a PMHNP order for a patient prior to starting them on lithium?

80. How often should a patient's lithium blood levels be checked?

81. What should a PMHNP be concerned about if a patient's serum lithium level is >2.0?

82. What are the symptoms of lithium toxicity?

83. A baby born to a mother on lithium is at risk of the cardiac defect, ________ ____________________________________.

84. Name five medications or factors that can increase Li + levels.

1.____
2.____
3.____
4.____
5.____

6.3 Stimulants

85. Stimulants increase the neurotransmitters __________________________ ______ and ______________________________________, which help improve focus, concentration, and motivation.

86. Stimulants increase the risk of developing cardiovascular side effects.

TRUE FALSE

87. The two categories of stimulants include __________________________ __ and __________________________________. However, efficacy and side effects do not differ much between the categories.

88. What are 3–5 side effects associated with the use of stimulants?

1.____
2.____
3.____
4.____
5.____.

89. Stimulant use in children has been linked to growth restriction later as adults.
TRUE FALSE

90. Complete the following table with the brand name or generic name of each stimulant medication, and identify if each is an amphetamine (A), methylphenidate (M), or other (O) category medication.

Generic name	Brand name	A, M, or O
	Adderall	
Atomoxetine		
	Ritalin, concerta	

Generic name	Brand name	A, M, or O
	Dexedrine	
Lisdexamfetamine		
	Intuniv	
Mixed amphetamine salts		
Dexmethylphenidate		
	Kapvay	

91. Because nonstimulants are significantly less effective at treating ADHD, what are some reasons why they might be prescribed?

92. The mechanism of action of atomoxetine is ______________________________ ______________________________.

93. ______________________________ and ______________________________ are α-2 receptor agonists used to treat ADHD. They help decrease impulsivity and hyperactivity by inhibiting the ______________________________ and can be sedating.

94. Norepinephrine inhibitors may ______________________________ blood pressure.

95. A patient with depression and mild ADHD symptoms could benefit from the antidepressant ______________________________ since, like stimulants, it also affects the neurotransmitters ______________________________ and ______________________________, albeit more mildly.

96. ______________________________ is a wake-promoting drug used in shift work disorder and narcolepsy. It was originally used by Air Force pilots to stay awake during long missions.

97. Since methylphenidates and amphetamines are similar in terms of efficacy, prescribers usually consider the ______________________________ _____ when choosing among the various medications.

6.4 Answers and Explanations to Chapter Activities

1. Pharmacodynamics studies medications' biochemical and physiological effects and mechanisms of action. Pharmacodynamics considers drug potency, effectiveness, toxicity, and concentration-response.
2. Drug absorption, distribution, metabolism, and excretion (ADME) are pharmacokinetics. These processes determine medication concentration and duration at its site of action. Therapeutic formulation, route of administration, bioavailability, and clearance are considered in pharmacokinetics to optimize therapeutic therapy and reduce side effects.
3. _____C_____1. Absorption
   _____B_____2. Distribution.
   _____D_____3. Metabolism.
   _____A_____4. Excretion
4. Pharmacokinetics helps us pick the optimal drug dose, route, and frequency for therapeutic efficacy. A medication with low oral bioavailability may require intravenous injection or a transdermal patch. Short-half-life drugs may require more frequent dosing to maintain therapeutic levels. Pharmacodynamics discusses how the drug interacts with the body at molecular, cellular, and organ levels to have the desired effect. The potency, efficacy, and affinity of a receptor-targeted drug can help determine its optimal dose and timing for therapeutic benefit.
5. Pharmacological potency is measured by the ED50 or response level. High-potency medications act at lower doses than low-potency ones. Effectiveness, a drug's highest effect regardless of dose, is different from potency. A powerful but ineffective drug requires a big dose.
6. The therapeutic index evaluates drug safety by comparing toxic and median effective doses. It is the ratio of a drug's median fatal dose (LD50) to its median effective dose (ED50) or minimal hazardous concentration to minimum effective concentration. Therapeutic index displays harmful and therapeutic dose ranges. Low therapeutic index drugs have a narrow margin of safety and may be harmful at therapeutic dosages, while high index drugs are relatively safe. Thus, the therapeutic index is essential for drug safety and hazard assessment in research and clinical practice.
7. Drugs with a higher therapeutic index are safer because their hazardous and therapeutic doses are farther apart. Therapeutically, a drug with a greater therapeutic index is safer. Thus, drugs with a significant therapeutic-to-toxic dose difference are safer and can be taken longer or at greater doses. However, narrow therapeutic index drugs are more dangerous and require tighter monitoring and precise dosing.
8. If a patient has had less restful sleep in the past two months, the PMHNP may need to increase the dose of a Z drug for insomnia due to tolerance. Drug tolerance occurs when the body adapts to a drug's effects, lowering its dose-response. Long-term Z medication use may have produced sedative tolerance, necessitating a higher dose. Tachyphylaxis and rebound insomnia may occur if the patient

does not respond within 2–3 nights. After a long time, abstaining from sleep medications like Z drugs might cause rebound insomnia. Stopping the drug can increase insomnia because the body needs it to sleep.

9. Some people and ethnic groups react differently to drugs due to pharmacogenetics. It examines genetic variations in drug metabolism, transport, and target receptors that affect drug response. Genetics can predict drug reactions and dosing. Carbamazepine can cause Stevens–Johnson Syndrome in Asians with HLA-B1502 alleles.
10. The liver bio transforms the most drugs through complex enzymatic mechanisms. In Phase I, enzymes like cytochrome P450s (CYPs) insert or expose a functional group to improve drug polarity and promote excretion. In Phase II, conjugation enzymes like glucuronosyltransferases (UGTs) add a larger, more polar molecule (e.g., glucuronic acid) to increase water solubility and prepare the drug or its Phase I metabolites for renal or bile removal. The liver metabolizes medicines, but the kidneys and lungs also remove them.
11. Agonists mimic neurotransmitters. They work like natural chemicals by binding to receptors. As agonists, partial agonists cause a lesser response even when all receptors are engaged.
12. Antagonists block neurotransmitter-receptor binding, inhibiting action. Antagonists prohibit neurotransmitters from binding to receptors like the normal neurotransmitter. It can calm an overactive neurotransmitter system or prevent medication effects. Antagonists are competitive or noncompetitive depending on receptor interaction. Endogenous neurotransmitters and competitive antagonists compete for receptors. Non-competitive antagonists change allosteric receptor conformation to prevent neurotransmitter binding. Antagonists treat anxiety, opioid addiction, and hypertension.
13. Inverse agonists connect to receptor sites but behave oppositely to agonists. Inverse agonists may aggravate illness symptoms or induce adverse effects depending on the receptor and drug. Inverse agonists are used in most receptor studies to study physiological function and therapeutic potential.
14. Partial agonists do not fully activate receptors. Even when completely occupied, partial agonists bind to the receptor site but elicit less physiologic response. Partial agonists have reduced affinity and efficiency than full agonists, resulting in sub-maximal receptor activation at high dosages. Partial agonists inhibit endogenous agonists at high-basal activity receptors. Some partial agonists have fewer negative effects or lessen tolerance or dependency. Buprenorphine reduces opioid abuse and overdose by causing less pleasure and respiratory depression than full agonists.
15. IV injection, subcutaneous injection, transdermal patch, inhalation, or rectal suppository prevent the first pass effect best. Avoiding the liver and gastrointestinal tract reduces the first-pass effect. IV drugs enter the circulation and target tissues without first passing through the liver. Inhalation and transdermal patch drugs enter the bloodstream immediately, avoiding first-pass effects. Prodrugs are another option. Metabolism converts prodrugs into active drugs. Prodrugs

can pass through the gastrointestinal tract without the first-pass impact by changing their chemical structure to increase lipid solubility or stability. Enzymes convert the prodrug into the active drug in target tissue, providing therapeutic advantages.

16. Pharmacology describes metabolism as the body's enzymatic biotransformation of drugs and xenobiotics. The body employs metabolism to convert food and other nutrients into energy and chemicals for tissue growth, maintenance, and repair. Catabolism breaks down complex molecules for energy, while anabolism synthesizes them to store energy and build tissues. Drug metabolism makes them water-soluble and excretable. The kidneys and lungs aid drug processing, but the liver is the major organ.
17. The first-pass metabolism of drugs is done by CYP450 enzymes. The liver's CYP450 enzymes oxidize, degrade, or hydrolyze the medicine into water-soluble metabolites that can be excreted in urine or bile Some drugs' first-pass metabolism can lower bioavailability and pharmacokinetics/dynamics. Most first-pass metabolism occurs in the liver and small intestines.
18. The gut absorbs oral medications. Before entering the small intestine, stomach acid and enzymes may break down the drug. Absorbable drug molecules reach the bloodstream through the small intestine wall. After liver processing, the drug reaches the target tissues via systemic circulation. Drug absorption depends on chemical properties, formulation, diet, other drugs, and gastrointestinal transit time.
19. FALSE. Most psychiatric medicines are lipophilic. High lipid solubility allows lipophilic medicines to cross the blood-brain barrier and enter the brain and central nervous system. Adipose tissue can inhibit the release of lipophilic medicines into the bloodstream, lengthening their duration of effect. Low lipid solubility and blood–brain barrier blockade limit hydrophilic medication mental therapy efficacy.
20. FALSE. Psychiatric medications are generally protein-bound but active. Drugs bind to blood plasma proteins like albumin or globulin reversibly. Only the unbound component of highly protein-bound drugs can pass cell membranes and interact with receptors or enzymes to work. Since most psychiatric drugs have a low therapeutic index, the modest plasma drug concentration changes can have large therapeutic or detrimental consequences.
21. Due to body composition, metabolism, and drug distribution, overweight and underweight patients may take psychiatric medicine differently. Underweight people have less body fat and muscle mass, therefore, lipophilic drugs may spread less. Lipophilic psychiatric drugs such as benzodiazepines and tricyclic antidepressants can cause drowsiness and respiratory depression due to high plasma concentrations and extended half-lives. An underweight person's higher metabolic rate and decreased liver and renal function may expedite drug clearance and shorten psychotropic drug effects. Overweight people may spread lipophilic drugs due to increased body fat and metabolism. Psychotropic drugs may have lower plasma concentrations and half-lives, limiting their efficacy. Overweight people may eliminate some psychiatric medicines faster due to

increased liver and renal function. Thus, underweight and overweight patients may need dose modifications to maximize therapeutic benefits and reduce side effects. Plasma drug levels help guide dosing and ensure therapeutic efficacy and safety.

22. Drug removal takes five half-lives. Each half-life destroys half the drug, and after five, almost 97%. For a steady state, where drug administration equals drug removal and plasma drug concentration is constant, the same number of half-lives is needed.
23. TRUE. A drug's half-life (t1/2) determines dose frequency to maintain therapeutic concentrations. The time it takes a drug's plasma concentration to decline by half after delivery indicates its clearance rate and elimination mechanism. Due to their quick metabolism and excretion, benzodiazepines may need higher doses to sustain therapeutic effects. Long-half-life drugs, like some antidepressants, are slowly eliminated and maintain therapeutic concentrations, requiring fewer doses. Dosing can be optimized using drug half-life, bioavailability, volume of distribution, and clearance rate. Patient age, weight, and renal/hepatic function may impact dose. Plasma medication monitoring may help maintain therapeutic concentrations.
24. Steady state occurs when drug administration matches elimination and plasma drug concentration is consistent. Drug pharmacokinetics, dosing schedule, and patient variables including age, weight, and renal or hepatic function affect steady-state time. Plasma medication concentration stabilizes after five doses after four to five half-lives. Steady-state concentrations maximize therapeutic efficacy and decrease toxicity and bad outcomes.
25. Children have faster first-pass metabolism due to hyperactive CYP450 enzymes 1A2, 2C9, 2C19, 2D6, and 3A4. This can alter treatment efficacy and safety in children and adults, necessitating dose adjustments or drug monitoring.
26. Drug metabolism is affected by hepatic drug-metabolizing enzyme inducers and inhibitors. Increased drug-metabolizing enzyme activity and clearance are caused by inducers. Inducers impair pharmacological efficacy and produce treatment failure and resistance. Prodrug metabolism is increased by inducers, limiting drug conversion and therapeutic efficacy. Inducers can reduce pharmacological efficacy, increase treatment failure or resistance, and lower the safety or toxicity of other enzyme-metabolized drugs. In contrast, inhibitors reduce drug metabolism and clearance by decreasing enzyme activity. Inhibitors improve drug efficacy and side effects. Plasma drug concentrations can also be increased by inhibitors, extending or worsening pharmacological effects. Inhibitors may increase pharmacological efficacy, toxicity, and other enzyme-processed medicines' safety and toxicity. Thus, drugs that boost or inhibit drug-metabolizing enzymes may need careful monitoring and dose modifications to improve efficacy and reduce side effects.
27. Patients with liver disease may need lower medication doses. Liver disease reduces liver function, blood flow, and enzyme activity, lowering medication metabolism. This can slow medication clearance, raise plasma concentrations, and prolong pharmacological effects, increasing toxicity and side effects.

28. Many physical changes render seniors more prone to pharmaceutical toxicity:

    1. Kidney function weakens with age, making medication and metabolite clearance tougher. This increases pharmaceutical exposure and toxicity, especially kidney-excreted drugs.
    2. Different body composition: Aging reduces lean body mass and increases body fat, affecting lipophilic drug distribution and metabolism. Higher plasma concentrations and longer pharmacological actions may enhance toxicity.
    3. Age reduces liver blood flow, enzyme activity, and medication metabolism. This reduces medicine clearance and raises plasma drug concentrations, raising toxicity risk.
    4. Aging reduces drug bioavailability and effectiveness by impairing gastrointestinal motility, stomach pH, and absorption.
    5. Multiple comorbidities and polypharmacy: Older people take more drugs, increasing drug interactions and negative effects. Drugs metabolized by the same enzymes or with cumulative or synergistic effects may be hazardous.

29. __D___Increases the activity of drug-metabolizing enzymes
__D___Leads to increased metabolism and clearance of other drugs.
__D___Decreases the effectiveness of other medications.
__D___Increases the risk of treatment failure or therapeutic resistance.
__D___Can decrease drug efficacy.
__D___Can decrease safety or increase toxicity of other drugs.
__D___Examples: rifampin, phenytoin, carbamazepine.
__H___Decreases the activity of drug-metabolizing enzymes.
__H___Leads to decreased metabolism and clearance of other drugs.
__H___Increases the effectiveness and toxicity of other medications.
__H___Increases the risk of adverse effects or toxicity.
__H___Can increase drug efficacy.
__H___Can decrease safety or increase toxicity of other drugs.
__H___Examples: cimetidine, fluconazole, grapefruit juice.

30.

Inhibitors	Inducers
Amiodarone	Barbiturates (e.g., phenobarbital)
Azole antifungals (e.g., ketoconazole)	Carbamazepine
Bupropion	Chronic alcohol use
Carbamazepine	Phenobarbital
Cimetidine	Phenytoin
Clarithromycin	Rifampin
Fluoroquinolones	Smoking tobacco
Grapefruit and grapefruit juice	St. John's Wort
Hypericum (St. John's Wort)	Tetracycline antibiotics (e.g., doxycycline)
Nefazodone	Glucocorticoids (e.g., dexamethasone)
Phenobarbital	
Phenytoin	
Protease inhibitors (e.g., ritonavir)	
Quinidine	
SSRIs (selective serotonin reuptake inhibitors)	
Verapamil	

31. Ion channels excite cells by letting sodium (Na^+) and calcium (Ca^{2+}) ions in. Depolarization raises the cell's membrane potential, making the inside more positive than the outside. This membrane potential change can cause an action potential, a fast electrical signal that passes along the neuron and allows neurons to communicate with neighboring cells. Neurotransmitter release, synaptic transmission, and neuronal signaling depend on Na^+ and Ca^{2+} ion channel inflow.
32. Hyperpolarization occurs when a cell's membrane potential becomes more negative than its exterior. Cl- and/or K+ ions enter and leave the cell, respectively. This membrane potential change can reduce neuron excitability and activity by lowering action potential firing.
33. Neuron presynaptic terminals have reuptake pumps. The presynaptic terminal releases neurotransmitters into the synaptic cleft, the small gap between the membranes. After neurotransmitter release, presynaptic membrane reuptake pumps actively carry neurotransmitter molecules back into the terminal for vesicularization or metabolism. Synaptic cleft neurotransmitter concentration and transmission duration and strength are regulated by reuptake pumps. Depression, anxiety, and addiction can result from reuptake pump dysfunction.
34.

Schedule I and Schedule II	High abuse and dependency
Schedule II	No refills
Schedule III	5 refill limit
Schedule III	Testosterone, suboxone
Schedule I	Research use only
Schedule IV	Wake-promoting drugs
Schedule V	Lowest abuse potential
Schedule IV	Benzodiazepines, Z drugs
Schedule III	Can telephone order, but follow with written prescription
Schedule II	Written prescription only
Schedule II	Opioids, stimulants
Schedule I	Heroin, marijuana
Schedule V	Cough syrups with codeine
Schedule III	Prescription renewal 6 months

35. __B___steroids
__M___antidepressants.
__D___Beta blockers.
___D__progesterone.
__D___benzodiazepines.
__M___disulfiram.
_D____interferon.
__D___antineoplastics.
__M___isoniazid.
__D___retrovirals.
__D___isotreretinoin
36. __A___Bupropion
__A___Fluoxetine.
__A___Nasal decongestants.

__A___Nefazodone.
__A___Pseudoephedrine.
__A___Ranitidine.
__A___Stimulants.
__A___Trazodone.
__B___Sertraline.
__C___Amoxicillin.
__C___Antibiotics.
__C___NSAIDs.
__E___Valium.
__H___Codeine.
__H___Poppy seeds.
__H___Quinolones.
__H___Rifampin.
__M___dextromethrophan

37. A reduced renal glomerular filtration rate (GFR) may increase medication serum levels, posing toxicity risks. Through glomerular filtration, kidneys filter blood and remove waste and drugs. Lower GFR due to kidney damage, aging, or other causes reduces medicine clearance, increases plasma concentrations, and prolongs pharmacological effects. Kidney-excreted or limited therapeutic window drugs may be more harmful.
38. Two major reasons medicine doses may need to be changed during pregnancy:

    - Physiological changes in mothers: Weight, composition, blood volume, and kidney function change throughout pregnancy. Drug pharmacokinetics affect absorption, distribution, metabolism, and elimination. Drug clearance declines with impaired renal function and raises plasma concentrations, while blood volume and cardiac output promote medication distribution and lower plasma concentrations. Drug doses may need to be adjusted during pregnancy to achieve therapeutic concentrations and reduce negative effects.
    - Drugs in the placenta can induce fetal toxicity, malformations, and other issues. Thus, pregnant drug safety and pharmacological therapy pros and disadvantages must be carefully considered. Some medications are prohibited during pregnancy, but others can be used if they are safe. For fetal safety and maternal health, lower drug doses or alternate treatments may be suggested.

39. Side effects encompass both positive and negative effects of a treatment, whereas adverse effects specifically refer to the harmful or serious negative effects that can occur as a result of a medication or medical treatment, often requiring medical attention. For example, if someone is taking a pain medication, a common side effect might be mild drowsiness or slight dizziness, which is generally tolerable. However, an adverse effect in this case could be a severe allergic reaction that causes difficulty breathing, swelling, and hives, which would require immediate medical attention due to its potentially life-threatening nature.

40. Failure to treat symptoms with medication is treatment resistance. Cancer, viral, and psychiatric problems can resist treatment. Treatment-resistant patients have not reacted to two or more adequate doses and durations of medication or other evidence-based treatments, according to psychiatry. Treatment-resistant patients may have persistent disability, lower quality of life, and higher health-care costs. Biology, genetics, environment, and behavior can create treatment resistance.
41. FALSE. Herbs, vitamins, and supplements can interact with prescription medicines and create negative effects. Natural remedies may not be safe or effective for everyone. Patients should also be informed about the risks and benefits of natural substances and encouraged to tell their doctors about all their supplements and pharmaceuticals for safe and effective treatment.
42. FALSE—subtherapeutic amounts can hurt also. Toxicity can result from overdose, medicine interactions, accumulation, inadequate drug metabolism or clearance, and idiosyncratic reactions. A narrow therapeutic index means the range between the therapeutic and hazardous doses is small, making even a little overdose dangerous.
43. FALSE. Although certain psychopharmacological adverse effects are irreversible or persist after medication cessation, proper care can correct many. Tardive dyskinesia, an involuntary muscle movement disorder, may persist despite antipsychotic medication. Weight gain, sexual dysfunction, and cognitive impairment may require additional therapies or lifestyle changes after medication cessation.
44. "Normal" metabolizers reach a steady state in 5 half-lives. Having a steady state in 4–5 half-lives suggests that the substance is being digested and eliminated as expected and that the person is neither an ultra-rapid nor a poor metabolizer.
45. The PMHNP should monitor sodium levels in antidepressant patients since some, notably SSRIs, can produce the rare but life-threatening condition of SIADH. SIADH causes increased ADH release, water retention, hyponatremia, convulsions, coma, and cerebral edema. ADH release and kidney water reabsorption increase with hypothalamic serotonin reuptake inhibition, generating antidepressant-induced SIADH. Older individuals, women, and those with hyponatremia or other water and electrolyte imbalances may develop SIADH.
46. Smoking is a risk factor for many medical and psychological problems and can improve health and quality of life, thus the PMHNP should help smokers quit in addition to cancer and respiratory infections. Diabetes, osteoporosis, heart disease, stroke, lung disease, and many malignancies are linked to smoking. Smoking worsens depression, anxiety, and schizophrenia and reduces psychotropic treatment efficacy. Smoking can potentially increase negative effects or decrease the efficacy of antidepressants and antipsychotics. Tobacco increases CYP450 and drug levels. It may accelerate psychotropic drug breakdown and elimination, risking subtherapeutic levels.

47.

Titration	Gradual increase in medication dose while monitoring for negative effects
Taper	Gradual decrease in medication dose while monitoring the return of signs or symptoms, or evidence of withdrawal

48. Titrating or "minimizing medication dose" addresses a patient's symptoms on the least effective dose. The lowest effective dose is crucial to pharmaceutical administration, especially in psychiatry, where many drugs have side effects and long-term impacts. PMHNPs may start with a low dose and titrate up carefully, employ combination therapies, and investigate non-pharmacological approaches including psychotherapy, exercise, and lifestyle changes to reduce drug dose.
49. Longer half-lives are simpler to wean patients off than shorter ones. Longer half-lives lessen withdrawal symptoms and rebound effects following dose reduction or termination due to their slower onset and offset. Longer half-lives may also allow for less frequent dosing and fewer drug level variations, which can reduce side effects and improve treatment adherence. Shorter-half-lived drugs may have a faster onset and offset of effect, a more frequent dosage, and larger drug-level variations. This can enhance withdrawal symptoms and rebound effects following dose decrease or termination, requiring more careful monitoring and longer tapering regimens.
50. SSRIs can cause hyperhidrosis. This may be treated with anticholinergics or antiperspirants. Glycopyrrolate and oxybutynin inhibit acetylcholine, which stimulates sweat glands, to reduce sweating. These drugs can treat hyperhidrosis off-label, although they can cause dry mouth, constipation, and impaired vision.

    - Antiperspirants like aluminum chloride constrict sweat ducts to reduce sweating. Topically applied, these products can treat mild to moderate hyperhidrosis but may induce skin irritation or allergic responses. Avoiding spicy foods, heat, and loose, airy clothing may help patients sweat less. Stress and anxiety can worsen hyperhidrosis, so relaxation exercises or cognitive-behavioral therapy may help.

51.

Side effect	Signs/aymptoms	Causes
Neuroleptic malignant syndrome (NMS)	Mental status change, fever, tachycardia, hypertension, tremor, elevated CPK, "lead pipe" rigidity	Long- or short-term use of antipsychotics
Tardive dyskinesia (TD)	Choreoathetoid muscle movements (mouth, tongue, neck, extremities)	Long-term antipsychotic use, especially first-generation
Hyperprolactinemia	Increased prolactin levels	First-generation antipsychotics and risperidone particularly
Extrapyramidal side effects (EPS)	Parkinsonism, akathisia, dystonia	First-generation antipsychotics, within hours or days of starting medication

Side effect	Signs/aymptoms	Causes
Hypertensive crisis	High BP	Buildup catecholamines caused by MAOIs and ingestion of tyramine-rich foods
Serotonin syndrome	Confusion, flushing, diaphoresis, tremor, myoclonic jerks, hyperthermia, hypertonicity, rhabdomyolysis, renal failure, death	Too much serotonin, often when SSRI and MAOI combined, or numerous SSRI medications at same time
HAM (antihistamine, antiadrenergic, antimuscarinic)	Sedation, weight gain; hypotension; dry mouth, blurred vision, urinary retention, constipation)	TCAs and antipsychotics

52. Anticholinergics can aggravate dementias. Anticholinergics disrupt acetylcholine, a neurotransmitter involved in learning, memory, and other cognitive functions. Since acetylcholine is already low in these conditions, stopping its activity may worsen cognitive impairment. Certain antihistamines, antidepressants, antipsychotics, bladder control medicines, and muscle relaxants are anticholinergic.
53. 4–6 weeks
54. Dizziness, headaches, nausea, insomnia, lethargy.
55. Symptoms, responses by family members to the medication, potential side effects, the patient's comorbidities, suicide risk, cost, and previously prescribed medications.
56. Increased.
57. __B___Fluoxetine
    __J___Sertraline.
    __D___Paroxetine.
    __I___Fluvoxamine.
    __F___(Es)Citalopram.
    __A___Venlafaxine.
    __C___Duloxetine.
    __K___Vortioxetine.
    __H___Desvenlafaxine.
    __E___Bupropion.
    __G___Mirtazapine
58. Histamine, adrenergic, muscarinic receptors.
59. Serotonin-norepinephrine reuptake inhibitors.
60. Bupropion can lower the seizure threshold. Eating disorders, such as anorexia nervosa and bulimia nervosa, can already carry a risk of electrolyte imbalances and other medical complications that may increase the risk of seizures. Bupropion, as a medication, can further elevate this risk by lowering the seizure threshold.
61. Decreased libido, erectile dysfunction, anorgasmia.
62. Priapism.
63. α2-adrenergic
64. Serotonin, norepinephrine.

65. Sodium bicarbonate.
66. __A___amitriptyline
  __F___imipramine.
  __G___clomipramine.
  __C___doxepin.
  __B___nortriptyline.
  __D___desipramine.
  __E___amoxapine
67. 1 week
68. Cardiotoxicity, convulsions, and coma.

  - Cardiotoxicity: TCAs can lead to significant cardiac complications, including arrhythmias (irregular heart rhythms), conduction disturbances, and even potentially life-threatening conditions like ventricular tachycardia or fibrillation. These effects can be particularly dangerous in overdose situations.
  - Convulsions: TCAs can lower the seizure threshold, increasing the risk of seizures, especially in individuals who are prone to seizures or have a history of epilepsy.
  - Coma: In cases of TCA overdose, patients may experience profound central nervous system (CNS) depression, leading to coma. Coma can be a severe and potentially life-threatening complication of TCA toxicity, and prompt medical intervention is essential to manage overdose cases.

69. ____A______Arrhythmias
  ____M______Blurred vision.
  ____M______Constipation.
  ____A______Dizziness.
  ____M______Dry mouth.
  ____M______Glaucoma exacerbation.
  ____A______Orthostatic hypotension.
  ____H______Sedation.
  ____M______Urinary retention.
  ____H______Weight gain.
  ____A______Widening of QRS, QT and PR intervals
70. Norepinephrine.
71. Phenelzine, tranylcypromine, and isocarboxazid.
72. Selegiline.
73. Cyproheptadine.
74. 2 weeks; 5–6 weeks if the patient was on fluoxetine
75. Hypertension, headache, diaphoresis, nausea, vomiting, photophobia, chest pain, arrhythmias, autonomic instability, and death.
76.

	SSRI	SNRI	TCA	MAOI	Other
Obsessive-compulsive disorder	X		X		
Panic disorder	X		X	X	
Eating disorder	X		X		

	SSRI	SNRI	TCA	MAOI	Other
Dysthymia (persistent depressive disorder)	X	X			
Social anxiety disorder	X	X		X	
Generalized anxiety disorder	X	X	X		
Posttraumatic stress disorder	X				
Irritable bowel syndrome	X		X		
Enuresis			X		
Neuropathic pain		X	X		
Chronic pain		X	X		
Fibromyalgia		X			
Migraines			X		
Smoking cessation					X (bupropion)
Premenstrual dysphoric disorder	X				
Insomnia			X		X (mirtazapine, trazodone)

77. Mood stabilizers.
78. Lithium.
79. ECG, BMP, thyroid function, CBC, pregnancy test, and creatinine.
80. After 5 days, then every 2–3 days until therapeutic.
81. Death.
82. Change in mental status, tremors, convulsions, delirium, coma, death, thyroid dysfunction, DI, GI disturbances, and sedation.
83. Ebstein's anomaly is a rare congenital heart defect that affects the structure and function of the tricuspid valve, one of the heart's four valves. In individuals with Ebstein's anomaly, the tricuspid valve is abnormally formed and positioned lower than normal in the right ventricle.
84. NSAIDs, Aspirin, thiazides, dehydration, hyponatremia, diaphoresis, decreased renal function.
85. Stimulants increase the neurotransmitters dopamine and norepinephrine, which help improve focus, concentration, and motivation.
86. FALSE. Research has shown that individuals without a preexisting cardiovascular ailment are not more likely to develop CV side effects. However, individuals with existing cardiovascular issues should be monitored for increased heart rate, elevated blood pressure, and in some cases, more serious cardiovascular complications.
87. Amphetamines; methylphenidates.
88. Abuse potential, irritability, restlessness, insomnia, GI disturbances, decreased appetite.
89. TRUE. Stimulant use in children, particularly for the treatment of attention deficit hyperactivity disorder (ADHD), has been associated with a potential risk of growth restriction or slower growth during childhood. Some children may experience a temporary slowing of growth while taking stimulant medications. However, it's important to note that this effect is usually modest, and growth typically catches up once the medication is discontinued or adjusted. The benefits of effectively managing ADHD symptoms often outweigh the potential for temporary growth restriction.

90.

Generic name	Brand name	A, M, or O
Amphetamine/Dextroamphetamine	Adderall	A
Atomoxetine	Strattera	O
Methylphenidate	Ritalin, Concerta	M
Dextroamphetamine	Dexedrine	A
Lisdexamfetamine	Vyvanse	A
Guanfacine	Intuniv	O
Mixed amphetamine salts	Mydayis	A
Dexmethylphenidate	Focalin	M
Clonidine	Kapvay	O

91. A non-stimulant may be preferred if a client can't tolerate stimulants, has concerns about abuse potential, doesn't want to take stimulants, is low weight or history of insomnia, preexisting cardiovascular condition.
92. Norepinephrine reuptake inhibitor.
93. Guanfacine; clonidine; sympathetic nervous system.
94. Lower.
95. Bupropion; dopamine; norepinephrine.
96. Modafinil.
97. Duration of action.

References and Resources

American Nurses Association. Role of the psychiatric-mental health nurse practitioner. American Nurses Association; 2015.

American Nurses Association, American Psychiatric Nurses Association, & International Society of Psychiatric-Mental Health Nurses. Psychiatric-mental health nursing: scope and standards of practice. 3rd ed. ANA.; 2022.

American Psychiatric Association, editor. Diagnostic and statistical manual of mental disorders: DSM-5-TR. 5th ed. American Psychiatric Association Publishing; 2022.

Goldin DS. Fast facts for psychopharmacology for nurse practitioners. Springer Publishing; 2022.

Johnson K, Vanderhoef D, Magrath N. Psychiatric-mental health nurse practitioner review and resource manual. American Nurses Association: American Nurses Credentialing Center; 2020.

Lewis J, Bachmann K. Drug interactions handbook: the new standard for drug and herbal interactions featuring a complete guide to cytochrome P450 enzyme substrates, inducers, and inhibitors. 2nd ed. Lexi-Comp; 2004.

Meyer JS, Quenzer LF. Psychopharmacology: drugs, the brain, and behavior. 2nd ed. Oxford University Press; 2018.

Okoli CTC, Kappi A, Wang T, Makowski A, Cooley AT. The effect of long-acting injectable antipsychotic medications compared with oral antipsychotic medications among people with schizophrenia: a systematic review and meta-analysis. Int J Ment Health Nurs. 2022;31(3):469–535. https://doi.org/10.1111/inm.12964.

Prus A. Drugs and the neuroscience of behavior: an introduction to psychopharmacology. 3rd ed. Sage Publications; 2020.

Swenson RS, Murphy-Ende K. Prolonged QT interval in patients receiving psychotropic medications. J Am Psychiatr Nurses Assoc. 2020;26(4):344–53. https://doi.org/10.1177/1078390319873049.

Zakhari R. The psychiatric-mental health nurse practitioner certification review manual. Springer Publishing Company; 2021.

Notes:

Notes:

7 Mood Disorders

Test your learning and check your understanding of this book's contents: Use the "Springer Nature Flashcards" app to access questions using ▶ https://sn.pub/62J0Ar.

To use the app, please follow the instructions in Chap. 1.

The American Psychiatric Association (2022) defines mood disorders as persistent mood alterations that impair daily life. Depression, sometimes known as unipolar depression, causes chronic sorrow, hopelessness, and a loss of interest in activities (American Psychiatric Association 2022). If untreated, these symptoms can impair daily life and lead to physical health issues and suicide (Fang et al. 2015). The NIMH estimates that 20.6 million US people (8.4% of the adult population) had a major depressive episode in the past year (NIH 2021).

Chronic depression called dysthymias is defined by a poor, persistent mood for at least 2 years (American Psychiatric Association 2022). Dysthymias' symptoms may not be as severe as major depression, but they can nevertheless affect daily living (Gabbay et al. 2016).

Symptoms of bipolar disorder include mania or hypomania and depression (American Psychiatric Association 2022). Bipolar I illness is defined by manic or mixed episodes lasting at least 7 days, while bipolar II disorder is characterized by hypomanic and depressed episodes (American Psychiatric Association 2022). Untreated bipolar disease can cost lives (Perlis et al. 2004).

The above should be differentiated from sadness and grief, which are normal emotional responses to loss. While they may be uncomfortable, they are a necessary part of the healing process (Stroebe et al. 2012). When these emotions persist and interfere with daily life, professional intervention may be needed. Medication, talk therapy, or both may be appropriate (Gabbay et al. 2016). Also, psychiatric-mental health nurse practitioners must be cognizant of cultural and individual variables that may affect an individual's experience and expression of these disorders (Fang et al. 2015).

T. Stewart, *Psychiatric-Mental Health Nurse Practitioner Program Companion and Board Certification Exam Review Workbook*,
https://doi.org/10.1007/978-3-031-60894-0_7

Psychiatric-mental health nurse practitioners should also understand mood disorder risk factors like heredity, stress, and medical illnesses (Kendler et al. 2003). By recognizing these risk factors, psychiatric-mental health nurse practitioners can prevent or minimize mood disorders in at-risk persons.

This chapter covers mood disorders. Depression, dysthymia, bipolar disorder I and II, and sadness and bereavement are discussed. Diagnostic criteria, relevant drugs, adverse effects such Stevens-Johnson syndrome and birth abnormalities, and treatments are presented.

7.1 Unipolar Depression Disorders

1. What are five chronic medical conditions associated with major depressive disorder?
    1.
    2.
    3.
    4.
    5.

2. Explain the diathesis-stress model of depression.

3. Why do many clients initially receive treatment for mood disorders from their primary care team?

4. The psychiatric disorder with the highest lifetime prevalence is ____________ ____.

5. When does sadness become pathological?

6. Episodic unipolar major depressive disorder is another term for ____________ ____.

7. Complete the following table of theories of the etiology of depression.

Category	Theory	Description/keywords
Psychodynamic	Object loss theory	Depression stems from loss of important people, things, or relationships
		Unresolved anger directed toward self leads to depression
Cognitive		Depression arises from negative thought patterns, dysfunctional beliefs, and cognitive distortions
	Learned helplessness-hopelessness theory	
Biological		Depression may have a hereditary component
	Endocrine	
	Neurotransmitters	
		Depression is linked to abnormalities in brain structures, such as the hippocampus and prefrontal cortex
	Chronobiology	

8. Name at least three screening tools for depression and their rating scales. What scores on each evidence normal and severe ranges?

Scale	Normal range	Severe range

Scale	Normal range	Severe range

9. The ____
_______ is a self-administered assessment that measures disability across cognitive, interpersonal, work, and social domains.

10. ________________________________ is the first objective for a patient having an acute episode of major depressive disorder.

11. Complete the following table for the mnemonic SIGECAPS for major depressive disorder.

	Symptom	Explanation
S		
I		
E		
C		
A		
P		
S		

12. __________ out of the nine above symptoms are required for a diagnosis of major depressive disorder.

13. For what minimum duration of time must depressive symptoms be present for a diagnosis of major depressive disorder?

14. What is meant by the term "nonreactive state"? What symptom makes it a nonreactive state?

15. ____ refers to an individual's thought patterns of rethinking and reconsidering.

16. SIGECAPS is a useful mnemonic for remembering primary diagnostic symptoms of major depressive disorder. However, depression can manifest with other signs and symptoms. Name at least five other signs and symptoms associated with depression.
    1.
    2.
    3.
    4.
    5.

17. Depression develops most often during which developmental period(s)? Why?

18. Are men or women diagnosed with depression at least two times more often than the other? Why?

19. An untreated episode of depression may last between _______________ months. With treatment, however, the length of a major depressive episode may be reduced to _____________ months or less.

20. The term for a normal reactive mood is ______________________________.

21. A patient who experiences a depressive episode is 50% more likely to have another episode in the future.
    TRUE FALSE

22. What is the most recommended treatment for depression?

23. Some individuals experience depression during certain times of the year. This is known as seasonal affective disorder. What are the three common symptoms of seasonal affective disorder and how is it treated?

24. Persistent depressive disorder, previously documented as dysthymia, may be diagnosed if an individual's depression is pervasive. To be considered pervasive, an individual must have experienced depression for __________ years, present with at least __________ symptoms, and have never been symptomatic for more than __________months.

25. Depression is born from chemical imbalance in the brain, specifically a lack of serotonin.
    TRUE FALSE

26. What is the role of the dysregulation of the hypothalamic-pituitary-adrenal (HPA) axis in depression?

27. Major depressive disorder can have episodes of mania, although very rare.
    TRUE FALSE

28. To be diagnosed with major depressive disorder, an individual must have at least 2 separate depressive episodes.
    TRUE FALSE

29. For individuals who experience multiple episodes of depression, we use the term ____________________.

30. What are some differentiating characteristics between typical and atypical depression?

Typical	Atypical

31. Another term for typical depression is ____________________ ________ depression.

32. Reactivity and severity help to distinguish pathological depression from normal emotional reactions to life events.
    TRUE FALSE

33. ____________________ captures depression or anxiety following a life stressor, but does not meet severity of diagnostic criteria for major depressive disorder.

34. Persistent depressive disorder is also known as ____________________ ____________. Being a chronic yet milder depressive disorder, the PMHNP would expect a patient to have symptoms for at least ____________________.

35. What is "double depression"?

36. Effects from which substances may mimic depression? Withdrawal from which substances can appear as depression?

37. What are three general medical conditions that may present as depression or depression-like symptoms?

38. What are the hallmark characteristics of borderline personality disorder?

39. What aspects of mood dysregulation link borderline personality disorder to depression?

40. What is a differentiating etiology between borderline personality disorder and major depressive disorder?

41. ____________________________ is mild depression. ____________________ ______________ is dissatisfaction with one's life. The former can have the latter.

42. Antidepressants are useful in treating borderline personality disorder.
TRUE FALSE

43. ____
__ therapy is first-line intervention for borderline personality disorder. It was developed by ____
___________.

44. ______________________ symptoms of schizophrenia may be mistaken as depression. However, depressed individuals retain functioning whereas there is noted deterioration in schizophrenia.

45. It is possible to have depression and ADHD simultaneously.
TRUE FALSE

46. What are three symptoms of PTSD that are shared with depression?

47. Almost two-thirds of individuals with depression also have a(n) ______________________________ disorder.

48. ____ may be used as a diagnosis for individuals who appear depressed and show little effort on cognitive tests even though they have the ability to engage. In addition, these individuals realize their memory loss.

49. What is the black box warning on antidepressants?

50. It is recommended that patients should be on antidepressants for a minimum of _____________ to _____________ months, even if their symptoms have abated. Indefinite use of antidepressants may be warranted for those individuals who have had multiple episodes of major depression.

51. Patients who abruptly stop taking antidepressants place themselves at risk for ____.

52. Antidepressants given to individuals who have bipolar disorder may induce ____.

53. Complete the following table on antidepressants.

Class	Mechanism of action	Examples	Adverse effects
Selective serotonin reuptake inhibitors (SSRIs)			
Tricyclic antidepressants (TCAs)			
Monoamine oxidase inhibitors (MAOIs)			
Serotonin-norepinephrine reuptake inhibitors (SNRIs)			

Class	Mechanism of action	Examples	Adverse effects
Norepinephrine-dopamine reuptake inhibitors (NDRIs)			
Serotonin agonist and reuptake inhibitors (SARIs)			

54. If an individual taking an MAOI consumes tyramine-rich foods/beverages, what may result? Why?

55. Place an X in front of each product below that should be avoided by individuals taking an MAOI.

_____Burrata mozzarella cheese.
_____Soft aged cheeses, such as Brie and Camembert.
_____Cured pastrami sandwich on rye bread.
_____Smoked sausage and sauerkraut.
_____Roasted chicken with lemon and rosemary.
_____Pickled herring.
_____Grilled salmon.
_____Iced tea.
_____Burgundy wine.
_____MSG.
_____Mango and papaya smoothie with almond milk.
_____Avocado toast.
_____Banana split.
_____Miso and soy marinated tofu.

56. ______________________________________ is a Category D SSRI medication for pregnancy due to an increased risk for cardiac defects.

57. The simultaneous use of ______________________, a weak μ-receptor opioid agonist, and serotonergic medications may increase the risk of serotonin syndrome as it increases concentrations of serotonin and noradrenaline within the limbic system of the brain.

58. ______________________ are antidepressants contraindicated within 2 weeks of a patient having used an MAOI due to increased risk of serotonin syndrome.

59. An individual with ADHD who is also looking to stop smoking may benefit from a trial of ______________________. However, this individual should not take this medicine if they have a history of ______________________.

60. When considering TCAs, ______________________ is the most selective for serotonin; ______________________ is the most selective for norepinephrine.

61. A baseline EKG is recommended prior to starting ______________ clients on a TCA.

62. A PMHNP should always ask about sleep. For example, a client newly established on ______________________, an antidepressant used for insomnia, might mention a reduction in their very vivid and weird nightmares at their next appointment. ______________________ is another medication used to abate nightmares, often prescribed to clients with PTSD.

7.2 Grief

63. Grief is a form of depression.

    TRUE FALSE

64. Grief usually develops within ________ months of a single, recurring, or developmental stressor.

65. How does a PMHNP differentiate between normal and pathological grief?

66. ______________________ disorder should be on the PMHNP's list of differential diagnoses when assessing grief response.

67. ____
__ was added as a diagnosis in the DSM 5-TR. It may be used for clients still grieving 1 year after experiencing a loss and unable to return to everyday activities.

7.3 Premenstrual Dysphoric Disorder and Postpartum Depression

68. ____
__ is a form of depression and dysphoria beginning in the luteal phase of a woman's menstrual cycle and lasts approximately 6 days or until menstruation begins. Patients should chart their mood and menstrual cycle for clearer associations.

69. Women who experience premenstrual dysphoric disorder may be prescribed antidepressants as a daily therapy or only during their menstrual cycle.
TRUE FALSE

70. What are the "baby blues"? Are they the same as postpartum depression?

71. ____ is a leading cause of infanticide. It requires psychiatric hospitalization.

72. Postpartum depression can be treated like major depressive disorder.
TRUE FALSE

73. If a woman previously experienced postpartum mania, It is not recommended that she be treated prophylactically with mood stabilizers during subsequent pregnancies.
TRUE FALSE

74. What treatment for pregnant women having a manic episode provides an alternative to potentially teratogenic medications and is overall relatively safe throughout pregnancy?

75. What are the three SSRIs with FDA approval to treat premenstrual dysphoric disorder?

7.4 Treatment of Unipolar Depressions

76. What type of anxiety is linked to major depressive disorder in children?

77. "Skill deficit" refers to an individual's physical inability to perform a skill. This is often seen in dementia patients. ______________________________ _____ deficit is seen in depression, when the individual lacks the drive to complete the skill.

78. What three elements are components of a functional assessment? When screening for depression, in which population should a functional assessment be completed?

79. What are five to seven symptoms of serotonin syndrome?
    1.
    2.
    3.
    4.
    5.
    6.
    7.

80. ________________ syndrome manifests in flu-like symptoms, insomnia, nausea, imbalance, paresthesias, and hyperarousal. It is caused not only by stopping SSRIs suddenly, but by using antidepressants irregularly, particularly those of high dosage and/or short half-life.

81. What is the intervention approach for serotonin syndrome?

82. ____________________________, an SSRI, has the least risk of discontinuation syndrome.

83. ___________________________, an MAOI, has the lowest risk of tyramine-associated hypertensive crisis.

84. __________________________________ is the antidepressant with the highest risk of liver failure. For this reason, liver function tests should be monitored closely.

85. The FINISH mnemonic is helpful for remembering symptoms of antidepressant discontinuation syndrome. These symptoms may present if a client abruptly stops an antidepressant after taking it for >6 weeks. Complete the table with these side effects.

F	
I	
N	
I	
S	
H	

86. Discontinuation syndrome is not life-threatening, but its effects can be experienced for ________week(s).

87. Patients on what TCAs should have serum blood levels checked to avoid toxicity?

88. For which populations are TCAs usually contraindicated?

89. Before switching a client from a TCA to a(n) ________________, a ______________ week washout period is required to avoid serotonin syndrome. If switching to fluoxetine, a washout period of ______________ weeks should be followed due to its long half-life.

90. The ________________________________ antidepressants can increase TCA concentrations if taken simultaneously.

91. What are common symptoms of a hypertensive crisis?

92. ____ is given during a hypertensive crisis to block the neurotransmitter ______________________________ ______________.

93. Name three to five medications and/or supplements that patients on MAOIs should avoid.
    1.
    2.
    3.
    4.
    5.

94. Children with persistent depressive disorder are more often described as ________________________, rather than sad.

95. ______________________________ is when neurons misfire freely, without electrical stimuli, due to membrane threshold desensitization.

96. Cognitive behavioral therapy focuses on ______________________________, ______________________________, and ______________________________.

97. While cognitive behavioral therapy may be the most recommended form of psychotherapy, what are other therapy models for use in treating depression?

98. What is the most popular class of antidepressants? Why?

99. In addition to increasing serotonin, other antidepressants often focus on the neurotransmitters ____________________ and ____________________.

100. A PMHNP should counsel their patient starting an SSRI that it may take ______________ weeks for full efficacy.

101. What is the "rule of thirds" regarding the treatment and prognosis of depression?

102. ______________________________ is a controversial, yet highly effective, non-pharmacological approach to treatment-resistant depression.

103. How would you explain electroconvulsive therapy to a patient? What side effects may they experience?

104. What class of antidepressants is useful for atypical depression?

105. A patient with major depressive symptoms plus paranoia, delusions, or hallucinations may be diagnosed with ____. In addition to antidepressants, ____ may be prescribed to address the latter symptoms.

106. What is catatonia? What are treatment options?

107. ____ uses magnetic fields to address treatment-resistant depression in an in-office setting. No anesthesia is required. Side effects are mild and include headache, scalp irritation, facial and trigeminal nerve stimulation in face, and hearing discomfort from the machine.

108. How many sessions of TMS is typical?

109. What are some side effects a patient may experience from a vagal nerve stimulation (VNS) procedure?

110. Bright light therapy may be used in ______________________________ disorder. "Light boxes" simulate sunshine missing during the winter months or geographies where there are less days of sunlight (e.g., farther from equator, gray-overcast environments).

111. It is recommended that bright light therapy should be used for a minimum of __________ minutes a day.

112. What treatment is recommended for adjustment disorder?

113. The ____ ___ and the ____ ______________ are both self-administered screening tools for bipolar disorder.

114. It is estimated that up to 50% of individuals with this type of depression, ___ ____ ________________, may be later diagnosed with bipolar disorder. Initial presentation later in life may evidence a medical etiology (e.g., multiple sclerosis).

115. In which cases would a PMHNP not initially recommend both medication and psychotherapy to a patient with MDD?

116. What are the recommended steps when getting a patient with MDD settled on pharmaco- and psychotherapies?

117. The PMHNP should schedule a follow-up appointment with a patient who has discontinued treatment for MDD approximately ____________ week(s) after the last appointment to check in.

118. Complete the table on antidepressants and adverse effects/risks.

Class	Mechanism of action	Generic drug (brand name)	Target diseases/ disorders	Adverse effects/risks
Selective serotonin reuptake inhibitors (SSRIs)				
Serotonin-norepinephrine reuptake inhibitors (SNRIs)				
Tricyclic antidepressants (TCAs)				
Monoamine oxidase inhibitors (MAOIs)				
Serotonin partial agonist reuptake inhibitor (SPARI)				

Class	Mechanism of action	Generic drug (brand name)	Target diseases/ disorders	Adverse effects/risks
Norepinephrine-dopamine reuptake inhibitor (NDRI)				
Atypical antidepressant				
Serotonin antagonist and reuptake inhibitor (SARI)				

7.5 Bipolar Disorders

119. Why is a manic episode considered a psychiatric emergency?

120. Mania and hypomania share common symptoms except for the duration of the mania itself.

TRUE FALSE

121. To be diagnosed with rapid cycling bipolar disorder, an individual must experience at least __________ mood episodes within 1 year.

122. What are the key symptoms of mania?

123. To receive a diagnosis of a manic episode, an individual has to present with at least _______________ symptoms over _______________ week.

124. An individual with a diagnosis of persistent depressive disorder who has a manic episode can retain the original diagnosis.

TRUE FALSE

125. The key symptom differentiating unipolar and bipolar depressions is _________________________.

126. Bipolar I disorder is associated with manic episodes. Bipolar II disorder has ____________________________ episodes. What is the difference between these episodes?

127. A helpful mnemonic for remembering the criteria for a manic episode is DIGFAST. Complete the following table with a description of each of the signs and symptoms of mania.

	Sign/symptom	Description
D		
I		
G		
F		

	Sign/symptom	Description
A		
S		
T		

128. A PMHNP must witness a patient in a manic episode in order to diagnose them with bipolar disorder.
TRUE FALSE

129. Bipolar symptoms, both depression and mania, that are lower in severity may qualify a patient for a diagnosis of ________________________________.

130. Why is making a diagnosis of bipolar disorder difficult at times?

131. Place an X before each of the following symptoms that may evidence a manic episode.
_____increased sleep
_____rapid speech pattern
_____grandiose self-concept
_____social avoidance
_____starting new projects and finishing them
_____decreased use of substances
_____excessive spending
_____sexual behaviors, risky departure from baseline
_____goal-oriented, focused thoughts and attention.

132. Most individuals with bipolar disorder type II have rapid cycling, which allows them to better manage mood changes and functioning.
TRUE FALSE

133. ______________________________ levels should be checked, as its dysfunction can result in mood dysregulation and ups and downs.

134. Name three prescription medications that can mimic mania symptoms.

135. As mania intensifies, individuals with bipolar I disorder may experience psychotic events, particularly ______________ hallucinations.

136. __________ with bipolar disorder report more illegal and violent acts. __________, in contrast, have higher rates of substance abuse, suicide, and thyroid disease.

137. The mean age of onset for bipolar disorders is between ________ and ________ years old.

138. Functional imaging among individuals with bipolar disorder has shown a loss of gray matter in the ______________________, ______________________, and ______________________. Executive function, decision-making, memory, and emotion are affected as a result.

139. What is the hypothesized connection between the hypothalamic-pituitary-thyroid-adrenal (HPTA) axis and bipolar disorder?

7.6 Treatment of Bipolar Disorders

140. What is lithium's mechanism of action?

141. ______________________________ is the only mood stabilizer shown to have antisuicidal effects.

142. Lithium is considered the gold standard for treating ___________________________ in bipolar disorder. But, it is not very effective in treating those with __________________________________ bipolar disorder.

143. The therapeutic window for lithium is ___________________ to ___________________ mEq/L.

144. When should lithium levels be drawn on a patient? How often?

145. When educating your patient about lithium toxicity and side effects, what key pieces of information would you include?

146. Match each of the following medications used to treat mood disorders/bipolar disorder with their adverse effects. Medications may have more than one choice.

Medication	Adverse effects
1. Lithium (Eskalith).	(a) Aplastic anemia
2. Carbamazepine (Tegretol)	(b) Agranulocytosis
3. Valproic acid/divalproex (Depakote, Depakene)	(c) Hepatotoxicity
4. Lamotrigine (Lamictal)	(d)Pancreatitis
	(e) Stevens-Johnson syndrome
	(f) GI distress
	(g) Vision changes/nystagmus
	(h) Delirium
	(i) Renal toxicity
	(j) Leukopenia
	(k) Hypothyroidism

147. Before starting a patient of ______________________________ ancestry on carbamazepine, the PMHNP should screen for the __________________ allele.

148. ________________________________ is a medication used to treat bipolar disorder that does not require blood level monitoring.

149. How would concomitant use of lamotrigine with either valproic acid or carbamazepine affect lamotrigine levels?

150. What is Stevens-Johnson syndrome? What are key signs and symptoms? What is the intervention?

151. Lithium and carbamazepine are excellent treatment options for bipolar disorder. However, they are teratogenic and carry significant risks to the developing fetus. Lithium can cause ____. Carbamazepine can cause ____.

152. Pregnant women should not take mood stabilizers.
TRUE FALSE

153. What is the Young Mania Rating Scale?

154. For which population is the Young Mania Rating Scale most appropriate due to its administration?

155. Patients with bipolar disorder should put into place a plan if they are to have a recurrence of mania.
TRUE FALSE

156. If a patient's acute mania is inadequately controlled after 2 weeks, what medications may be added or changed?

157. In addition to lithium or lamotrigine, an antidepressant should be prescribed for a patient with bipolar disorder in acute depression.
TRUE FALSE

158. What are the common symptoms of metabolic disorder, a common side effect of mood stabilizer medications?

159. Which two atypical antipsychotics have FDA approval to treat bipolar depression?

160. Name two support groups for individuals with bipolar disorder and their families and friends.

161. ______________________________ and ______________________________ are anticonvulsants used as mood stabilizers, particularly for rapid cycling bipolar disorder and bipolar disorder with mixed features.

162. What are the signs and symptoms of lithium toxicity?

163. What is the treatment for lithium toxicity?

164. What is Epstein's anomaly?

165. What laboratories should be ordered for patients taking lithium?

166. ______________________________ are used to treat bipolar disorder, based on the theory that mania may be due to neuronal hyperactivity.

167. What is the mechanism of action of valproic acid?

168. What are the most serious side effects associated with valproic acid use?

169. ______________________________ require genetic screening for the ______________________________ allele prior to starting carbamazepine as they are at increased risk for developing Stevens-Johnson syndrome.

170. In addition to Stevens-Johnson syndrome, what are other side effects associated with carbamazepine use?

171. The therapeutic range of valproic acid is ____—_____ μg/mL.

172. The most serious side effect of lamotrigine is ______________________, a medical emergency.

173. What is the mechanism of action of carbamazepine?

174. The therapeutic range of carbamazepine is ____—_____ μg/mL.

175. Which mood stabilizer can induce its own metabolism in the liver, leading to a decreased concentration of the drug over time?

176. __________________________ is an anticonvulsant used for mood stabilization and impulsivity. It is known for weight loss and mental dulling.

177. ____ and ________________________________ are first-line medications for acute mania.

178. Name the three antipsychotics that are effective for bipolar depression since they work more on serotonin.

179. Why is the use of antidepressants limited to treating unipolar depression?

7.7 Suicide

180. Determine if each of the following statements about suicide is TRUE (T) or FALSE (F).

__________A suicidal individual usually wants to live, but thinks they have no other alternative to relieve their pain.

__________ Most suicides are spontaneous.

__________An individual contemplating suicide does not usually give any clues of their intent.

__________Suicidal persons are not typically psychotic.

__________Asking a client about suicidal intent increases the likelihood of subsequent suicidal behavior.

__________Men attempt suicide more frequently and are also more successful than women.

__________ Suicide incidence is lower in married adults.

181. According to Seligman, what is "learned helplessness" and how might it explain suicidal ideation?

182. Place an X before each of the following if it can be considered a risk factor for suicide.

_____Female.

_____New job.

_____Owns pets.

_____Previous suicide attempt.

_____Married.

_____Chronic illness.

_____Member of a religious organization.

_____African American.

_____White.

_____Single, separated.

_____2–4 weeks after starting an antidepressant, particularly among pediatric patients.

183. Entering into "safety contracts" or "no-harm" agreements have been found to mitigate suicide attempts among individuals voicing suicidal ideation.
TRUE FALSE

184. What is the Columbia-Suicide Severity Rating Scale (C-SSRS)?

7.8 Answers and Explanations to Chapter Activities

1. Possible answers include cardiovascular illness, diabetes mellitus, chronic pain, obesity, chronic fatigue syndrome, multiple sclerosis, inflammatory bowel disease, COPD, Cushing's, syphilis, HIV, thyroid and parathyroid diseases, liver dysfunction (hepatitis, cirrhosis), and malignancies.
2. The diathesis-stress concept explains that depression is caused by genetic or biological vulnerabilities (diathesis) and stressful life events. Genetic differences in neurotransmitter function or neuroplasticity may raise depression risk. Negative cognitive biases and low self-esteem can also increase depression risk. Acute or chronic stressors include major life events like the death of a loved one or continuous work or relationship issues. High-vulnerability people may not acquire depression if they don't face stress. Stress can cause depression in low-vulnerability people.
3. Many clients obtain mood disorder treatment from their primary care team for numerous reasons:

   - Accessibility: Primary care providers are accessible and many people have a relationship with them.
   - Comorbidity: Cardiovascular disease, diabetes, and chronic pain typically accompany mood problems. Primary care physicians are educated to address various medical issues and coordinate physical and mental health care. The PCP also sees patients with somatic complaints.
   - Stigma: Mental health therapy is still stigmatized, which may deter people. Mental health care is generally considered regular by primary care doctors, making it a less stigmatized entrance point.
   - Screening: Primary care physicians can screen for mood disorders during normal medical visits to identify at-risk or affected patients. Early detection and intervention improve treatment outcomes.
   - Treatment: Primary care doctors can treat mild to moderate mood disorders with medicines and brief counseling. When needed, they might send patients to professional mental health providers for more intense treatment.

4. Major depressive disorder has the highest lifetime prevalence. MDD causes persistent depression, hopelessness, and loss of interest in previously enjoyable activities. The World Health Organization (WHO) estimates lifetime prevalence of MDD at 10% to 15% in the general population. It is more common among women and peaks in young adulthood. MDD can lower quality of life and impede social and occupational functioning.
5. Sadness is a typical reaction to loss, disappointment, and other life challenges. It becomes pathological when it lasts too long, is disproportionate, or disrupts daily life. Pathological melancholy is associated with mood disorders such as major depressive disorder (MDD) or persistent depressive disorder (PDD). These diseases are characterized by persistent unhappiness, hopelessness, and loss of interest in previously enjoyable activities. Changes in food and sleep, weariness, low self-esteem, difficulties focusing, and suicidal thoughts are other MDD or PDD symptoms.

   - Sadness and depression differ from person to person, so what is pathological for one may not be for another. Cultural and socioeconomic influences also affect sadness and depression perception.

6. Episodic unipolar major depressive disorder is another term for clinical depression.
7.

Category	Theory	Description/keywords
Psychodynamic	Object loss theory	Depression stems from loss of important people, things, or relationships
	Aggression-turned-inward theory	Unresolved anger directed toward self leads to depression
Cognitive	Cognitive theory	Depression arises from negative thought patterns, dysfunctional beliefs, and cognitive distortions
	Learned helplessness-hopelessness theory	Belief that no matter what one does, the outcome will be negative, leading to helplessness and hopelessness
Biological	Genetic	Depression may have a hereditary component
	Endocrine	Depression can be caused by dysregulation of hormones such as cortisol or thyroid hormone
	Neurotransmitters	Depression is associated with imbalances in neurotransmitters such as serotonin, norepinephrine, and dopamine
	Neuroanatomy	Depression is linked to abnormalities in brain structures, such as the hippocampus and prefrontal cortex
	Chronobiology	Disruptions in circadian rhythms can contribute to the development of depression

8.

Scale	Normal range	Severe range
Beck depression inventory (BDI)	0–13	29–63
Edinburgh postnatal depression scale (EPDS)	<10	>10
Hamilton depression rating scale (HAM-D)	0–7	>20
Montgomery-Asberg depression rating scale (MADRS)	<15	>44
Patient health questionnaire 9 (PHQ-9)	<5	20–27
Zung depression scale	20–49	>70

9. The WHO Disability Assessment Schedule may assess a person's functionality and disability regardless of health state or situation. WHODAS 2.0 assesses disability in six areas: understanding and communicating, getting around, self-care, getting along with people, living activities (home and work), and societal engagement. WHODAS 2.0 is used in research and therapy and translated into numerous languages for cross-cultural use.
10. Assessing and managing patient suicide or self-harm risk is paramount. Depression, hopelessness, despair, suicide history, and social support are often assessed during suicide risk assessment. Hospitalization or intense outpatient treatment may be needed for significant suicide risk for patient safety. Assess the patient's physical condition and medical needs to manage comorbidities. After establishing patient safety and health, a comprehensive depression assessment should lead to diagnosis and treatment.
11.

S	Sleep	May manifest as a disruption in the amount and or quality of sleep, patients may have difficulty with sleep initiation or sleep maintenance
I	Interest	Refers to anhedonia, or inability to feel pleasure, leading to decreased interest in socializing or other normally pleasurable activities. It is a lack of joy
G	Guilt	Overfocusing on negative thoughts. May manifest as feelings of worthlessness or hopelessness
E	Energy	Decrease in energy is a common symptom. Patients may complain not wanting to get out of the bed each morning
C	Concentration	Affected by other symptoms associated with depression. Will improve as depression lifts.
A	Appetite	Many find that appetite decreases, finding food unappetizing or flavorless, although some may eat more during a depressive episode
P	Psychomotor	The general slowing down as reported by the patient. This may include speech patterns and gross motor movements, considered a sign of more severe depression, which could develop into catatonia
S	Suicidal ideation	An extreme exacerbation of hopelessness and worthlessness experienced by some individuals with depression often born out of myriad phenomena and symptoms

12. Five out of the nine above symptoms are required for a diagnosis of major depressive disorder.

13. Depressed mood or loss of interest or pleasure in daily activities for at least 2 weeks, known as "two blue weeks," is required by the DSM-5. Other symptoms include changes in appetite or sleep patterns, feelings of worthlessness or guilt, difficulty concentrating or making decisions, and recurrent thoughts.
14. Depression often causes a "nonreactive state"—emotional indifference to good or harmful stimuli. The person does not react emotionally to situations or experiences like most others. Blunting or numbness is emotional inaction. A person in a nonreactive state may appear apathetic and lose interest in previously appreciated activities. The voice and face may not match their emotions, causing a blunted effect. Depressed people may feel hopeless and miserable since they cannot enjoy or be driven. Since patients may not feel good or perceive the usefulness in therapy, mental health practitioners may have trouble motivating them.
15. Rumination is rethinking and focusing on negative thoughts, memories, and experiences. Depressed people may feel helpless and despair due to ruminating thoughts about past mistakes. It can deepen depression, raise relapse risk, and inhibit social and professional functioning. Rumination, which emphasizes negatives rather than solutions, can hamper problem-solving and decision-making.
16. Answers may include anxiety, stomach pain, headaches, motivation, feelings of disassociation, hygiene changes, loss of eye contact, slouched posture, and slower or slurred speech.
17. Depression can happen at any age, but teens and young adults are frequently affected. In this period, physical, emotional, and social changes might cause depression. Teens can develop depression due to peer pressure, academic demands, or interpersonal concerns. Depression and mood swings might result from puberty hormones. Financial stability, family and relationship commitments, and independence might stress early adulthood. These demands can cause depression.
18. Women. This gender discrepancy in depression frequency is consistent across cultures and countries. Gender inequality may be caused by complex biological, psychological, and social variables. The gender gap in depression may be due to hormone swings during menstruation, pregnancy, and menopause and brain shape and function. Rumination, low self-esteem, and negative cognitive processes and coping techniques may also affect gender variations in depression. Gender discrimination, role tension, and socialization may contribute.
19. Untreated depression lasts 6–12 months. Major depression can last 3 months or less with treatment.
20. Euthymia is a balanced emotional state without depression, mania, or other mood disorders. Patients with euthymia are happy and can handle daily tasks and socializing.
21. TRUE. One bout of depression increases the risk of another by 50% and two episodes by 70%. Each episode of depression increases the risk of recurrence, especially in persons with a family history, chronic or severe depression, or physical or mental issues. The necessity to monitor and manage depression following recovery is stressed to prevent recurrence.

22. The best depression treatment is medicine and psychotherapy. Antidepressants alleviate depression by regulating serotonin and norepinephrine. CBT helps depression too. Identifying and challenging negative thought patterns and learning adaptive coping strategies is CBT. Psychodynamic and interpersonal therapy may also be effective. In addition to medication and psychotherapy, exercise, mindfulness-based therapies, and lifestyle changes (e.g., good eating, appropriate sleep, stress management) may help manage depression symptoms.
23. Three typical SAD symptoms are:

    - Depressed and Irritable: SAD sufferers feel empty for days or weeks. Negativity typically leads to hopelessness and worthlessness.
    - SAD sufferers may have problems waking up due to hypersomnia. All-day fatigue may also occur.
    - Carb cravings, especially for sugary or starchy foods, may trigger SAD weight gain.
    - Fall and winter, with less sunlight and shorter days, cause SAD. Lack of sunlight can affect mood, sleep, and appetite by altering the circadian cycle. Medical, psychotherapeutic, and light treatments for SAD are common. Daily morning light therapy exposes patients to bright light. The light simulates sunlight and regulates mood and circadian rhythm. Depression can be treated with SSRIs. Psychotherapy, especially CBT, can help SAD sufferers change negative thought patterns and improve coping. SAD self-help includes exercise, social support, stress management, and a healthy diet.

24. Dysthymia is 2 years of depression, two symptoms, and 2 months of symptomatology.
25. FALSE. Although neurotransmitter imbalances, including serotonin, may induce depression, the causes are complex. Genetics, environment, and psychology can cause depression. Family history of depression may increase depression risk. Environmental variables such as stress, chronic illness, and trauma can produce depression. Negative thinking, low self-esteem, and poor coping may increase depression risk. Depression may be caused by neurotransmitter imbalances, but medications may not work.
26. Depression may be caused by HPA axis dysregulation. Stress is controlled by the HPA axis, which includes the brain, pituitary gland, and adrenal glands. Stress releases CRH from the hypothalamus, which stimulates ACTH secretion from the pituitary gland. To prepare the body for stress, ACTH stimulates adrenal glands to produce cortisol. Depression elevates cortisol and stress sensitivity due to HPA axis dysregulation. Nighttime cortisol levels in depressed people might impair sleep and increase depression. In mood-regulating brain regions, HPA axis dysregulation may also induce depression.
27. FALSE. Chronic sadness, emptiness, and hopelessness are symptoms of MDD. It seldom produces mania, which causes irritability, activity, and sleeplessness. MDD patients may develop bipolar disorder and cyclothymia, which cause depression and mania or hypomania.

28. FALSE. MDD is diagnosed after one major depressive episode. For 2 weeks, symptoms must be present practically every day. Repeated significant depressive episodes may suggest MDD.
29. Recurring MDD involves two or more major depressive episodes with remission. With each depressive episode, recurrent MDD patients' risk of recurrence increases.
30.

Typical	Atypical
• Melancholic depression • Chronic sorrow, emptiness, or hopelessness, changes in eating or sleep patterns, exhaustion, feelings of worthlessness or guilt, and difficulties concentrating or making decisions • May cause psychomotor agitation or retardation • SSRIs and tricyclics may help	• Mood symptoms match experience—Less depression during happy events that worse after sad ones • Interpersonal sensitivity, hunger, weight gain, hypersomnia, and leaden paralysis • Neurovegetative symptoms reversed • Generalized anxiety or social phobia • May benefit from MAOIs, CBT, or interpersonal therapy

31. Normal depression is melancholy depression, characterized by chronic sorrow, emptiness, or hopelessness, changes in eating or sleep patterns, exhaustion, feelings of worthlessness or guilt, and difficulties concentrating or making decisions. Melancholy can cause psychomotor agitation or retardation.
32. TRUE. Depression often impairs receptivity, so nice things do not boost mood. Pathological depression is insensitive, unlike typical emotional reactions to life experiences, which can include both positive and negative emotions. The symptoms of pathological depression are harsher and linger longer than typical emotional reactions.
33. Adjustment disorder can develop from death, divorce, job loss, or illness. Anxiety, depression, hunger, sleep disturbances, attention issues, and social withdrawal might result from adjustment disorder. Adjustment disorder symptoms endure 6 months. Major depressive disorder and other mood disorders have more severe symptoms than adjustment disorder.
34. Persistent depression persists as dysthymia. Chronic, milder depression produces low mood for at least 2 years in adults and one in children and adolescents. In addition to a persistently bad mood, persistent depression can cause eating or sleep problems, fatigue, low self-esteem, trouble concentrating or making decisions, and hopelessness. Persistent depression symptoms can influence daily living and quality of life despite being less severe than serious depression.
35. In "double depression" a person experiences persistent low-grade depression symptoms such as dysthymia plus periodic episodes of more severe depressive symptoms such as MDD. More severe than PDD or MDD, double

depression is hard to treat. Drugs and psychotherapies such as CBT or IPT can treat chronic and episodic depression.

36. Depression-Imitating Drugs.

    - Brain chemistry alterations from persistent alcohol usage may cause low mood, apathy, decreased energy. Alcoholism can produce depression due to social, economic, and physical effects.
    - Drugs: Chronic opioid use affects brain chemistry, causing sadness, apathy, and weariness. Opioids can cause depression due to social, financial, and physical effects.
    - Similar to depression, sedatives, and tranquilizers cause drowsiness, apathy, and energy loss.
    - Cannabis: Chronic marijuana usage changes brain chemistry, causing sadness, apathy, and weariness. The social, economic, and physical implications of cannabis use disorder can create depression.
    - Depression may mimic substance withdrawal:
    - Alcohol: Alcohol withdrawal causes melancholy, anger, anxiety, and tiredness.
    - Detoxing from opioids can produce melancholy, anxiety, and tiredness.
    - Depression-like symptoms such as anger, anxiety, and tiredness can result from benzodiazepine withdrawal.
    - Cocaine and methamphetamine withdrawal can cause depression-like mood fluctuations, lethargy, and apathy.

37. Depression can result from several common medical issues.

    - Thyroid Abnormalities: Fatigue, depression, concentration issues, and weight gain can result.
    - Chronic Pain: Arthritis, fibromyalgia, and migraines cause fatigue, depression, and insomnia.
    - Neurological Disorders: MS, Parkinson's disease, and Alzheimer's disease disrupt brain chemistry and function, producing depression, apathy, and attention problems.
    - Diseases such as heart attack and stroke can change brain chemistry and function, causing mood, apathy, and concentration problems.
    - Chronic fatigue syndrome causes extreme fatigue, low mood, trouble concentrating, and sleep problems.
    - Diabetes: Blood sugar alterations can cause weariness, depression, and attention problems.
    - Fatigue, low mood, and attention impairments can result from vitamin B12 and vitamin D shortages.

38. Relationships, self-image, and emotions are unstable with BPD. BPD patients' self-images change. Those with BPD may experience sudden emotional changes. They may miscontrol their emotions and respond excessively to tiny causes. They may use drugs, binge eat, drive recklessly, or have unprotected sex. Impulse control may be difficult. Rejection and abandonment may worry

these individuals. Due to this fear, they may isolate or overdepend on certain individuals. Those with BPD may quickly idealize and downgrade others. Those with BPD may struggle to find meaning in life. They may cut, burn, or attempt suicide.

39. BPD is a complex mental illness that causes mood dysregulation and severe feelings including depression. Depression-like despair, wrath, and anxiety can result from BPD. Minor events can trigger these sentiments, which alter fast. As with depression, BPD can cause poor mood, hopelessness, and high exhilaration or energy. BPD can cause persistent emptiness or boredom, which can mirror depression. Separation from people or emotions may accompany these sensations. Depression-related suicide may increase with BPD. Life meaninglessness, hopelessness, and worthlessness may create this.
40. The etiology of BPD and MDD differ. BPD is thought to result from multiple genetic, environmental, and psychological factors. Childhood trauma such as abuse or neglect and early attachment disorders are often linked to it. Some research suggests BPD affects the amygdala, prefrontal brain, and other emotional processing and regulation areas. MDD may be caused by brain chemistry changes, particularly serotonin and other mood-regulating neurotransmitter defects. A chemical imbalance in the brain may induce MDD, along with genetic and environmental factors. Although BPD and MDD symptoms overlap, their diagnostic criteria differ. MDD causes melancholy or hopelessness, changes in eating, sleep habits, energy levels, and other physical or emotional symptoms, while BPD causes relational, self-image, and emotional instability.
41. Mild depression is dysthymia. Life dissatisfaction is existential unhappiness.
42. FALSE. Antidepressants rarely are used initially in BPD treatment. Antidepressants can help control occasional depression or anxiety, but they cannot treat BPD's core symptoms, such as emotional dysregulation, impulsivity, and relational difficulties. Dialectical behavior therapy, mentalization-based treatment, and transference-focused psychotherapy are the main BPD treatments. These therapies train emotional regulation, distress tolerance, interpersonal effectiveness, and mindfulness in a safe and supportive environment.
43. Dialectical behavior therapy is the first-line treatment for BPD. Marsha Linehan developed it in the 1980s to treat BPD's core symptoms, including emotional dysregulation, impulsivity, and relationship difficulties. DBT incorporates mindfulness, distress tolerance, emotion regulation, and interpersonal effectiveness. Weekly group treatment, individual therapy, and phone coaching deliver it in a regulated and supportive environment. Depressive, anxious, and drug use disorder symptoms are reduced with DBT. In a customized treatment plan, it is used with medicine and other psychotherapies.
44. In early schizophrenia, negative symptoms may resemble depression. Negative symptoms include diminished motivation, emotion, social engagement, and cognition. Unlike sadness, schizophrenia can impair function during remission. The issues can include work, school, relationships, and social interactions.

45. TRUE. Both ADHD and depression are possible. Research shows these two illnesses often coexist. Depression can affect 50% of those with ADHD and vice versa. Both can alter mood, motivation, and concentration.
46. Depressive and PTSD symptoms can create hopelessness and despair. Memory, concentration, and other cognitive difficulties might result from PTSD and depression. Depression and PTSD can cause insomnia, nightmares, and night sweats.
47. Anxiety and depression often share symptoms such as chronic sadness, trouble concentration, and sleep problems.
48. Depression or anxiety can create pseudodementia. Presumed dementia causes memory loss, confusion, mood swings, and concentration problems. Pseudodementia patients can do cognitive tasks and may improve with depression or other mental health treatment.
49. All FDA-mandated antidepressants must have black box warnings. In children, teenagers, and young adults (up to 24 years old) taking antidepressants for major depressive disorder or other mental disorders, the prominent label on packaging and product information materials cautions that suicidal thoughts or actions may rise.
50. Patients should take antidepressants for 6–12 months after symptoms are resolved. A long-term antidepressant can prevent depression return.
51. Discontinuing antidepressants abruptly or without tapering can cause antidepressant discontinuation syndrome. The flu-like symptoms of antidepressant discontinuation syndrome include headaches, nausea, muscle aches, and mood disturbances such as anxiety, irritability, and agitation. Discontinuing antidepressants suddenly can induce dizziness, electric shock ("brain zaps"), and confusion.
52. Antidepressants may cause mania or hypomania in those with bipolar disorder. To treat depression and mania, bipolar illness patients commonly use mood stabilizers.
53.

Class	Mechanism of action	Examples	Adverse effects
Selective serotonin reuptake inhibitors (SSRIs)	Inhibit presynaptic reuptake of serotonin	Fluoxetine (Prozac), sertraline (Zoloft), citalopram (Celexa), escitalopram (Lexapro), paroxetine (Paxil)	Sexual dysfunction, weight gain, gastrointestinal disturbances, anxiety, insomnia, serotonin syndrome (rare)
Tricyclic antidepressants (TCAs)	Inhibit serotonin and norepinephrine presynaptic reuptake	Amitriptyline (Elavil), nortriptyline (Pamelor), imipramine (Tofranil)	Sedation, anticholinergic effects (dry mouth, blurred vision, constipation, urinary retention), orthostatic hypotension, weight gain, cardiac toxicity (rare)

Class	Mechanism of action	Examples	Adverse effects
Monoamine oxidase inhibitors (MAOIs)	Block MAO enzyme from breaking down serotonin and norepinephrine	Phenelzine (Nardil), tranylcypromine (Parnate)	Hypertensive crisis (with ingestion of tyramine-containing foods), sexual dysfunction, weight gain, gastrointestinal disturbances, insomnia, serotonin syndrome (with concomitant use of other serotonergic agents)
Serotonin-norepinephrine reuptake inhibitors (SNRIs)	Selectively inhibit presynaptic reuptake of serotonin and norepinephrine	Venlafaxine (Effexor), duloxetine (Cymbalta)	Nausea, headache, hypertension, sexual dysfunction, weight gain, insomnia, serotonin syndrome (rare)
Norepinephrine-dopamine reuptake inhibitors (NDRIs)	Selectively inhibit presynaptic reuptake of norepinephrine and dopamine	Bupropion (Wellbutrin)	Agitation, anxiety, insomnia, dry mouth, headache, seizures (rare)
Serotonin agonist and reuptake inhibitors (SARIs)	Selectively inhibit presynaptic reuptake and agonism of serotonin	Trazodone (Desyrel)	Sedation, dizziness, headache, dry mouth, gastrointestinal disturbances, priapism (rare)

54. Tyramine-rich foods and drinks might cause a life-threatening hypertensive crisis in MAOI users. MAOIs block monoamine oxidase, which breaks down tyramine in the liver and intestines. Unbroken tyramine can release too much norepinephrine, raising blood pressure dangerously. Tyramine-induced hypertension crises can cause headaches, palpitations, chest pain, perspiration, nausea, and vomiting. In severe circumstances, it might cause stroke, heart attack, or convulsions.
55. __x___Soft aged cheeses, such as Brie and Camembert.
    __x___Cured pastrami sandwich on rye bread.
    __x___Smoked sausage and sauerkraut.
    __x___Pickled herring.
    __x___Burgundy wine.
    __x___MSG.
    __x___Avocado toast.
    __x___Banana split.
    __x___Miso and soy marinated tofu.
56. Category D drugs have been demonstrated to harm the fetus in human trials, although they may be taken if the benefits outweigh the risks. Paroxetine, an

SSRI, treats major depressive disorder, anxiety, and other mental health issues. Studies have linked first-trimester paroxetine use to fetal congenital heart abnormalities.

57. Tramadol increases limbic system serotonin and noradrenaline due to its opioid and serotonergic characteristics. Combining serotonergic drugs such as SSRIs or MAOIs may raise the risk of serotonin syndrome. Agitation, confusion, rapid heart rate, high blood pressure, dilated pupils, muscle rigidity, and convulsions are symptoms of serotonin syndrome.
58. Due to the danger of serotonin syndrome, SSRIs are contraindicated within 2 weeks after MAOI usage. Extreme central nervous system serotonin buildup can cause serotonin syndrome. Agitation, confusion, rapid heart rate, high blood pressure, dilated pupils, muscle rigidity, and convulsions are symptoms of serotonin syndrome.
59. Bupropion may help clients to quit smoking. Seizure and eating disorder sufferers should not take bupropion. Bupropion may lower the seizure threshold and increase seizure risk. Bupropion may also cause weight loss and worsen eating disorder symptoms.
60. The most selective TCAs for serotonin and norepinephrine are clomipramine (Anafranil) and desipramine (Norpramin), respectively. Since it has strong noradrenergic effects, desipramine is used to treat depression and other mental health issues, while clomipramine treats OCD due to its serotonergic activity.
61. Pediatrics and elderly. A TCA can lengthen the QT interval, increasing the risk of life-threatening cardiac arrhythmias in sensitive populations including children and elderly people with preexisting heart problems. They may be more susceptible to TCAs' anticholinergic effects, which can induce dry mouth, constipation, and urine retention. They may also be more susceptible to orthostatic hypotension, which can cause falls and other complications.
62. A client starting trazodone, an insomniac antidepressant, may report fewer intense and strange nightmares. Prazosin, an α-1 adrenergic receptor antagonist, blocks noradrenaline's brain effects to lower nightmare frequency and severity.
63. FALSE. Grief is a normal response to a major loss such as a death, divorce, or job loss. Grief is not depression, yet it can produce extreme sadness, loneliness, and despair.
64. A single, recurring, or developmental stressor usually causes grief within 6 months. While sorrow can produce tremendous sadness, loneliness, and despair, it usually fades as the person adjusts to the loss and moves forward. Complex grieving, also known as extended grief disorder, lasts longer than 6 months and is marked by strong and persistent longing, yearning, and melancholy that interfere with daily life. Psychotherapy or medication may help handle complicated grieving.
65. Complex grieving can endure longer and be more intense than normal grief, which usually lasts 6 months. Normal mourning involves sadness, loneliness, and despair, yet people may work. Complex grieving can make these

sentiments too intense for daily life. Complex grieving can cause suicide thoughts, concern with the deceased, and guilt or self-blame.

66. Adjustment disorder should be a differential diagnosis. Adjustment disorder can result from a major life stressor such as the death of a loved one, a breakup, or a job loss. Adjustment disorder can include depression, hopelessness, anxiety, insomnia, and mood or behavior changes.
67. Prolonged grief disorder, which can occur after a loved one dies, is characterized by intense yearning and longing for the deceased, disruptive preoccupation with thoughts of the deceased, and difficulty accepting the loss. To be diagnosed with PGD, a person must have lost a loved one and had grief symptoms for 12 months or more that cause considerable anguish or functional impairment.
68. Premenstrual dysphoric disorder (PMDD) is a severe form of PMS that causes mood swings, anger, anxiety, melancholy, exhaustion, and bloating. At least five of the following symptoms must be present during the luteal phase of the menstrual cycle and severe enough to interfere with everyday life to be diagnosed with PMDD:

    - Frequent mood swings.
    - High irritation or anger.
    - Depression, hopelessness, or self-criticism.
    - Feeling tense, anxious, or on edge.
    - Disinterest in job, education, friends, and interests.
    - Subjective concentration difficulty.
    - Fatigue, lethargy, or low energy.
    - Increased appetite, overeating, or food cravings.
    - Oversleeping.
    - The feeling of being overpowered.
    - Breast discomfort, joint or muscle pain, bloating, or weight gain.

69. TRUE. SSRIs reduce PMDD symptoms and are routinely given. Some women use the drug daily to prevent symptoms, while others only during the luteal phase, when symptoms are worse.
70. Women often suffer moderate emotional reactions in the first few days after giving birth, known as the "baby blues." Depression, anxiety, and fatigue are thought to be caused by hormonal changes and physical exhaustion during childbirth. Baby blues usually go away in a week or two without treatment. Some women get postpartum depression, a more serious and long-lasting form of depression. Symptoms include chronic depression, anxiety, and irritability, as well as hunger, sleep, and energy problems. Postpartum depression can start any time in the first year following childbirth and may require therapy or medication.
71. Postpartum psychosis is rare but dangerous. It affects 1–2 per 1000 new mothers and is a medical emergency that requires rapid treatment. Postpartum psychosis can cause mood changes, hallucinations, delusions, confusion, disorientation, and suicidal or homicidal thoughts. Postpartum psychosis can

cause infanticide or suicide, thus early detection and treatment are crucial for mother and child safety. Hospitalization and medication and therapy are common treatments for postpartum psychosis.

72. FALSE. Mothers who are breastfeeding should choose drugs cautiously because some can pass to the baby through breast milk. Some drugs, such as SSRIs, are safe for breastfeeding moms and their babies, but others may need close monitoring.
73. FALSE. A woman with a history of postpartum mania or bipolar disorder should be monitored during subsequent pregnancies and postpartum periods and take mood stabilizers to prevent relapse. Some medications may not be safe to use during pregnancy and nursing, so the expectant mother should weigh the risks and benefits.
74. Electroconvulsive therapy (ECT) may be an alternate treatment for pregnant women with manic episodes when medication is risky. ECT reduces mania symptoms quickly by sending regulated electrical shocks to the brain under general anesthesia. It is normally safe and effective when administered by a professional healthcare team in a controlled setting.
75. The three FDA-approved SSRIs for PMDD are fluoxetine, paroxetine, and sertraline.

    - PMDD is a severe version of PMS that causes emotional and physical symptoms before menstruation. PMDD is often treated with SSRIs because they regulate brain serotonin levels, improving mood and reducing symptoms including irritability, anxiety, and depression.

76. In youth, separation anxiety disorder causes severe distress and impairment in everyday functioning due to excessive worry and fear over being removed from attachment figures such as parents or caregivers. Children with separation anxiety disorder may also have sleep difficulties and somatic complaints (e.g., headaches, stomach aches) and avoid school or other activities that involve caregiver separation. Some children with separation anxiety disorder may have depression symptoms such persistent melancholy, decreased interest in activities, and changes in eating or sleep.
77. Depression causes "motivational deficit" or "reduced behavioral activation." This is a loss of drive or energy to do things that were once pleasant or vital. Even with the talents and abilities, it might make starting or finishing tasks difficult. In contrast, "skill deficit" is the inability to perform a task or activity owing to physical or cognitive constraints. Dementia, stroke, traumatic brain injury, and other cognitive or motor diseases can cause skill deficiencies.
78. A functional evaluation evaluates an individual's activities of daily living (ADLs), instrumental activities of daily living (IADLs), and social functioning. ADLs include bathing, dressing, eating, and toileting, while IADLs include finances, transportation, and medication management. Social functioning measures an individual's capacity to socialize, establish relationships, and participate in community activities. Since late-life depression often causes functional impairment, older persons should undergo a functional

examination when screening for depression. Chronic medical diseases such as heart disease or diabetes can affect functional status and raise depression risk, thus a functional assessment may be appropriate. Functional assessments can assist detect impairments that may cause depression, guide treatment planning, and identify actions to improve functioning.

79. Serotonin overload can cause life-threatening serotonin syndrome. It can be induced by antidepressants and illegal narcotics such as MDMA. Common serotonin syndrome symptoms include:

    1. Restlessness/agitation.
    2. Confused or lost.
    3. Rapid heartbeat or hypertension.
    4. Pupil dilation.
    5. A stiff or trembling muscle.
    6. A fever or sweat.
    7. Nausea and diarrhea.
    8. Unconsciousness, respiratory failure, seizures, and coma.

80. Flu-like symptoms, sleeplessness, nausea, unbalance, paresthesias, and hyperarousal characterize discontinuation syndrome.
81. Serotonin syndrome treatment usually entails stopping medications that cause excess serotonin and providing supportive care. This may include:

    - Anti-dehydration intravenous fluids.
    - Blood pressure and heart rate medications.
    - Benzodiazepines for agitation and stiffness.
    - Cyproheptadine as a serotonin antagonist.
    - Extreme fevers may require cooling blankets or other remedies.
    - Mechanical ventilation or oxygen treatment for respiratory distress.
    - Treatment of any underlying medical issues that may cause the syndrome.
    - Hospitalization may be needed for close monitoring and vigorous treatment in severe cases.

82. Fluoxetine (Prozac) has a long half-life and causes less withdrawal syndrome than other SSRIs. Its lengthy half-life means it lingers in the body longer than other SSRIs, preventing the abrupt drop in serotonin levels that might occur with withdrawal.
83. Selegiline is less likely to cause tyramine-associated hypertensive crises than other MAOIs.
84. Cymbalta (duloxetine) has the highest liver failure risk. It is an SNRI used to treat depression, anxiety, and chronic pain. Since duloxetine might cause liver damage, liver function tests should be constantly monitored.
85.

F	Flu-like symptoms
I	Insomnia
N	Nausea

I	Imbalance
S	Sensory paresthesias
H	Hyperarousal and headache

86. One week, but can last weeks depending on antidepressant use.
87. The typical therapeutic range for nortriptyline is 80–200 ng/mL. Tricyclic antidepressant imipramine is 150–250 ng/mL therapeutic.
88. TCAs are contraindicated in the following groups:

    - Patients with MI histories.
    - Heart block and arrhythmia patients.
    - Glaucoma sufferers.
    - Experienced seizure patients.
    - Urine retention patients.
    - Overactive thyroid patients.
    - Patients taking MAOIs.
    - Suicide-prone and heart disease/dysrhythmia patients.

89. Avoid serotonin syndrome by following a 2-week washout period before transitioning from a TCA to an SSRI. Switching to fluoxetine requires a 5-week washout period due to its long half-life.
90. If used together, MAOIs can raise TCA levels.
91. Significant headache, chest discomfort, palpitations, perspiration, nausea, vomiting, shortness of breath, and anxiety are hypertensive crisis symptoms. It can cause stroke, heart attack, and organ damage if neglected.
92. A hypertensive crisis is treated with phentolamine, which blocks norepinephrine.
93. St. John's wort, TCAs, second-generation antipsychotics, decongestants, stimulants, asthma medicines, meperidine opioid, tryptophan, dextromethorphan, and others may be answers.
94. Irritable or grouchy children with chronic depression illness are more common than sad ones.
95. Membrane threshold desensitization causes neurons to misfire without electrical stimulation, forming kindling.
96. Cognitive behavioral therapy addresses thoughts, emotions, and behaviors.
97. Other depression therapies include:

    - Interpersonal Therapy: This therapy addresses interpersonal difficulties that cause depression. We want better communication and relationships.
    - Psychodynamic treatment helps people understand how past events and unconscious ideas and feelings cause their symptoms. Identify and resolve underlying tensions.
    - Behavior Activation Therapy: This therapy promotes positive behavior and mood.
    - Mindfulness-based cognitive therapy combines cognitive behavioral therapy with mindfulness. Learning to recognize and respond to thoughts and feelings without judgment is the goal.

- Acceptance and Commitment Therapy (ACT): This therapy helps people recognize and accept conflicting emotions and commit to good life changes. Increase psychological flexibility and resilience.

98. SSRIs are the most prescribed antidepressants due to their mild side effects, great efficacy in treating depression and anxiety, and reduced overdose danger.
99. Dopamine and norepinephrine.
100. A PMHNP should advise SSRI users that full efficacy may take 4–6 weeks or even 8 weeks.
101. "Rule of thirds" describes depression treatment response. Within 4–6 weeks, one-third of depressed individuals respond to a placebo. Depression is gone. One-third of antidepressants work within 4–6 weeks. One-third of patients will not respond to the first medication and require a modification, combination, or other treatments such as psychotherapy or electroconvulsive therapy.
102. ECT are controversial but effective non-pharmacological treatments for treatment-resistant depression.
103. Electroconvulsive therapy (ECT) sends an electrical current through the brain to cause a short seizure. A muscle relaxant and anesthesia will reduce pain throughout the procedure. Your scalp will have electrodes that send a small amount of electricity to your brain. You will have a brief seizure and be closely monitored by doctors. Soon after ECT, headache, muscle discomfort, nausea, and confusion may occur. Memory loss may occur, especially for events around treatment. These adverse effects normally alleviate over time. For some mental health issues, ECT is safe and effective. For treatment-resistant depression, psychosis, and catatonia, the seizure is used to reanimate synapses and neuronal connections, theoretically increasing dopamine, serotonin, norepinephrine, endorphins, and hormones to treat depression and anhedonia. Typically, 6–12 treatments are required.
104. Atypical depression benefits from MAOIs.
105. Paranoia, delusions, or hallucinations may accompany significant depressive symptoms in psychotic depression. Antidepressants and antipsychotics may treat the latter symptoms.
106. Catatonia is an unresponsiveness to external stimuli or increased reluctance to movement or verbalization. The symptoms of major depressive disorder, bipolar disorder, schizophrenia, and neuroleptic malignant syndrome are possible. In situations of metabolic imbalance, treating the underlying medical illness may cure catatonia. For mental catatonia, benzodiazepines and ECT may be utilized. Some antipsychotics may increase catatonic symptoms.
107. Treatment-resistant depression can be treated in-office using transcranial magnetic stimulation (TMS).
108. Transcranial magnetic stimulation (TMS) for depression typically requires 20–30 sessions over 4–6 weeks.
109. Hoarseness, sore throat, cough, shortness of breath, difficulty swallowing, neck pain, headache, nausea, and vomiting may result from vagal nerve stimulation (VNS). In rare situations, VNS might induce nerve injury, infection, or bleeding.

110. SAD can be treated with bright light at 10,000 lux.
111. Use bright light treatment for 30 min, one to two times a day.
112. Psychotherapy and medicines often address adjustment disorder. CBT, IPT, and supportive treatment are psychotherapy options. For symptoms, antidepressants or anti-anxiety drugs may be administered. Lifestyle changes including exercise, diet, and stress reduction can also help. Since psychotherapy may take action before antidepressants, the event may pass.
113. Self-administered bipolar disorder screening techniques include the Mood Disorder Questionnaire (MDQ) and Bipolar Spectrum Diagnostic Scale (BSDS).
114. Up to 50% of people with persistent depressive disorder (cyclothymia) may develop bipolar disorder.
115. If the patient has mild depression and symptoms are not severely impairing daily functioning, a PMHNP may not offer both medication and psychotherapy. Similarly, if the patient favors one treatment. The PMHNP must consider the patient's values and interests when choosing a treatment. Finally, if a client has a medical condition or takes medications that contraindicate antidepressants, the PMHNP may suggest psychotherapy or another medication.
116. Take antidepressant and begin therapy.

    - Increase drug dosage or therapy frequency.
    - Try greater doses or switch therapies.
    - Usually switch to SSRI or SNRI.
    - Try TCA or MAOI.
    - Addition of atypical antipsychotics (aripiprazole, quetiapine).
    - Supplement with a different antidepressant such as bupropion.
    - Assess lithium or atypical antipsychotics.
    - Treat-resistant patients receive ECT, TMS, ketamine, or vagus nerve stimulation.

117. A patient who has stopped MDD treatment should see the PMHNP 4–6 weeks later to check in.

118.

Class	Mechanism of action	Generic drug (brand name)	Target diseases/disorders	Adverse effects/risks
Selective serotonin reuptake inhibitors (SSRIs)	Inhibits serotonin reuptake	Fluoxetine (Prozac), sertraline (Zoloft), paroxetine (Paxil), citalopram (Celexa), escitalopram (Lexapro)	Major depressive disorder, anxiety disorders, OCD, PTSD, panic disorder, social phobia	Sexual dysfunction, gastrointestinal disturbances, withdrawal syndrome, QTc prolongation, activation
Serotonin-norepinephrine reuptake inhibitors (SNRIs)	Inhibits serotonin and norepinephrine reuptake	Venlafaxine (Effexor), duloxetine (Cymbalta), desvenlafaxine (Pristiq)	Major depressive disorder, anxiety disorders, neuropathic pain, fibromyalgia	Hypertension, dose-related elevation of blood pressure, hepatotoxicity, discontinuation syndrome, serotonin syndrome
Tricyclic antidepressants (TCAs)	Blocks the reuptake of norepinephrine and serotonin	Amitriptyline (Elavil), clomipramine (Anafranil), desipramine (Norpramin), doxepin (Sinequan), imipramine (Tofranil), nortriptyline (Pamelor), protriptyline (Vivactil), trimipramine (Surmontil)	Major depressive disorder, neuropathic pain, migraines, anxiety disorders, enuresis, ADHD, OCD	Sedation, anticholinergic effects, cardiac arrhythmias, tremor, weight gain
Monoamine oxidase inhibitors (MAOIs)	Blocks the breakdown of monoamine neurotransmitters	Phenelzine (Nardil), tranylcypromine (Parnate), isocarboxazid (Marplan), selegiline (Emsam), moclobemide (Aurorix)	Major depressive disorder, anxiety disorders, PTSD	Hypertensive crisis with tyramine-containing foods, serotonin syndrome, hepatotoxicity, gastrointestinal symptoms, application site reactions
Serotonin partial agonist reuptake inhibitor (SPARI)	Blocks serotonin transporter, partial agonist at 5-HT1A receptor	Vilazodone (Viibryd)	Major depressive disorder	Reduced risk of sexual dysfunction

Class	Mechanism of action	Generic drug (brand name)	Target diseases/disorders	Adverse effects/risks
Norepinephrine-dopamine reuptake inhibitor (NDRI)	Inhibits norepinephrine and dopamine reuptake	Bupropion (Wellbutrin)	Major depressive disorder, seasonal affective disorder, smoking cessation, ADHD	Seizures, lowers seizure threshold
Atypical antidepressant	α2/5-HT2 receptor antagonist, H1 receptor antagonist, and inhibits the reuptake of norepinephrine and serotonin	Mirtazapine (Remeron)	Major depressive disorder, generalized anxiety disorder, insomnia, and nausea associated with chemotherapy	Sedation, weight gain, anticholinergic effects
Serotonin antagonist and reuptake inhibitor (SARI)	Blocks serotonin transporter, antagonizes 5-HT2A/2C receptors	Trazodone (Desyrel)	Major depressive disorder, insomnia	Monitor liver function, priapism risk, QTc prolongation possible

119. A manic episode is an emergency since it can lead to unsafe driving, substance addiction, excessive spending, and risky sexual activity. Individuals can also be irritable, aggressive, or violent. In severe cases, psychosis can cause hallucinations or delusions.
120. FALSE. Symptom severity and duration vary between mania and hypomania. Mania lasts at least 1 week and is more severe than hypomania, which lasts at least 4 days. Hypomanics rarely require hospitalization, have no significant social or occupational impairment, and do not have psychotic symptoms.
121. Rapid cycling bipolar illness requires four mood episodes in a year.
122. Key mania symptoms

    - High or irritated mood.
    - Increased energy and restlessness.
    - Rapid speech and racing ideas.
    - Increased self-esteem and decreased sleep needs.
    - Impulsivity and risk-taking.
    - Bad judgment.
    - Distractibility.
    - Psychomotor agitation.

123. Three symptoms over a week are required to diagnose a manic episode.
124. FALSE. During a manic or hypomanic episode, the patient is diagnosed with bipolar or cyclothymic disorder.
125. The main difference between unipolar and bipolar depressions is mania.
126. Hypomanic; longer, more severe manic episodes necessitate immediate hospitalization and treatment. Patients can function during shorter hypomanic episodes.
127.

Sign/symptom	Description
Distractibility	Easy distractibility, attention being pulled from one thing to the next
Insomnia	Difficulty sleeping, feeling rested on only a few hours of sleep
Grandiosity	Inflated sense of self-esteem or ability, exaggerated belief in one's accomplishments or talents
Flight of ideas	Rapid, often tangential, thought processes, or speech
Activity increase	Increased energy level, hyperactivity, or agitation
Speech (pressured)	Fast, pressured, or difficult to interrupt speech
Thoughtlessness (risky behavior)	Engaging in activities with potentially painful consequences, such as unrestrained buying sprees, sexual indiscretions, or foolish business investments

128. FALSE. A PMHNP can diagnose bipolar illness based on a patient's symptoms, history of episodes, and observed symptoms such as increased activity, poor sleep, and heightened mood or energy. Patients rarely seek help during manic episodes.
129. Symptoms of sadness and mania that are milder may indicate cyclothymia.
130. Bipolar illness symptoms can mimic other psychiatric conditions such major depressive disorder and borderline personality disorder, making diagnosis

challenging. Bipolar illness patients may not seek treatment during manic or hypomanic episodes, making it harder for doctors to diagnose. Finally, bipolar illness may have periods of stability between episodes, making it difficult to diagnose if the doctor only sees the patient during those times. Manic patients rarely seek help. Diagnosis of manic episodes is usually based on self-report or supporting evidence. For many psychiatric comorbidities, depressive symptoms are more common.

131. __x___Rapid speech pattern.
   __x___Grandiose self-concept.
   __x___Excessive spending.
   __x___Sexual behaviors, risky departure from baseline.
132. FALSE. Rapid cycling is a small subset only and carries a poorer prognosis.
133. Thyroid hormone imbalance can cause mood swings and dysregulation.
134. Answers may include ACE inhibitors, corticosteroids, isoniazid, disulfiram, cimetidine, cyclosporine, hydralazine, stimulants, fluoroquinolones, calcium channel blockers, and B-blockers.
135. Bipolar I patients may experience auditory hallucinations as mania worsens.
136. Men with bipolar disorder commit more crimes and violence. Females have higher incidences of substance misuse, suicide, and thyroid disease.
137. Bipolar disorders usually start between 18 and 22 years old.
138. Bipolar disorder patients have gray matter reduction in the prefrontal cortex, hippocampus, and amygdala, according to functional MRI.
139. Studies have shown that bipolar disorder may affect the HPTA axis, which regulates stress. Research suggests that bipolar disorder patients may have higher cortisol levels during manic episodes and lower cortisol during depressed periods. Thyroid imbalance can also affect mood and energy.
140. While its precise mode of action remains incompletely understood, lithium is believed to stabilize mood swings by modulating neurotransmitters such as serotonin, norepinephrine, and dopamine. Additionally, lithium may exhibit neuroprotective effects, influence intracellular signaling pathways by inhibiting enzymes such as glycogen synthase kinase-3 (GSK-3), impact ion transport processes, and modulate neurotransmitter release and reuptake. Lithium may decrease second messenger signaling inositol availability by inhibiting inositol monophosphatase, an enzyme in the phosphatidylinositol signaling pathway. Lithium may modulate intracellular signaling cascades and increase neurotrophic factor expression to impact neurotransmitter release and reuptake and protect the brain.
141. Only lithium has antisuicidal properties.
142. Lithium is the benchmark for bipolar mania treatment. However, it does not treat rapid cycling bipolar disorder well.
143. Lithium therapy is 0.5–1.2 mEq/L.
144. Draw trough level 12 h after dosage. Patients' lithium levels should be drawn in the morning 8–12 h following the last medication. Patient stability and treatment phase determine monitoring frequency. The acute phase requires lithium levels every 2–3 days until stable, then weekly for 2–4 weeks. After that, monitor levels every 2–3 months. Dose, symptoms, renal function, and other factors that affect lithium levels should be considered while adjusting the monitoring schedule. Weekly until therapeutic range, then every 3 months unless negative effects arise.

145. When teaching a patient about lithium toxicity and side effects, include these critical points

- It is crucial to take lithium as prescribed and have regular blood tests to monitor lithium levels to avoid life-threatening lithium toxicity.
- Lithium poisoning can cause diarrhea, vomiting, tremors, confusion, and seizures, which require emergency medical intervention.
- Discuss lithium side effects such hand tremors, increased thirst and urination, weight gain, and thyroid dysfunction with the patient.
- Dehydration can worsen lithium toxicity; thus, patients should avoid it and be careful when taking any lithium-interacting drugs or supplements.
- Caffeine and alcohol can reduce lithium's efficacy and increase negative effects; therefore, patients should avoid them.
- Mild: severe nausea, vomiting, hand tremors, confusion, visual disturbances, and unsteadiness standing or walking (1.5–2.5 mEq/L).
- Moderate: confusion, agitation, delirium, tachycardia, and hypertonia (2.5–3.5 mEq/L).

146. 1/fghijk, 2/abe, 3/cd, and 4/egj.
147. Before starting a patient of Asian ancestry on carbamazepine, the PMHNP should screen for the HLA-B*1502 allele.
148. Lamotrigine (Lamictal) treats bipolar illness without blood tests.
149. The concomitant use of Lamotrigine with either Valproic Acid or Carbamazepine can have significant effects on Lamotrigine levels in the body. When used with Valproic Acid, Lamotrigine levels tend to increase due to Valproic Acid inhibiting Lamotrigine metabolism enzymes, potentially raising the risk of side effects. Conversely, combining lamotrigine with carbamazepine can decrease lamotrigine levels as carbamazepine induces the enzymes responsible for its metabolism, potentially reducing its therapeutic effectiveness.
150. Stevens-Johnson syndrome (SJS), an uncommon skin disorder, causes painful, blistering, and necrotic skin and mucous membrane lesions, including the eyes, mouth, and genitals. For certain people, inflammation of the eyes, mouth, and genitals causes considerable pain and suffering. The first step in treating SJS is stopping the problematic drug and supporting the sufferer. Hospitalization, hydration and electrolyte replenishment, wound treatment, pain management, and infection or respiratory distress management may be required. Patients may need ICU or burn unit treatment in severe circumstances.
151. Carbamazepine with lithium can induce neural tube malformations, craniofacial deformities, and developmental delay in fetuses.
152. FALSE. Managing bipolar disease during pregnancy may require mood stabilizers because untreated bipolar disorder can harm both mother and fetus. Medication hazards and advantages during pregnancy should be carefully considered with the patient's PMHNP.
153. The Young Mania Rating Scale (YMRS) measures bipolar disorder manic episodes' severity. It includes 11 items: heightened mood, motor activity/energy,

sexual interest, sleep, irritability, speech, language, content, disruptive/aggressive behavior, appearance, and insight. Higher scores indicate more severe manic symptoms on the 0–60 scale.

154. The Young Mania Rating Scale (YMRS) is best for inpatient use with individuals with bipolar illness or other disorders including manic or hypomanic episodes.
155. TRUE. Patients with bipolar disorder should have a relapse prevention plan in place, not only for mania but also for depressive episodes. This plan typically involves working closely with healthcare providers to identify early warning signs of mood episodes, understanding triggers, adhering to medication regimens, and implementing strategies to manage symptoms if they start to worsen.
156. Valproic acid, carbamazepine, risperidone, olanzapine, quetiapine, and atypical antipsychotics may be added or altered.
157. FALSE. Antidepressants for bipolar depression are controversial and require rigorous risk-benefit analysis. Antidepressants may improve some bipolar disorder subtypes but increase the risk of mania/hypomania or rapid cycling, according to some research. Antidepressants should be chosen based on the patient's history, symptoms, and other considerations.
158. Answers may include excessive blood pressure, glucose, waist circumference, and abnormal cholesterol levels, weight increase, hyperlipidemia, hyperglycemia, and insulin resistance.
159. Lurasidone (Latuda) with Seroquel. Most other antipsychotics only treat acute mania.
160. There are numerous support groups. Answers may include Depression and Bipolar Support Alliance (DBSA), National Alliance on Mental Illness (NAMI), National Mental Health Association (NMHA), and Mood Disorders Association (MDA).
161. Anticonvulsants such as carbamazepine and valproic acid regulate mood in rapid cycling and mixed-feature bipolar disorder.
162. Symptoms include:

    - Nausea, vomiting, and diarrhea.
    - Hand tremors and muscle weakness.
    - Coordination issues or walking problems.
    - Sleepiness, disorientation, agitation, or slurred speech.
    - Tremors, hyperreflexia, and seizures.
    - Vision or hearing problems.
    - Reduced or no urine output.
    - Arrhythmias or hypotension.

163. Symptom severity determines lithium toxicity treatment. Reduced lithium dosing may be enough in moderate situations. Hospitalization may be needed in extreme situations. Sodium polystyrene sulfonate or hemodialysis can quickly remove lithium from the circulation.
164. Fetus <5 weeks old with low tricuspid valve implantation and atresia.

- Epstein's abnormality is an uncommon congenital cardiac defect that affects the tricuspid valve, which separates the right atrium and ventricle. Epstein's abnormality causes blood to leak back into the right atrium due to the tricuspid valve being pushed downward into the right ventricle. This can cause right atrium and ventricular hypertrophy and heart failure or arrhythmias.

165. Serum monitor lithium levels every 3 months once stable.
    - BUN, creatinine, GFR testing.
    - Thyroid function tests (TSH, free T4).
    - Sodium, potassium, and calcium electrolytes.
    - A complete blood count.
    - As needed, HCG pregnancy test.
166. Neuronal hyperactivity may cause mania; hence, anticonvulsants treat bipolar illness.
167. Valproic acid's mechanism of action is not completely understood. It may boost brain GABA, an inhibitory neurotransmitter. Reduced neuron excitability helps regulate mood and lessen mania and hypomania symptoms. Valproic acid may also affect mood-regulating neurotransmitters including dopamine and serotonin.
168. Liver failure, pancreatitis, and thrombocytopenia are the most dangerous valproic acid side effects. Teratogenicity, hyperammonemia, and hypersensitivity reactions are rare but dangerous adverse effects.
169. Asians at risk for Stevens-Johnson syndrome should be screened for the HLA-B*1502 allele before commencing carbamazepine.
170. Carbamazepine can cause sleepiness, dizziness, headache, ataxia, disorientation, hepatotoxicity, hyponatremia, and leukopenia in addition to Stevens-Johnson syndrome. It interacts with other drugs and can cause birth abnormalities including Spina Bifida in fetuses.
171. Valproic acid has a therapeutic range of 50–100 μg/mL.
172. Stevens-Johnson syndrome is lamotrigine's worst adverse effect.
173. Carbamazepine blocks voltage-gated sodium channels in neurons to regulate hyper-excited neural membranes and diminish neuronal activity. It also enhances GABA transmission.
174. Carbamazepine has a therapeutic range of 4–12 μg/mL.
175. Carbamazepine's own metabolism in the liver lowers its concentration with time.
176. Topiramate stabilizes mood and impulsivity. This causes weight loss and mental dulling.
177. Antipsychotics and mood stabilizers are first-line treatments for acute mania.
178. Seroquel, Latuda, and olanzapine-fluoxetine (Symbyax).
179. Antidepressants can provoke manic or hypomanic episodes in bipolar disorder, hence they are only used to treat unipolar depression. Antidepressants may cause bipolar patients to flip from depression to mania or hypomania, worsening symptoms and perhaps worsening episodes. Thus, mood stabilizers are the main treatment for bipolar disorder, and antidepressants are only used in conjunction or for unipolar depression.

180. ____T______A suicidal individual usually wants to live, but thinks they have no other alternative to relieve their pain.
 ___F_______ Most suicides are spontaneous.
 ___F_______An individual contemplating suicide does not usually give any clues of their intent.
 ___T_______Suicidal persons are not typically psychotic.
 ___F_______Asking a client about suicidal intent increases the likelihood of subsequent suicidal behavior.
 ___F_______Men attempt suicide more frequently and are also more successful than women.
 ___T_______ Suicide incidence is lower in married adults.
181. Seligman defines learned helplessness as the idea that one's actions are fruitless and will not achieve desired results, resulting in depression. Helplessness can contribute to suicidal ideation because people may believe they can do nothing to change their condition.
182. __x___Previous suicide attempt.
 __x___Chronic illness.
 __x___White.
 __x___Single, separated.
 __x___2–4 weeks after starting an antidepressant, particularly among pediatric patients.
183. FALSE. Safety contracts and no-harm agreements may help reduce suicide attempts, although research has shown they are not always effective. Mental health practitioners must assess suicide risk and create patient-specific safety measures.
184. The Columbia-Suicide Severity Rating Scale (C-SSRS) screens for suicidal ideation and conduct. It measures suicide risk across the lifespan and is extensively used and evidence-based. The C-SSRS can be used in mental health clinics, emergency departments, and primary care to assess suicidal thoughts, actions, and plans. Identifying high-risk suiciders allows for effective treatments to prevent suicide attempts and completion.

References and Resources

American Psychiatric Association, editor. Diagnostic and statistical manual of mental disorders:DSM-5-TR. 5th ed. American Psychiatric Association Publishing; 2022.

Brieler JA, Keegan-Garrett E. Diagnosis and treatment of bipolar illness in the primary care office. Mo Med. 2022;119(3):213–8.

Chen Y, Bennett D, Clarke R, Guo Y, Yu C, Bian Z, Ma L, Huang Y, Sun Q, Zhang N, Zheng X, Chen J, Peto R, Kendler KS, Li L, Chen Z. Patterns and correlates of major depression in Chinese adults: a cross-sectional study of 0.5 million men and women. Psychol Med. 2017;47(5):958–70. https://doi.org/10.1017/S0033291716002889.

Dols A, Sienaert P, van Gerven H, Schouws S, Stevens A, Kupka R, Stek ML. The prevalence and management of side effects of lithium and anticonvulsants as mood stabilizers in bipolar disorder from a clinical perspective: a review. Int Clin Psychopharmacol. 2013;28(6):287–96.

Fang L, Cheng Z, Tan Z, He W. An exploration of cultural variables in suicide among Chinese rural youth. J Affect Disord. 2015;183:68–74. https://doi.org/10.1016/j.jad.2015.04.030.

Gabbay V, Ely BA, Li Q, Bangaru SD, Panzer AM, Alonso CM, et al. Striatum-based circuitry of adolescent depression and anhedonia. J Am Acad Child Adolesc Psychiatry. 2016;55(10):770–81. https://doi.org/10.1016/j.jaac.2016.05.018.

Grover S, Sahoo S, Rabha A, Koirala R. ECT in schizophrenia: a review of the evidence. Acta Neuropsychiatrica. 2019;31(3):115–27.

Johnson K, Vanderhoef D, Magrath N. Psychiatric-mental health nurse practitioner review and resource manual. American Nurses Association: American Nurses Credentialing Center; 2020.

Kendler KS, Prescott CA, Myers J, Neale MC. The structure of genetic and environmental risk factors for common psychiatric and substance use disorders in men and women. Arch Gen Psychiatry. 2003;60(9):929–37. https://doi.org/10.1001/archpsyc.60.9.929.

Kristensen P, Weisæth L, Heir T. Bereavement and mental health after sudden and violent losses: a review. Psychiatry. 2012;75(1):76–97. https://doi.org/10.1521/psyc.2012.75.1.76.

McIntyre RS, Berk M, Brietzke E, Goldstein BI, López-Jaramillo C, Kessing LV, Malhi GS, Nierenberg AA, Rosenblat JD, Majeed A, Vieta E, Vinberg M, Young AH, Mansur RB. Bipolar disorders. Lancet. 2020;396(10265):1841–56.

Monroe SM, Harkness KL. Life stress, the "kindling" hypothesis, and the recurrence of depression: considerations from a life stress perspective. Psychol Rev. 2005;112(2):417–45.

Muneer DA. Mood disorders: practical issues in diagnosis and management. Routledge; 2018.

National Institute of Mental Health (NIMH). (2021). Major Depressive Disorder. https://www.nimh.nih.gov/health/topics/depression/index.shtml.

Nock MK, Hwang I, Sampson NA, Kessler RC. Mental disorders, comorbidity and suicidal behavior: results from the National Comorbidity Survey Replication. Mol Psychiatry. 2010;15(8):868–76. https://doi.org/10.1038/mp.2009.29.

Patel RK, Rose GM. Persistent depressive disorder. In: StatPearls [internet]. Treasure Island (FL): StatPearls publishing; 2023. https://www.ncbi.nlm.nih.gov/books/NBK541052/.

Perlis RH, Smoller JW, Mysore JS, Sun M, Trivedi MH, Fava M, et al. Prevalence and clinical correlates of irritability in bipolar I disorder: Results from the first 1000 STEP-BD participants. Biol Psychiatry. 2004;55(9):948–54. https://doi.org/10.1016/j.biopsych.2004.01.016.

Schoeyen HK, Kessler U, Andreassen OA, Auestad BH, Bergsholm P, Malt UF, Vaaler A. Treatment-resistant bipolar depression: a randomized controlled trial of electroconvulsive therapy versus algorithm-based pharmacological treatment. Am J Psychiatry. 2015;172(1):41–51. https://doi.org/10.1176/appi.ajp.2014.13111517.

Segal ZV, Bieling P, Young T, MacQueen G, Cooke R, Martin L, et al. Antidepressant monotherapy vs. sequential pharmacotherapy and mindfulness-based cognitive therapy, or placebo, for relapse prophylaxis in recurrent depression. Arch Gen Psychiatry. 2010;67(12):1256–64.

Shibasaki C, Takebayashi M. Advances in electroconvulsive therapy for psychiatric disorders. Adv Modern Med. 2017;233:233–41.

Socci C, Medda P, Toni C, Lattanzi L, Tripodi B, Vannucchi G, Perugi G. Electroconvulsive therapy and age: age-related clinical features and effectiveness in treatment resistant major depressive episode. J Affect Disord. 2018;227:627–32. https://doi.org/10.1016/j.jad.2017.11.064.

Stroebe M, Schut H, Stroebe W. Health outcomes of bereavement. Lancet. 2012;380(9852):1960–73.

Svensson TK, Miller L, Hurd C. Expanding the nurse practitioner role in treatment resistant major depression. J Hosp Med Manag. 2016;2:100009. https://doi.org/10.4172/2471-9781.100009.

Tajika A, Hori H, Iga JI, Koshikawa Y, Ogata H, Ogawa Y, Watanabe K, Kato T, Matsuo K, Kato M. Mood stabilizers and antipsychotics for acute mania: systematic review and meta-analysis of augmentation therapy vs monotherapy from the perspective of time to the onset of treatment effects. Int J Neuropsychopharmacol. 2022;25(10):839–52. https://doi.org/10.1093/ijnp/pyac050.

Zakhari R. The psychiatric-mental health nurse practitioner certification review manual. Springer Publishing Company; 2021.

Notes:

Notes:

Anxiety Disorders and Obsessive-Compulsive Disorder 8

Test your learning and check your understanding of this book's contents: Use the "Springer Nature Flashcards" app to access questions using ▶ https://sn.pub/62J0Ar.

To use the app, please follow the instructions in Chap. 1.

Anxiety disorders are the most common mental health disorders, affecting approximately 18.1% of the adult population in the United States (Kessler et al. 2005). Anxiety disorders are characterized by persistent, excessive, and irrational fear or worry about everyday situations (American Psychiatric Association 2022). These disorders can significantly impact an individual's quality of life, as they may experience physical symptoms such as racing heart, shortness of breath, and muscle tension. Common types of anxiety disorders include generalized anxiety disorder, social anxiety disorder, specific phobias, and panic disorder.

OCD, a type of anxiety disorder, affects approximately 2.2% of the adult population in the United States (Kessler et al., 2005). OCD is characterized by repetitive, obsessive thoughts and behaviors that an individual feels compelled to perform (American Psychiatric Association 2022). These obsessions and compulsions often interfere with daily functioning and can be time-consuming and distressing.

PMHNPs must recognize the signs and symptoms of anxiety disorders and OCD, as early diagnosis and treatment can lead to improved outcomes. It is also paramount to consider cultural and individual differences when working with clients, as these factors can influence the presentation and experience of anxiety disorders and OCD.

Effective treatment for anxiety disorders and OCD often involves a combination of pharmacotherapy and psychotherapy. Cognitive behavioral therapy (CBT) has been shown to be effective in the treatment of anxiety disorders and OCD (Barlow, 2014). CBT involves helping clients identify and modify negative thoughts and

T. Stewart, *Psychiatric-Mental Health Nurse Practitioner Program Companion and Board Certification Exam Review Workbook*,
https://doi.org/10.1007/978-3-031-60894-0_8

behaviors that contribute to their anxiety or obsessive-compulsive symptoms. In addition to traditional treatment approaches, psychiatric-mental health nurse practitioners can also consider alternative and complementary treatments, such as mindfulness-based therapies and relaxation techniques (Barlow, 2014).

By recognizing the signs and symptoms, considering cultural and individual differences, and utilizing a combination of pharmacotherapy, psychotherapy, and alternative treatments, we can help clients manage their anxiety and obsessive-compulsive symptoms and improve their overall quality of life. This chapter presents anxiety and its various associated disorders. Among those are generalized anxiety disorder, panic disorder, and phobias. Obsessive-compulsive disorder also is included in this chapter, along with behavioral manifestations of anxiety (e.g., hairpulling, hoarding, skin picking). Diagnostic criteria, pertinent medications, along with side effects, and therapies are presented.

8.1 Stress

1. What is stress?

2. Name three to five ways to reduce stress.

    1.
    2.
    3.
    4.
    5.

3. Chronic, severe stress can lead to physiological illness.

    TRUE FALSE.

8.2 Anxiety

4. What are some common physical manifestations of stress and anxiety, which often mimic sympathetic nervous system activation?

5. ______________________________ is the most common psychopathology.
6. Define anxiety. What are anxiety disorders?

7. When is anxiety considered pathological? When would psychiatric providers consider diagnosing someone with an anxiety disorder?

8. Most anxiety is ______________________________ and ______________________________, meaning that it will pass particularly once the individual removes themself from the environment/setting.
9. Determining a specific cause of anxiety is difficult, as there is often a multifactorial etiology involved. What are some potential causes of anxiety?

10. A primary anxiety disorder is those with signs and symptoms linked to substance use, medications, or a medical condition.
    TRUE FALSE
11. The three neurotransmitters most implicated in anxiety are: (1) ______________________________, (2) ______________________________, and (3) ______________________________.
12. In general, females experience anxiety disorders more than males.
    TRUE FALSE

13. A patient who presents with first-time anxiety symptoms later in life should be assessed for what causes?

14. Individuals who endorse anxiety should be evaluated for ________________________________ consumption and may need to reduce or eliminate their intake.

15. For each of the body systems, provide at least three signs and symptoms of anxiety.

Body system	Signs and symptoms of anxiety
Constitutional	
Cardiac	
Respiratory	
Neurologic	
Musculoskeletal	
Gastrointestinal	
Sensory	
Integumentary	

Body system	Signs and symptoms of anxiety
Endocrine	
Immunologic	
Renal/urinary	
Reproductive	
Ophthalmologic	

16. Name five common behavioral manifestations of anxiety.

    1.
    2.
    3.
    4.
    5.

17. List common effects for each degree of anxiety.

Ability to deal with stress, ability to learn is reduced →			
Mild	Moderate	Severe	Panic
Perceptual field, ability to focus is reduced →			

18. Individuals who do not possess adequate coping skills may abuse substances and medications to help mitigate their anxiety and somatic symptoms.
    TRUE FALSE

19. Name five medications and substances that can cause anxiety.
    1.
    2.
    3.
    4.
    5.

20. For each of the body systems, provide at least three medical conditions that can cause, or present as, anxiety.

Body system	Medical conditions
Neurologic	
Endocrine	
Metabolic	
Respiratory	
Cardiovascular	
Gastrointestinal	
Hematologic	
Oncologic	
Musculoskeletal	
Dermatologic	

21. Provide a summary of each of the following anxiety rating scales.

Zung's Self-Rating Anxiety Scale	Hamilton Rating Scale for Anxiety (HAM-A)	Yale-Brown Obsessive-Compulsive Scale (Y-BOCS)

8.3 Panic Disorder

22. What is a panic attack? When does a panic attack present?

23. What are common sequelae of panic attacks and for how long might these last?

24. Most panic disorders subside within ________________ minutes.

25. Complete the following table, which presents the symptoms of panic attacks in the mnemonic Da PANICS.

Da	
P	
A	
N	
I	
C	
S	

26. In addition to caffeine, the use of ____________________________________ ______, a legal substance, increases one's risk for panic attacks.

27. An individual with panic attacks is at (increased/decreased) risk for suicide attempts.

28. What are some medical conditions that should be ruled out when a patient presents with a panic attack?

29. Per DSM criteria, a diagnosis of panic disorder means that an individual has ____ and ________________ ________________________ panic attacks, followed by at least __________ month(s) of continuous worry about experiencing another. This type of anxiety is known as ______________________________________.

8.4 Phobias

30. Define phobia.

31. What is agoraphobia? How does it relate to panic disorder?

32. For a diagnosis of agoraphobia, symptoms must last a minimum of ______________________, and cause significant occupational or social dysfunction.

33. Give an explanation and examples for each of the following common subtypes of specific phobias.

Subtype	Description	Examples
Animal		
Blood-injection-injury		
Natural environment		
Situational		
Other		

8.5 Social Anxiety and Performance Anxiety

34. A fear of scrutiny by others or fear of acting in an embarrassing manner would be termed ______________________. It can include speaking in public, using public restrooms, or eating in public. The symptoms must have a duration of ______________________.

35. First-line medication for performance anxiety is ______________________ ______________________, recommended 30 min to 1 h before the performance. Other useful medications would include ______________________ or ______________________, but taken on a daily basis.

36. Social anxiety disorder is often comorbid with selective mutism.
TRUE FALSE

37. ______________________________ is the failure to speak in certain situations. The individual must have this deficit for at least ______________________________.

38. Selective mutism usually develops in adulthood among those individuals with language delay.

    TRUE FALSE.

8.6 Separation Anxiety

39. ______________________________ is inappropriate fear/anxiety experienced by an individual when not with their attachment figs. A diagnosis may be made if the condition lasts for longer than __________ weeks in children or __________ months in adults.

40. Why do some individuals with separation anxiety disorder report somatic symptoms?

8.7 Generalized Anxiety

41. A useful mnemonic for generalized anxiety disorder (GAD) is worry warts. Complete the table below with the missing symptoms/keywords.

W	
A	
R	
T	
S	

42. To receive a diagnosis of generalized anxiety disorder, a patient must show excessive anxiety or worry about various daily activities for at least __________ months. This anxiety or worry must be difficult to control and may be associated with physical symptoms such as muscle tension, restlessness, fatigue, irritability, or sleep disturbance.

43. There is a genetic risk of developing generalized anxiety disorder.

    TRUE FALSE

44. While symptoms of worry may begin in childhood, the median age of onset of generalized anxiety disorder is __________ years old.

8.8 Obsessive-Compulsive Disorder and Associated Disorders

45. What are obsessions?

46. What are compulsions?

47. Obsessive-compulsive disorder and obsessive-compulsive personality disorder have similar clinical presentations.
    TRUE FALSE

48. Explain body dysmorphic disorder.

49. ________________________ Disorder is when an individual retains items regardless of value. The individual experiences distress when attempting to discard possessions. This disorder is more prevalent in the elderly and has a very strong genetic component.

50. ____ is the repetitive pulling out of one's hair from the scalp, eyebrows, or eyelashes typically. It is 10 times more common in women and has an onset often after a stressful event.

51. ________________________________ disorder is recurrent skin picking, often resulting in lesions. These individuals do attempt to stop their behavior. Women with OCD and family members with this disorder are most at risk.

8.9 Post-Traumatic Stress Disorder

52. Use the mnemonic trauma to remember key signs and symptoms of PTSD.

T	
R	
A	
U	
M	
A	

53. What is the key difference between the stressful event leading to adjustment disorder and the stressful event resulting in PTSD?

54. PTSD is not curable.

TRUE FALSE

55. For each of the disorders, identify if it is an anxiety disorder (A), obsessive-compulsive disorder (OC), or a trauma-related disorder (T).

	Agoraphobia
	Generalized anxiety
	Panic
	Post-traumatic stress
	Reactive attachment
	Selective mutism
	Social anxiety (social phobia)
	Specific phobia
	Trichotillomania (hairpulling)
	Hoarding
	Excoriation (skin picking)
	Body dysmorphic
	Depersonalization or derealization
	Acute stress
	Dissociative identity
	Disinhibited social engagement
	Dissociative amnesia

56. Complete the crossword puzzle on anxiety-related disorders.

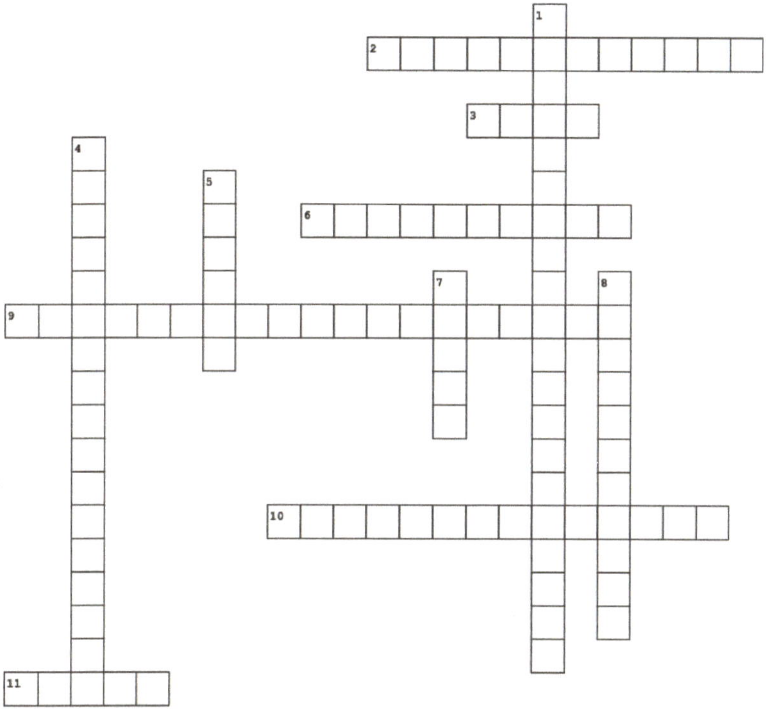

Across		Down	
2.	History of multiple physiologic complaints with no associated demonstrable organic pathology	1.	Existence of two or more distinct personalities within a person
3.	Recurrently experience thoughts and feelings associated with a severe, specific trauma	4.	Altered self-perception in which one's own reality is temporarily lost or changed
6.	Loss of or altered physical function suggesting a physiological disorder be caused by psychological factors	5.	Persistent, irrational fear of a specific object, activity, or situation
9.	Recurring, disturbing fault that cannot be dismissed from awareness without completing an uncontrollable, persistent behavior of ritualistic nature	7.	Sudden, unexpected travel away from home with an inability to recall the past
10.	Preoccupation with the fear of serious disease	8.	Anxiety pervasive, persistent anxiety of at least 6 months duration
11.	Unpredictable, recurrent attacks of intense anxiety that interfere with normal functioning		

8.10 Medication and Psychotherapeutic Management of Anxiety

57. To rule out a comorbid medical condition, what laboratories should the PMHNP order when assessing anxiety?

58. It is recommended that patients achieve symptomatic relief for at least ____________________ before titrating off of anxiolytic medications.

59. First-line medications for panic disorder are ________________________ ________________. They should be titrated slowly to avoid initiating anxiety symptoms.

60. ____________________________________ medications are seldom used for anxiety as they can exacerbate anxiety symptoms.

61. Since antidepressants can take 4-6 weeks to become effective, however, _____ ________________________________ can be used as a bridge medication temporarily.

62. If first-line agents are not successful against anxiety symptoms, other antidepressants, such as ______________________ and ______________________, can be used. However, they have side effects which must be monitored more closely.

63. Psychotherapy should accompany medication to address panic disorders.
    TRUE FALSE

64. What is behavioral therapy? Name at least three types of behavioral therapy and explain why this type of therapy is useful for clients with anxiety disorders.

65. Compare and contrast cognitive behavioral therapy (CBT) and psychodynamic psychotherapy as modalities to use with individuals with anxiety.

	Cognitive-behavioral therapy (CBT)	Psychodynamic psychotherapy
Focus		
Duration		
Techniques		
Goal		
Evidence		

66. For pediatric clients with anxiety disorder, ________________________________ ________________ is recommended as the first treatment approach.

67. ______________________________ may be prescribed for panic attacks and performance anxiety.

68. It is recommended that benzodiazepines be prescribed if a patient presents with both anxiety and depressive features.
    TRUE FALSE

69. Benzodiazepines primarily act on the ____________________ neurotransmitter receptor.

70. Compare how benzodiazepines and barbiturates affect the inhibitory effects in the brain.

	Benzodiazepines	Barbiturates
Mechanism of action		
Duration of ion channel open		
Onset of sedative effects		
Risk of respiratory depression		
Risk of overdose		
Risk of dependence and addiction		

71. Medications ending in the suffix -barbital are a first-line treatment for anxiety.
    TRUE FALSE

72. Common suffixes for benzodiazepines include ____________ and ____________.

73. What are the most common side effects of long-term use of benzodiazepines?

74. Benzodiazepines are not recommended for patients over __________ years old.

75. Complete the following chart of benzodiazepines by t1/2 and onset of action.

Benzodiazepine	Half-life	Duration
Triazolam		
Oxazepam		
Midazolam		
Diazepam		
Chlordiazepoxide		
Lorazepam		
Clonazepam		
Alprazolam		
Temazepam		

76. Rapid-onset benzodiazepines are most commonly used for ______________ ________________, while long-acting benzodiazepines are useful when patients are detoxing off __________________________.

77. Which three benzodiazepines are safe to give patients with hepatic dysfunction? Why?

    1.
    2.
    3.

78. ______________________________ is a non-benzodiazepine anxiolytic. It is used primarily as an adjunct to other medications, particularly in the treatment of GAD. It acts as a partial agonist on 5-HT1A and takes several weeks to take effect.

79. The α-receptor antagonist ________________________________ may be used to target nightmares and hypervigilance in individuals with PTSD.

80. Along with psychotherapy, the two α-agonists, ______________________ and ______________________, may be used for anxiety in pediatric populations.

81. Which medications are most recommended for the treatment of OCD?

82. What aspect of cognitive behavioral therapy is particularly useful in treating OCD?

83. Complete the following table on common non-benzodiazepine anxiolytics for adults.

Generic	Brand	Dose	Side effects
Buspirone			
	Gabitril		
			Dizziness, somnolence, peripheral edema, ataxia, asthenia, nystagmus, tremor, dysarthria, headache
	Inderal	60-80 mg daily	

84. ________________________________ is a 1- and 2-blocker used for performance anxiety. It crosses the blood-brain barrier, but does not act on neurotransmitters such as GABA.

85. Prazosin is a(n) ________________________________, blocking the sympathetic response and reducing nightmares. One side effect of this medication is ________________________________, so patients are at increased risk for falls.

86. What is the mechanism of action of gabapentin, which makes it prescribed off-label for anxiety?

87. ______________________________ is an antihistamine used as an anxiolytic, but should be used carefully due to sedating effects.

88. ______________________________ acts at GABA receptors but patients do not develop tolerance. It does share other side effects common to benzodiazepines and should be used only as a muscle relaxant.

89. In addition to cognitive behavior therapy, which medications may be used in the treatment of hairpulling and skin picking disorders?

90. Benzodiazepines should be used in the treatment of PTSD.
TRUE FALSE

91. What are some of the side effects associated with Z-drug hypnotics?

92. Z-drugs act more at the GABA-A receptor subtype. These drugs include ______________________________, ______________________________, and ______________________________. List these Z-drugs from shortest to longest half-life (t1/2).

93. ______________________________ and ______________________________ are two over-the-counter antihistamines useful as occasional hypnotics. Long-term use should be avoided (> 3 days) as they can alter the sleep cycle.

94. ______________________________ is an exogenous prescription form of the naturally occurring hormone ______________________________, which may be useful for the elderly and sufferers of jet lag.

95. Trazodone is an antidepressant used solely for sleep problems. It has the notable side effects of leaving patients with the feeling of a ______________________________ and men at increased risk of ______________________________.

8.11 Answers and Explanations to Chapter Activities

1. Stress occurs when demands exceed coping resources and capacities, creating harm. Stress is always present but intensifies during change, a perceived threat, or challenge causing physiological and psychological stress. Stress releases hormones such as adrenaline and cortisol that prepare the body for "fight or flight."
2. Answers may include:
   - Exercise regularly to release endorphins, which enhance mood and lessen discomfort.
   - Deep breathing, meditation, and gradual muscle relaxation can reduce stress and increase relaxation.
   - Sleep: Get 7–8 h a night to reduce stress.
   - Eat a balanced diet: A healthy diet gives the body the nutrients it needs to function well, reducing stress.
   - Connect with others: Social support reduces stress. Visiting family or joining a support group can help you feel connected.
   - Break tasks into smaller, more manageable steps and prioritize them to lessen stress.
   - Enjoyable hobbies alleviate stress and boost pleasure and contentment.
   - Seek professional help: If stress is interfering with daily life, a mental health expert can offer assistance and coping skills.
3. TRUE. Chronic, severe stress can cause heart disease, obesity, diabetes, immune system dysfunction, digestive issues, depression, and anxiety.
4. Many physical signs of stress and anxiety might mimic sympathetic nervous system activation. Stress and anxiety can cause physical symptoms like:
   - Palpitations or rapid heartbeat.
   - Rapid or shallow breathing.
   - Tightness or chest discomfort.
   - Tense or painful muscles.
   - Headaches.

- Sweating.
- Nausea and digestive issues.
- Exhaustion or fatigue.
- Nighttime sleep issues.
- Unsteadiness.
- Visual blurring or strain.
- Changes in weight or appetite.

5. The most frequent psychopathology in the United States is anxiety disorders, impacting one in five persons. Generalized anxiety disorder, panic disorder, social anxiety disorder, and particular phobias are anxiety disorders.
6. Anxiety is a typical human emotion that involves fear, concern, or uncertainty about an imminent event or uncertain consequence. This natural response to perceived threats or danger can motivate people to act and prepare for prospective challenges. However, excessive or persistent worry can disrupt normal life and constitute a problem. Generalized anxiety disorder, panic disorder, social anxiety disorder, and particular phobias are anxiety disorders. Some anxiety disorders cause physical symptoms such as rapid heartbeat, perspiration, and shortness of breath, as well as psychological symptoms such as persistent concern, difficulty concentrating, and anger. Treatment for anxiety disorders can include therapy, medication, or both.
7. Pathological anxiety is excessive, chronic, and life-interfering. Psychiatric providers may diagnose anxiety disorders if symptoms fulfill DSM-5 criteria. These criteria usually involve excessive and persistent concern or fear about numerous circumstances or occurrences, which can cause severe distress or impairment in social, occupational, or other areas of functioning. Symptoms must last at least 6 months and not be explained by another medical or mental health condition. If someone has excessive worry or fear, restlessness, irritability, difficulty concentrating, muscle tension, sleep disturbances, and physical symptoms such as heart palpitations, sweating, and shortness of breath, psychiatric providers may diagnose them with an anxiety disorder.
8. Most anxiety is fleeting and situational, meaning it is produced by a specific scenario or incident and usually goes away as the person leaves the surroundings. A person may feel anxious before a public speech, but thereafter, it usually goes away.
9. Possible anxiety causes include:

   - Genetics: Certain genes may increase the likelihood of anxiety disorders, according to research.
   - Brain Chemistry: Serotonin and dopamine imbalances can cause anxiety disorders.
   - Environmental Factors: Abuse, death, and financial problems can cause anxiety.
   - Personality: Perfectionists and worriers may be more prone to anxiety disorders.
   - Medical Conditions: Thyroid issues and heart disease can create anxiety.

- Alcohol and drug addiction can increase anxiety symptoms.
- Childhood Experiences: Neglect, abuse, and trauma can raise the incidence of adult anxiety disorders.

10. FALSE. Primary anxiety disorder symptoms are unrelated to substance usage, medications, or medical conditions. Generalized anxiety disorder, panic disorder, social anxiety disorder, and particular phobias are examples of these disorders, which cause excessive and persistent worry or terror about daily events. However, substance use, medications, or physical conditions might create secondary anxiety disorders.
11. The three main anxiety-causing neurotransmitters are:

    - Serotonin: This neurotransmitter regulates mood, anxiety, and sleep. Serotonin deficiency increases anxiety.
    - Gamma-aminobutyric acid (GABA): GABA calms the brain by inhibiting other neurotransmitters. Low GABA levels cause anxiety.
    - Norepinephrine: This neurotransmitter stimulates the "fight-or-flight" response to stress. Norepinephrine excess increases anxiety symptoms.

12. TRUE. Women report anxiety disorders about twice as often as males. Generalized anxiety disorder, panic disorder, and specific phobias show the greatest gender difference. This gender difference may be caused by a complex interaction of biological, psychological, and societal variables.
13. Patients who develop first-time anxiety symptoms later in life should be evaluated for substance use, physical disorders, prescription side effects, and psychological variables. Thyroid issues, heart disease, and respiratory disorders can cause anxiety. Medication adverse effects can include anxiousness. Life events such as retirement or divorce, as well as psychological reasons such as bereavement or sadness, can cause anxiety in older persons. In order to design an effective treatment strategy, it is necessary to evaluate the medical, psychological, and social anxiety symptoms.
14. Caffeine raises heart rate, blood pressure, and other physiological responses, worsening anxiety. In sensitive people, increasing caffeine intake might enhance anxiety symptoms, and limiting caffeine intake can reduce them. Thus, doctors may advise anxiety sufferers to cut less on caffeine.
15.

Body system	Signs and symptoms of anxiety
Constitutional	Fatigue, diaphoresis (sweating), shivering, or trembling
Cardiac	Chest pain, palpitations (irregular heartbeats), tachycardia (rapid heart rate), and hypertension (high blood pressure)
Respiratory	Shortness of breath, hyperventilation (rapid breathing), rapid breathing, and sighing
Neurologic	Vertigo (dizziness or a spinning sensation), lightheadedness, paresthesias (tingling or numbness in the extremities), tremors, insomnia (difficulty sleeping), and headaches
Musculoskeletal	Muscle tension, muscle aches or soreness, restlessness, or fidgeting

Body system	Signs and symptoms of anxiety
Gastrointestinal	Abdominal discomfort or pain, anorexia (loss of appetite), nausea or vomiting, diarrhea, or constipation
Sensory	Pupil dilation (widening of the pupils), sensitivity to light or sound, and visual disturbances
Integumentary	Sweating, flushing, dry mouth, cold or clammy hands, skin rash, or hives
Endocrine	Increased or decreased appetite, weight changes, and increased or decreased libido
Immunologic	Increased susceptibility to infections or allergies, and exacerbation of autoimmune conditions
Renal/urinary	Increased or decreased urinary frequency, and incontinence
Reproductive	Dysmenorrhea (painful periods), irregular periods, erectile dysfunction, premature ejaculation, and decreased sexual desire
Ophthalmologic	Blurred vision, eye strain, light sensitivity, and eye twitching

16. Common Anxiety Behaviors

- Avoidance: Anxious people may avoid social interactions, crowds, and flights.
- Restlessness or Fidgeting: Anxious people may pace, tap their feet, or fidget with objects.
- Hypervigilance: Anxiety can make people hypervigilant and continually monitor for threats.
- Irritation: Anxiety can make people more irritable and reactive to environmental stimuli.
- Anxiety can impair concentration because people are distracted by worry or fear.
- Sleep Disturbances: Anxiety can make it hard to fall or stay asleep, causing exhaustion and other symptoms.
- Excessive Reassurance-Seeking: Anxious people may seek reassurance from others to feel better, but this can develop into dependency.
- Substance Abuse: Anxious people may abuse alcohol or drugs to self-medicate, which can lead to addiction and other problems.

17.

Ability to deal with stress; ability to learn is reduced →			
Mild	Moderate	Severe	Panic
• Increased alertness • Enhanced learning ability • Enhanced stress management • Maximized problem-solving • Ability to focus on central concerns • Can lead to increased motivation and productivity • Can lead to improved performance and creativity • Can be a normal and adaptive response to stress • Can help individuals prepare for challenging situations	• More difficulty staying attentive and being able to learn • Selective inattention • Problem-solving possible with assistance • Relaxation techniques helpful • Can still allow individuals to function and complete tasks • Can be a warning sign of escalating anxiety • May require intervention to prevent further escalation • Can lead to increased stress and impairment	• Inability to focus or problem-solve • Sympathetic nervous system activity • News structured activities and large muscle activities • Complete inability to focus • Disintegrated ability to cope • Can significantly impair daily functioning • Can lead to avoidance behaviors and isolation • Can cause significant distress and impairment • May require immediate intervention	• Environmental stimuli should be decreased • Direction and structure should be provided • Can lead to physical symptoms such as chest pain and shortness of breath • Can lead to feelings of terror or impending doom • Can cause individuals to feel out of control • Can require immediate medical attention
→ Perceptual field, ability to focus is reduced			

18. TRUE. Abuse of alcohol, caffeine, nicotine, and anti-anxiety drugs is prevalent. Lack of coping skills may lead to self-medication for anxiety and physical symptoms. Substance misuse, addiction, physical and mental health issues, social and vocational issues, and legal and financial issues can result. Thus, anxiety sufferers must seek treatment and learn healthy coping skills to manage their symptoms and improve their quality of life.
19. Medications and substances that trigger anxiety include:

   - Alcohol: Alcohol is a depressant that can produce relaxation but also rebound anxiety and other mental health issues.
   - Nicotine: Nicotine raises heart rate and blood pressure and may worsen anxiety in vulnerable people.
   - Stimulants: Amphetamines and methylphenidate, used to treat ADHD and narcolepsy, might cause anxiety in certain people. Stimulants such as caffeine can raise heart rate, blood pressure, and other physiological responses,

worsening anxiety symptoms. Cocaine and methamphetamine can worsen anxiety and lead to addiction and other problems.

- Steroids: Anxiety and other psychological issues can result from corticosteroids, which treat inflammation, autoimmune disorders, and other ailments.
- Antidepressants: Some antidepressants might create or worsen anxiety before improving mood.
- Thyroid medications: Abnormal thyroid hormone levels and thyroid problem treatments can cause anxiety.
- Weight Loss Supplements: Caffeine or ephedrine can worsen anxiety.
- Decongestants: Pseudoephedrine can raise heart rate and blood pressure and worsen anxiety.

20.

Body system	Medical conditions
Neurologic	Epilepsy, migraines, multiple sclerosis, brain tumors, Huntington's disease, traumatic brain injury
Endocrine	Hyperthyroidism, hypothyroidism, hypoglycemia, pheochromocytoma, Addison's disease, Cushing's syndrome
Metabolic	Vitamin B12 deficiency, electrolyte abnormalities, porphyria, Wilson's disease, hepatic encephalopathy, hypoxia
Respiratory	Asthma, chronic obstructive pulmonary disease (COPD), pulmonary embolism, pulmonary hypertension, sleep apnea, lung cancer
Cardiovascular	Congestive heart failure, arrhythmia, myocardial infarction, aortic dissection, mitral valve prolapse
Gastrointestinal	Crohn's disease, irritable bowel syndrome (IBS), peptic ulcers, gastroesophageal reflux disease (GERD), pancreatitis
Hematologic	Anemia, sickle cell disease, thrombocytopenia, polycythemia vera, hemophilia
Oncologic	Breast cancer, prostate cancer, lung cancer, lymphoma, leukemia
Musculoskeletal	Rheumatoid arthritis, fibromyalgia, systemic lupus erythematosus (SLE), osteoarthritis, osteoporosis
Dermatologic	Eczema, psoriasis, hives, rosacea, acne

21.

Zung's Self-Rating Anxiety Scale	Hamilton Rating Scale for Anxiety (HAM-A)	Yale-Brown Obsessive-Compulsive Scale (Y-BOCS)
This self-report questionnaire measures adult anxiety severity. The 20-item scale measures physical and psychological symptoms such as anxiousness, worry, and restlessness. A 4-point scale rates each item, with higher ratings indicating more intense anxiety	This clinician-administered questionnaire measures adult anxiety severity. The 14-item scale measures physical and psychological symptoms such as tension, dread, and insomnia. A 5-point scale rates each item, with higher ratings indicating more intense anxiety	This clinician-administered questionnaire measures obsessive-compulsive symptoms in adults and children. The 10-item scale measures obsessions and compulsions' frequency, intensity, and resistance or neutralization. Each item is assessed on a 5-point scale, with higher scores indicating more severe OCD

22. Panic attacks are abrupt, acute bouts of terror or discomfort that last minutes to an hour. Palpitations, sweating, trembling, chest pain, shortness of breath, feelings of choking or suffocation, nausea, dizziness or lightheadedness, feelings of unreality or detachment from oneself or one's surroundings, and fear of losing control, going crazy, or dying may occur during a panic attack. Panic episodes occur in many scenarios. They may occur spontaneously or in response to activities such as driving, flying, speaking in public, or being in a crowded or enclosed place. Panic disorder involves recurrent, unexpected panic attacks, and prolonged worry about them and their repercussions. Generalized anxiety disorder, social anxiety disorder, post-traumatic stress disorder, and medical issues including cardiac or respiratory diseases can also cause panic attacks.
23. Panic episodes may cause anticipatory worry, avoidance of circumstances or places that may trigger them, and disturbance of normal life. These symptoms can affect social, vocational, and other functioning. Panic attacks can potentially lead to agoraphobia, severe depressive illness, and substance use disorders. The length of these consequences depends on the patient and treatment.
24. Panic attacks usually last 20-30 min, but their strength and duration vary. Even a 5-min panic episode can be upsetting and disruptive, affecting an individual's well-being and functioning.
25.

Da	Dizziness, disconnectedness, derealization, depersonalization
P	Palpitations, paresthesias
A	Abdominal distress
N	Numbness, nausea
I	Intense fear of dying, losing control, or "going crazy"
C	Chills, chest pain
S	Sweating, shaking, shortness of breath

26. Nicotine is legal but increases panic attack risk. Nicotine raises heart rate, blood pressure, and other physiological responses including panic episodes.
27. Increased. Panic episodes can interrupt social, vocational, and other functioning and cause severe suffering. Panic attacks can also be linked to psychological disorders including major depressive disorder and post-traumatic stress disorder that raise suicide risk.
28. Rule out any underlying medical issues that may be causing or contributing to a panic attack. Consider and rule out these medical conditions:

    - MI, angina, arrhythmia, and heart failure.
    - Respiratory diseases such asthma, COPD, and pulmonary embolism.
    - Neurological disorders such epilepsy, MS, and brain tumors.
    - Hyperthyroidism, hypoglycemia, thyrotoxicosis, and pheochromocytoma.
    - GERD, peptic ulcers, and inflammatory bowel disease.
    - Blood disorders such anemia and thrombocytopenia.
    - Hypoxia and electrolyte imbalances: metabolic problems.

29. The DSM defines panic disorder as recurring and sudden panic attacks followed by at least 1 month of persistent worry about having more attacks or their effects. Anticipatory anxiety can affect social, vocational, and other functions.

30. A phobia is an excessive or illogical fear of an object, event, or activity that causes avoidance or severe distress. Fear is usually disproportionate to the stimulus's risk and can interfere with normal life. Many people dread heights, spiders, snakes, enclosed areas, and social situations.
31. Agoraphobia is an anxiety condition that causes fear of being in situations where escape or aid may be difficult or embarrassing or where help may not be available in the event of a panic attack or other incapacitating symptoms. This dread makes people avoid crowds, public transit, and leaving home alone. Panic disorder sufferers may develop agoraphobia to avoid circumstances they think would cause panic attacks. Over 50% of people acquire agoraphobia after a panic attack.
32. Agoraphobia requires 6 months of symptoms and considerable occupational or social impairment.
33.

Subtype	Description	Examples
Animal	Fear of specific animals or insects	Snakes, spiders, dogs, bees
Blood-injection-injury	Fear of medical procedures, needles, or injections; may include fainting or a drop in blood pressure	Injections, blood draws, surgery
Natural environment	Fear of natural disasters or situations in nature	Thunderstorms, earthquakes, heights
Situational	Fear of specific situations or activities	Flying, driving, elevators, enclosed spaces
Other	Fear of other specific stimuli	Clowns, balloons, bridges

34. A fear of public scrutiny or embarrassment is called social anxiety disorder or social phobia. Diagnostic criteria require 6 months of symptoms.
35. Beta-blockers such as propranolol are indicated for performance anxiety 30 min to an hour before the performance. Beta-blockers can lessen anxiety symptoms including fast heart rate and shaky hands without harming cognition. Performance anxiety may be treated with SSRIs such as sertraline or fluoxetine or benzodiazepines such as clonazepam or lorazepam. However, these drugs are usually used daily rather than before a performance and have a higher risk of side effects and dependence.
36. TRUE. Selective mutism typically occurs with social anxiety disorder. Selective mutism causes a persistent refusal to speak in specific social contexts. Selective mutism can cause social anxiety and avoidance of speaking settings. As many as 90% of children with selective mutism have social anxiety disorder or other anxiety disorders.
37. Selective mutism must last at least 1 month and not be related to a lack of spoken language understanding or comfort.
38. FALSE. Selective mutism usually begins between 2 and 5 years old and can last into adulthood if untreated. Selective mutism is not usually linked to language delay, although it can make expressive language and social communication challenging. Selection mutism may be linked to social anxiety disorder or other anxiety disorders.

39. Separation anxiety disorder is inappropriate fear/anxiety without attachment figures such as parents or caregivers. It may include persistent reluctance or refusal to attend school or work, recurrent nightmares about separation, physical symptoms such as headaches or stomach aches, or intense worry about harming oneself or one's loved ones. Children can be diagnosed with separation anxiety disorder if the problem lasts longer than 4 weeks, while adults must have symptoms for 6 months.
40. Due to their great emotional discomfort when separated from their attachment figures, some people with separation anxiety disorder may have physiological symptoms including headaches, stomachaches, or nausea. This bodily response may be related to stress and worry, which stimulate the sympathetic nervous system and cause symptoms. Others may report these symptoms to avoid school or job to be near their attachment figure. This can cause severe social and vocational disruption.
41.

W	Wound up, worn out
A	Absent-minded
R	Restless
T	Tense
S	Sleepless

42. Six months. Generalized anxiety disorder causes excessive worry or anxiety about everyday circumstances, events, and activities. This worry may be disproportionate to the situation's threat and interfere with normal life.
43. TRUE. A family history of anxiety disorders has been linked to generalized anxiety disorder, suggesting a genetic risk. Genetics alone do not cause anxiety disorders; stress, trauma, and life experiences also contribute.
44. The median age of onset for GAD is 30. Although worry or anxiety may start in infancy or adolescence, generalized anxiety disorder is usually diagnosed in adulthood. Generalized anxiety disorder is also more common among women.
45. Obsessions are unwelcome, intrusive, and persistent thoughts, impulses, or pictures that cause severe anguish or anxiety. The person may try to ignore or repress these unreasonable or improper thoughts or pictures, but they keep coming back. OCD is characterized by obsessions; however, other anxiety disorders including GAD and PTSD can also have obsessions.
46. Obsessions or dreaded outcomes cause compulsions. Excessive, time-consuming compulsions can disrupt daily life. Compulsions include excessive washing or cleaning, checking actions, repetitive counting, sorting objects, or seeking reassurance. These compulsions can temporarily relieve obsession-related anxiety but can also reinforce the cycle.
47. FALSE. OCD patients are upset by their symptoms, or ego-dystonic. Individuals with OCPD consider them ego-syntonic.
48. Body dysmorphic disorder (BDD) is an OCD that involves obsessing over minor imperfections in one's appearance. These perceived flaws or defects usually concern the skin, hair, nose, eyes, or body shape. BDD sufferers often spend a lot of time inspecting, grooming, or camouflaging the perceived fault or

seeking confirmation that it is not evident. They may also shun social interactions, employment, and school to hide the fault. The apparent imperfection might cause severe distress or hamper daily functioning.

49. Hoarding disorder is characterized by repeated difficulties discarding belongings, regardless of their value, due to a felt desire to save them or an excessive emotional attachment. These items can create congested living areas that disrupt daily life and offer health and safety risks. Hoarding is more common among the elderly, and those with first-degree relatives are more likely to be diagnosed.
50. Trichotillomania, an obsessive-compulsive disorder, involves repeatedly pulling hair from the scalp, eyebrows, and eyelashes, causing hair loss and bald areas. The activity usually begins with tension or worry and ends with comfort or pleasure. Approximately 1-2% of the population has trichotillomania. Stressful events such as trauma or disease often cause the disorder.
51. Excoriation disorder is an obsessive-compulsive disorder that causes skin lesions, scarring, and discolouration by picking at one's skin. Excoriation disorder sufferers may hide their skin picking out of shame, humiliation, or remorse.
52.

T	Traumatic event
R	Reexperience
A	Avoidance
U	Unable to function
M	Month or more of symptoms
A	Arousal increased

53. The severity of the stressor and its symptoms distinguish adjustment disorder from PTSD. Adjustment disorder is a stress-related disorder that follows a substantial life change, loss, or sickness. The stressor may be low or severe, yet the symptoms cause distress or impairment in daily life. After removing the stressor, symptoms such as anxiety, depression, irritability, and physical complaints usually disappear within 6 months.
In contrast, PTSD is a more severe stress-related disorder that can result from death, major injury, or sexual violence. The stressor is usually more severe, and the symptoms persist longer. PTSD symptoms include intrusive thoughts or recollections of the traumatic incident, avoidance of reminders, negative mood or cognition changes, and hyperarousal, such as difficulties sleeping, impatience, or hypervigilance. PTSD symptoms can last months or years and lower quality of life.
54. FALSE. 50% of PTSD patients recover within 3 months. CBT, EMDR, and antidepressants or anti-anxiety medicines are effective PTSD therapies.
55.

A	Agoraphobia
A	Generalized anxiety
A	Panic
T	Post-traumatic stress
T	Reactive attachment
A	Selective mutism
A	Social anxiety (social phobia)

A	Specific phobia
OC	Trichotillomania (hairpulling)
OC	Hoarding
OC	Excoriation (skin picking)
OC	Body dysmorphic
T	Depersonalization or derealization
T	Acute stress
T	Dissociative identity
T	Disinhibited social engagement
T	Dissociative amnesia

56.

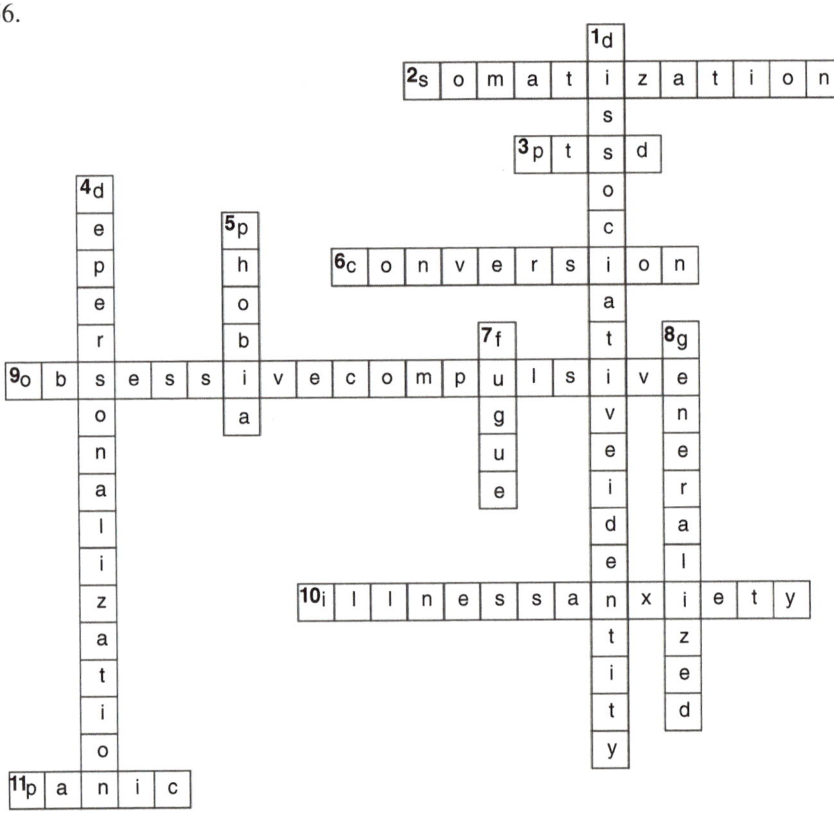

57. Laboratory testing may vary depending on the patient's history and symptoms. Some frequent tests include:

- Complete Blood Count (CBC): This test monitors blood cell count and type to detect anemia or infection that may be causing symptoms.
- Thyroid function tests examine thyroid hormone levels in the blood and can detect anxiety-causing hypothyroidism or hyperthyroidism.
- The basic metabolic panel (BMP) examines blood levels of electrolytes, glucose, and other substances to assist diagnose illnesses including diabetes or kidney disease.

- Urinalysis: This test analyzes urine to detect urinary tract infections and kidney damage.
- Drug Screen: This test can identify substance use that may be causing symptoms.
- Imaging examinations such as MRI or CT scans and heart function tests such as ECGs or echocardiograms may be conducted depending on the patient's symptoms and medical history.

58. Before tapering anxiolytics such as benzodiazepines, patients should have symptomatic relief for 6-12 months. This stabilization period can help the patient manage their anxiety symptoms and build appropriate coping mechanisms and behavioral methods.
59. SSRIs and SNRIs are first-line panic disorder treatments. These drugs reduce panic episodes, anxiety, and sadness.
60. Stimulants. Medications such as amphetamines, used primarily for attention deficit hyperactivity disorder (ADHD), can exacerbate anxiety symptoms due to their stimulating effects.
61. Benzodiazepines are typically used to treat anxiety problems while antidepressants or other long-term drugs work. Benzodiazepines can relieve anxiety quickly, but they might cause tolerance, dependence, and other side effects. Benzodiazepines can be prescribed for 2-4 weeks to treat acute anxiety, but they should be discontinued gradually.
62. TCAs and MAOIs may be used if SSRIs and SNRIs fail to address a client's anxiety. TCAs such as imipramine and clomipramine alleviate anxiety but have higher negative effects than SSRIs and SNRIs. MAOIs such as phenelzine and tranylcypromine may alleviate anxiety, but they have greater dietary and pharmaceutical restrictions and may interact with other drugs. TCA and MAOI users must be monitored for adverse effects, medication interactions, and overdose. Thus, these drugs are usually reserved for patients who have not responded to conventional treatments or who have severe comorbidities.
63. TRUE. Psychotherapy such as CBT is typically suggested for panic disorder patients in addition to pharmaceutical management. CBT can teach patients coping skills and relaxation techniques to minimize panic attack frequency and intensity. CBT can also uncover and change panic disorder-related negative thoughts and behaviors. Psychotherapies such as exposure therapy may also cure panic disorder.
64. Behavioral psychotherapy teaches new skills and techniques to change harmful behaviors and thoughts. The learning theory-based approach stresses environmental influences and conditioning in psychological disease development. Behavioral therapy helps anxiety sufferers identify and change dysfunctional ideas, feelings, and actions by building coping and problem-solving skills. New behaviors and cognitive patterns can help clients manage stress, reduce anxiety, and improve their quality of life. Behavioral therapy is also a flexible and effective treatment for anxiety disorders because it is short-term and customizable. Types of behavioral therapy include:

- Cognitive Behavioral Therapy (CBT): Changes negative thought patterns and actions that cause anxiety.
- Exposure Therapy: The client is gradually exposed to anxiety-provoking stimuli or events to diminish anxiety and terror.
- Relaxation Training: Teaching clients deep breathing, progressive muscular relaxation, and guided imagery to soothe and reduce anxiety.
- Systematic Desensitization: Relaxation and anxiety-provoking stimuli are used to lessen anxiety.
- Behavioral Activation Treatment: Improves mood and reduces anxiety by enhancing positive and lowering negative behaviors.

65.

	Cognitive behavioral therapy (CBT)	Psychodynamic psychotherapy
Focus	Changing negative thought patterns and behaviors	Exploring unconscious conflicts and emotions
Duration	Short-term (12-20 sessions)	Longer-term (several months to years)
Techniques	Cognitive restructuring, exposure therapy, relaxation training	Free association, interpretation, analysis of transference
Goal	Developing coping strategies and problem-solving skills	Gaining insight into unconscious conflicts and emotions
Evidence	Supported by a large body of research and effective for anxiety disorders	Less well-researched but shown to be effective for some anxiety disorders

66. For pediatric clients with anxiety disorder, cognitive behavioral therapy (CBT) is recommended as the first treatment approach.
67. Beta-blockers.
68. FALSE. Benzodiazepines can aggravate depression and cause dependence and addiction; hence, they should not be prescribed to individuals with anxiety and depression. Antidepressants or non-benzodiazepine anxiolytics may work better.
69. GABA-A.
70.

	Benzodiazepines	Barbiturates
Mechanism of action	Enhances the affinity of GABA for its binding site on the receptor, thereby increasing the frequency of the chloride ion channel opening	Directly open the chloride ion channel
Duration of ion channel open	Shorter duration of the chloride ion channel being open	Longer duration of the channel being open
Onset of sedative effects	Faster	Slower
Risk of respiratory depression	Lower	Higher
Risk of overdose	Lower	Higher
Risk of dependence and addiction	Lower	Higher

71. FALSE. Barbiturates or -barbitals are not recommended for anxiety treatment due to their significant risk of dependence and addiction and other side effects. Anxiety disorders should be treated first with SSRIs or SNRIs.
72. Common suffixes for benzodiazepines include "-azepam" and "-azolam."
73. Long-term benzodiazepine use may cause:

- Physical Dependence: Benzodiazepines are addictive and can cause physical dependence. Abrupt benzodiazepine withdrawal might cause life-threatening seizures.
- Cognitive Impairment: Long-term benzodiazepine use can impair memory, attention, and focus.
- Benzodiazepines can cause sleepiness and sedation, which can impair motor coordination and increase fall risk.
- Depression: Benzodiazepines can aggravate depression and increase suicide risk.
- Respiratory Depression: High benzodiazepine dosages might cause deadly respiratory depression.
- Tolerance: Long-term benzodiazepine use can cause tolerance, requiring greater dosages to get the same effect and increasing overdose risk.

74. 65 years old.
75.

Benzodiazepine	Half-life (h)	Duration
Triazolam	1-12	Short
Oxazepam	4-15	Short
Midazolam	1.5-2.5	Short
Diazepam	20-50	Long
Chlordiazepoxide	24-48	Long
Lorazepam	10-20	Intermediate
Clonazepam	18-50	Intermediate
Alprazolam	6-20	Intermediate
Temazepam	8-22	Intermediate

76. Rapid-onset benzodiazepines are utilized for acute panic episodes, sleep onset, and short medical operations, whereas long-acting ones help patients detox from short-acting benzos or alcohol.
77. Hepatic dysfunction patients can safely use oxazepam, temazepam, and lorazepam (OTL). They create no active metabolites and are processed mostly outside the liver. With reduced liver function, they are less likely to accumulate and cause harm.
78. Buspirone.
79. Prazosin can treat PTSD nightmares and hypervigilance.
80. Clonidine and guanfacine are pediatric anxiety alpha-agonists.
81. Sertraline, fluvoxamine, and clomipramine are the most prescribed OCD medications.
82. Cognitive behavioral therapy's exposure and response prevention (ERP) is effective for OCD. ERP gradually exposes the patient to anxiety-provoking

stimuli while preventing obsessive behaviors or rituals. Repeated exposure to frightening circumstances and prevention of compulsive responses can help OCD sufferers lessen anxiety and resist compulsions.

83.

Generic	Brand	Dose	Side effects
Buspirone	Buspar	20-60 mg daily	Dizziness, insomnia, tremors, akathisia, stomach upset, dry mouth
Tiagabine	Gabitril	2-8 mg twice daily	Dizziness, drowsiness, nervousness, tremors, difficulty concentrating, gastrointestinal discomfort
Gabapentin	Neurontin	900-3600 mg daily	Dizziness, somnolence, peripheral edema, ataxia, asthenia, nystagmus, tremor, dysarthria, headache
Propranolol	Inderal	60-80 mg daily	Dizziness, fatigue, bradycardia, bronchospasm, hypotension, impotence, exacerbation of Raynaud's phenomenon

84. Propranolol.
85. Prazosin blocks sympathetic response and reduces nightmares as an α-1 adrenergic receptor antagonist. This medicine can cause orthostatic hypotension, increasing fall risk.
86. Gabapentin controls seizures by binding to the brain's voltage-gated calcium channel α-2-δ subunit. This decreases glutamate, norepinephrine, and substance P release, which are involved in anxiety and other mental diseases. Gabapentin calms anxiety by regulating these neurotransmitters.
87. Hydroxyzine.
88. Baclofen reduces muscular spasms and spasticity by boosting GABA in the central nervous system. It is rarely used as an anxiolytic; however, there is evidence that it may help alcohol users. Although it can produce dizziness, sleepiness, and weakness, Baclofen is generally well-tolerated.
89.

- SSRIs: These drugs are widely used to treat these diseases because they reduce obsessive-compulsive symptoms.
- Naltrexone and other opioid antagonists reduce hairpulling and skin picking.
- Topiramate, an anticonvulsant, reduces hair and skin tugging.
- N-acetylcysteine (NAC): This amino acid supplement may reduce hair and skin tugging.
- Lithium and pimozide are used to treat hairpulling and skin picking problems when other treatments fail.

90. FALSE. Due to its abuse and dependence risk and limited efficacy in treating PTSD symptoms, benzodiazepines are not suggested. It may increase feelings of detachment. Instead, SSRIs and SNRIs are recommended as first-line therapies. Psychotherapy such as CBT is also beneficial for PTSD treatment.

91. Z-drugs' common negative effects include:
    - Drowsiness.
    - Dizziness.
    - Headache.
    - Nausea and vomiting.
    - Mouth dry.
    - Fatigue.
    - Tiredness during the day.
    - Trouble remembering and anterograde amnesia.
    - Increased sadness and suicide risk due to behavioral changes.
    - Rebound insomnia (after medication discontinuation).
    - Addiction and withdrawal symptoms such as anxiety, irritability, and insomnia.
    - Somnambulism.
    - Sleep-eating.
92. Zaleplon (Sonata)—t1/2 of about 1 h → Zolpidem (Ambien)—t1/2 of about 2.5 h → Eszopiclone (Lunesta)—t1/2 of about 6 h.
93. Diphenhydramine and doxylamine succinate are two over-the-counter antihistamines useful as occasional hypnotics.
94. Ramelteon; melatonin.
95. Trazodone's notable side effects include leaving patients with the feeling of a dry mouth (i.e., hangover-like symptoms) and men at increased risk of priapism (prolonged and painful erection).

References and Resources

American Psychiatric Association. Diagnostic and statistical manual of mental disorders:DSM-5-TR. 5th ed. American Psychiatric Association Publishing; 2022.

Baker HJ, Lawrence PJ, Karalus J, Creswell C, Waite P. The effectiveness of psychological therapies for anxiety disorders in adolescents: a meta-analysis. Clin Child Fam Psychol Rev. 2021;24(4):765–82. https://doi.org/10.1007/s10567-021-00364-2.

Barlow DH. Anxiety and its disorders: the nature and treatment of anxiety and panic. 2nd ed. Guilford Press; 2014.

Barlow DH, Conklin LR, Bentley KH. Psychological treatments for panic disorders, phobias, and social and generalized anxiety disorders. In: Nathan PE, Gorman JM, editors. A guide to treatments that work. 4th ed. Oxford Academic; 2015. https://doi.org/10.1093/med:psych/9780199342211.003.0014.

Borkovec TD, Ray WJ, Stöber J. Worry: a cognitive phenomenon intimately linked to affective, physiological, and interpersonal behavioral processes. Cogn Ther Res. 1998;22(6):561–76. https://doi.org/10.1023/A:1018790003416.

Carl E, Witcraft SM, Kauffman BY, Gillespie EM, Becker ES, Cuijpers P, Van Ameringen M, Smits JAJ, Powers MB. Psychological and pharmacological treatments for generalized anxiety disorder (GAD): a meta-analysis of randomized controlled trials. Cogn Behav Ther. 2020;49(1):1–21. https://doi.org/10.1080/16506073.2018.1560358.

Del Casale A, Sorice S, Padovano A, Simmaco M, Ferracuti S, Lamis DA, Rapinesi C, Sani G, Girardi P, Kotzalidis GD, Pompili M. Psychopharmacological treatment of obsessive-compulsive disorder (OCD). Curr Neuropharmacol. 2019;17(8):710–36. https://doi.org/10.2174/1570159X16666180813155017.

Hofmann SG, Asnaani A, Vonk IJ, Sawyer AT, Fang A. The efficacy of cognitive behavioral therapy: a review of meta-analyses. Cogn Ther Res. 2012;36(5):427–40. https://doi.org/10.1007/s10608-012-9476-1.

Hofmann SG, Gómez AF. Mindfulness-based interventions for anxiety and depression. Psychiatr Clin N Am. 2017;40(4):739–49. https://doi.org/10.1016/j.psc.2017.08.008.

Hofmann SG, Smits JA. Cognitive-behavioral therapy for adult anxiety disorders: a meta-analysis of randomized placebo-controlled trials. J Clin Psychiatry. 2008;69(4):621–32.

James AC, James G, Cowdrey FA, Soler A, Choke A. Cognitive behavioural therapy for anxiety disorders in children and adolescents. Cochrane Database Syst Rev. 2013;6:CD004690. https://doi.org/10.1002/14651858.CD004690.pub3.

Johnson K, Vanderhoef D, Magrath N. Psychiatric-mental health nurse practitioner review and resource manual. American Nurses Association: American Nurses Credentialing Center; 2020.

Kessler RC, Chiu WT, Demler O, Walters EE. Prevalence, severity, and comorbidity of 12-month DSM-IV disorders in the National Comorbidity Survey Replication. Arch Gen Psychiatry. 2005;62(6):617–27.

Lack CW. Obsessive-compulsive disorder: evidence-based treatments and future directions for research. World J Psychiatry. 2012;2(6):86–90. https://doi.org/10.5498/wjp.v2.i6.86.

Murphy DL, Timpano KR, Wheaton MG, Greenberg BD, Miguel EC. Obsessive-compulsive disorder and its related disorders: a reappraisal of obsessive-compulsive spectrum concepts. Dialogues Clin Neurosci. 2010;12(2):131–48. https://doi.org/10.31887/DCNS.2010.12.2/dmurphy.

Rapp AM, Bergman RL, Piacentini J, McGuire JF. Evidence-based assessment of obsessive-compulsive disorder. J Cent Nerv Syst Dis. 2016;8:13–29. https://doi.org/10.4137/JCNSD.S38359.

Stein DJ, Costa DLC, Lochner C, Miguel EC, Reddy YCJ, Shavitt RG, van den Heuvel OA, Simpson HB. Obsessive-compulsive disorder. Nat Rev Dis Primers. 2019;5(1):52. https://doi.org/10.1038/s41572-019-0102-3.

Sturm R. Obsessive-compulsive disorder in children: the role of nurse practitioners. J Am Acad Nurse Pract. 2009;21:393–401. https://doi.org/10.1111/j.1745-7599.2009.00414.x.

Zakhari R. The psychiatric-mental health nurse practitioner certification review manual. Springer Publishing Company; 2021.

Notes:

Notes:

9 Schizophrenia, Psychosis, and Delusions

Test your learning and check your understanding of this book's contents: use the "Springer Nature Flashcards" app to access questions using ▶ https://sn.pub/62J0Ar.

To use the app, please follow the instructions in Chap. 1.

PMHNPs are essential in the diagnosis and treatment of schizophrenia, psychosis, and delusions. They are responsible for conducting comprehensive assessments, formulating treatment plans, and providing support to individuals with these conditions.

Psychosis is a term used to describe a group of symptoms that affect an individual's ability to perceive reality. It can be a symptom of various mental health disorders, including schizophrenia, bipolar disorder, and substance abuse. Psychotic symptoms may include delusions, hallucinations, disorganized thinking, and abnormal behaviors.

Schizophrenia is a severe and chronic mental health disorder characterized by a wide range of symptoms, including delusions, hallucinations, disorganized thinking, and abnormal behaviors. It is estimated to affect around 1% of the global population, with a peak onset age of 20–30 years (World Health Organization 2021). Schizophrenia can have a significant impact on an individual's ability to function in daily life and can lead to significant disability if left untreated.

Delusions are false beliefs that an individual holds despite evidence to the contrary. They can be a symptom of various mental health disorders, including schizophrenia and psychosis. Delusions can be categorized into different types, including persecutory delusions (believing that one is being persecuted or harassed), grandiose delusions (believing that one has exceptional abilities or talents), and somatic delusions (believing that one has a physical ailment or illness).

T. Stewart, *Psychiatric-Mental Health Nurse Practitioner Program Companion and Board Certification Exam Review Workbook*,
https://doi.org/10.1007/978-3-031-60894-0_9

Effective treatment for schizophrenia, psychosis, and delusions typically involves a combination of pharmacological and psychosocial interventions. Antipsychotic medications, such as clozapine and risperidone, are often used to manage psychotic symptoms, while cognitive-behavioral therapy (CBT) and other psychosocial interventions can be effective in addressing delusions and improving coping skills (American Psychiatric Association 2022).

This chapter focuses on the schizophrenia spectrum and other psychoses. Differentiations between delusions and hallucinations are highlighted. Brief psychotic disorders, with respect to substance use, and Folie à Deux are mentioned. Diagnostic criteria, pertinent medications, along with side effects, and therapies are presented.

9.1 Psychosis

1. Psychosis is a distorted perception of ____________________ and an inability to process ____________________ accurately.
2. Three characteristics of psychosis include: (1) ____________________, (2)____________________,and(3)____________________.
3. Name 5 psychiatric disorders in which psychosis may be a symptom.

    1.
    2.
    3.
    4.
    5.

4. Name 5 medical disorders which psychosis may accompany.

    1.
    2.
    3.
    4.
    5.

5. Place an X next to those behaviors which may be present as a symptom of psychosis.

	Playful silliness, child-like
	Predictable anger outbursts
	Well-kempt, fulfills self-hygiene needs
	Bizarre dress, make-up, hair
	Slowed, varying movements
	Needs assistance with ADLs
	Inappropriate comments or behaviors, particularly sexual

	Misinterprets environmental stimuli, placing significance on mundane
	Able to organize information, interpretation, thoughts, speech, behavior

6. To be diagnosed with brief psychotic disorder, a patient must show signs of at least two elements of psychosis for a duration of at least ________________ day(s), but less than ________________ month(s), with eventual full return to premorbid level of functioning.

7. Match each of the perceptual disturbances with its most common association.

1. ____Auditory hallucinations	A. False perception upon waking
2. ____Visual hallucinations	B. Most common hallucination; associated with schizophrenia
3. ____Olfactory hallucinations	C. Least common hallucination, associated with epilepsy
4. ____Tactile hallucinations	D. Present in psychoses as well as substance use and delirium
5. ____Gustatory hallucinations	E. False perception when falling asleep
6. ____Hypnopompic hallucinations	F. Secondary to withdrawal from substances
7. ____Hypnogogic hallucinations	G. Reported most prior to an epileptic seizure

8. Individuals who hear nonexistent voices telling them to do certain acts are experiencing ________________________ auditory hallucinations.

9. Label each definition with the correct type of disorganized thinking.

	Jumping from one idea to another without a clear connection between them.
	Going off on a tangent and talking about something unrelated to the topic at hand.
	Providing excessive and unnecessary detail when answering a question or describing a situation, without ever getting to the main point.
	Using words and phrases that do not make sense or are not related to one another.
	Creating new words or using words in a way that is not consistent with their usual meaning.
	Suddenly stopping in the middle of a sentence or thought, often because of an interruption in the person's thought process.
	Repeating a particular word, phrase, or idea over and over again, even if it does not make sense in the context.

10. A(n) ________________________ is a misinterpretation of an existing stimulus.

11. Complete the following crossword with types of disorganized thinking. Examples of client quotes are provided in each clue.

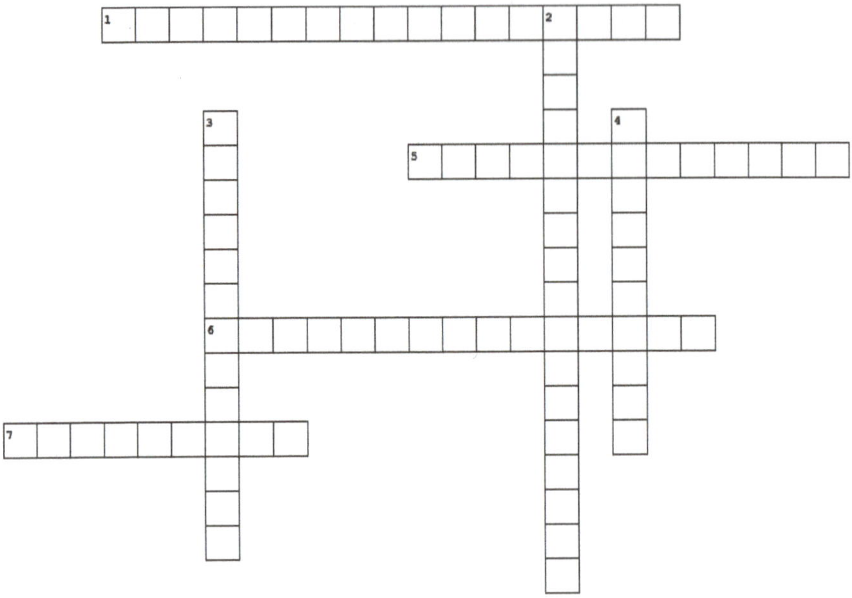

Across		Down	
1.	"Well, first I got up this morning and I brushed my teeth. I use Colgate toothpaste, it's the only kind I like. Then I took a shower and I used the lavender soap my sister gave me. She's always giving me soap. Anyway, after that, I got dressed and came here."	2.	"I want to go to the store and buy some apples. Apples are healthy. I need to be healthy so I can climb a mountain. Mountains are beautiful. I wish I could paint a mountain."
5.	"I saw a red car on the way here. It was really red, you know? Like fire engine red. Red is my favorite color. When I was a kid, I had a red bike. I rode it everywhere. I loved that bike."	3.	"I'm feeling really anxious today. Did I tell you about my dog? He's a poodle. I had a poodle when I was a kid. My mom loved poodles. She used to make me wear a bow in my hair like a poodle. But that's not why I'm anxious, it's because of the test I have to take tomorrow."
6.	"I was going to tell you about my day, but... I can't remember what I was going to say. Sorry."	4.	"I was out 'apeaching' yesterday. Peach and preaching, you know, like talking about god and nature."
7.	"Purple rhinoceros hippopotamus buttercup. I'm not sure about the soap. It smells like my aunt's shoes."		

9.2 Delusions

12. What are delusions?

13. Distinguish bizarre vs. nonbizarre delusions. Provide an example of each.

Bizarre delusion	Nonbizarre delusion
Example:	Example:

14. To be diagnosed with delusional disorder, an individual must have nonbizarre delusions for at least ___________ and their life is not significantly impaired.

15. Risk for delusional disorder increases after the age of _______.

16. Match the following categories of delusions with the best example patient statement.

Category	Example statement
1. ____ persecutory	A. "I can feel something moving inside my body, like there are insects crawling under my skin."
2. ____Ideas of reference	B. "My partner is cheating on me and I can see the signs everywhere."
3. ____ thought broadcasting	C. "Every time I hear a car honk, I think it's a message meant specifically for me."
4. ____ grandeur	D. "I believe that a famous celebrity is in love with me and is sending me secret messages."
5. ____ thought insertion	E. "Someone is following me everywhere I go and is trying to harm me. They are watching my every move."
6. ____ guilt	F. "I am the chosen one, destined for greatness. I am here to save the world."

Category	Example statement
7. ____ somatic	G. "I am being watched by the government and they are trying to take me down."
8. ____ paranoid	H. "I am responsible for all the suffering in the world. I have committed terrible sins."
9. ____ Erotomanic	I. "I can hear my thoughts being transmitted to everyone around me."
10. ____ religious	J. "I have been chosen by god to carry out a special mission. I have been given divine guidance."
11. ____ jealous	K. "I keep having these thoughts that are not my own. It's like someone else is putting them in my head."

17. Explain folie à deux.

9.3 Schizophrenia

18. To be diagnosed with schizophrenia per the DSM, an individual must have symptoms for ____________months. Less than this period of time would qualify them for a diagnosis of ______________________________________disorder. Brief psychotic disorder lasts for ____________________ or less.

19. Schizophrenia exists in both acute and chronic forms.
    TRUE FALSE

20. Prevalence of schizophrenia among men and women is mostly equal/similar.
    TRUE FALSE

21. __________________ tend to present with symptoms of schizophrenia from 18–25 years old.

22. ___________________ with schizophrenia tend to have poorer outcome prognoses and ______________________ symptoms, while __________________ with schizophrenia experience more _______________________ symptoms.

23. In the following table, identify which characteristic of schizophrenia is associated more with men (M) or women (W).

	Age of onset 18–25 years
	Age of onset 25–35 years
	More negative symptoms
	More paranoid delusions and hallucinations
	Fewer prodromal symptoms
	Poorer prognosis
	Poorer response to medications
	Fewer neurostructural abnormalities
	More cognitive impairment

24. In the following table, define and then list examples of positive and negative symptoms of schizophrenia.

	Positive symptoms	Negative symptoms
Definition		
Example		

25. Do positive or negative symptoms often appear first as schizophrenia develops?

26. What is catatonia? What is its relationship to schizophrenia?

27. Complete the table below with example findings that a PMHNP might expect when conducting a mental status exam on a client with schizophrenia.

Aspect	Examples of findings in schizophrenia
Appearance	
Speech	
Affect	
Mood	

Aspect	Examples of findings in schizophrenia
Thought process	
Thought content	
Cognition	
Orientation	
Memory	
Concentration	
Abstraction	
Judgment	

28. There are commonly three phases to schizophrenia symptomatology. For each of these phases, provide a definition and some examples.

	Definition	Example 1	Example 2
Prodromal			
Psychosis			
Residual			

29. What does "downdrift" refer to when discussing the functionality of individuals with schizophrenia?

30. Which non-prescription substance is used/abused most commonly by individuals with schizophrenia?

31. The pathophysiology of schizophrenia is linked strongest to an increase in the neurotransmitter ______________________________.

32. Which classes of substances can lead to schizophrenia-like symptoms?

33. For each dopamine pathway, explain their trek through the brain, list the symptoms of adverse events when antipsychotics are used to address these symptoms.

Pathway	Trek in brain	Symptoms of adverse events
Mesocortical/prefrontal cortex		
Mesolimbic		
Tuberoinfundibular		
Nigrostriatal		

34. Positive symptoms of schizophrenia originate within the ______________ dopamine pathway.

35. Negative symptoms of schizophrenia are associated with the ____________________________ dopamine pathway.

36. When the nigrostriatal dopamine pathway is blocked, this can lead to ____________________________ symptoms.

37. A patient complains that they cannot sit still. They have continuous feelings of restlessness and need to move. They explain the sensation as they are about "to jump out of their skin" and need to move to settle down the sensation. This continuous feeling of needing to move is referred to as ___________________________.

38. What are four other neurotransmitters that are implicated in schizophrenia?

39. Schizophrenia has a strong genetic component. It is estimated that if one twin develops schizophrenia then the risk to their sibling will be ______________. Children of parents with schizophrenia also have higher incidence of schizophrenia than those children without.

40. For each of the prognostic factors of schizophrenia, decide if it is associated with better or worse prognosis over time. Label each with a B for better, or W for worse prognosis.

	Later onset
	Early onset
	Poor social support
	Positive symptoms
	Family history
	Few relapses
	Gradual onset
	Good social support
	Male gender
	Poor premorbid functioning
	Many relapses
	Negative symptoms
	Female gender
	Acute onset
	Good premorbid functioning
	Comorbid substance use
	Mood symptoms

41. The etiology of schizophrenia is considered to be multifactorial. However, there are some neurodevelopmental and neurobiological events that are considered to be linked to the development of schizophrenia. CT and MRI scans of the brains of individuals with schizophrenia are most likely to show enlargement of the ________________________ and atrophy of the ____________________________. This results in overall reduced brain volume.

42. In the table below, use the definition and patient example to label each speech issue that may manifest in schizophrenia with the correct term.

Speech issue	Definition	Patient example quote
	Newly invented words or phrases that have no meaning	"I'm trying to find my zimmerhoodle so I can go to the store"
	Repetition of words or phrases spoken by someone else	Interviewer: "What is your name?" patient: "Name... Name...Name."
	Speech patterns based on the sound of words rather than meaning	"I'm as jumpy as a rumble-tumble, it's time to fumble"
	Reduction in the amount of speech or a lack of spontaneous speech	Interviewer: "Tell me about your interests" patient: "Nothing"
	Increase in rate and volume of speech, often with urgency or pressure	"I need to tell you everything that's happened, and I need to tell you now"
	Speech that is disorganized and difficult to follow	"I want to be the future and the past, the present is the present so we must stay fast"
	Complete lack of speech	No verbal response from patient
	Illogical or tangential speech	"I need to buy some apples, but the sky is blue today"

43. A patient experiencing a depressive or manic episode concurrently with psychosis may be diagnosed with ____ __________.

44. What is schizophreniform disorder?

45. Order the following psychotic disorders from mild to severe in terms of overall prognosis: schizophrenia, brief psychotic disorder, schizoaffective, schizophreniform.

46. What specific lab studies might a provider expect to find when diagnosing schizophrenia?

9.4 Antipsychotics and Nonpharmacological Management

47. Typical antipsychotics are synonymous with neuroleptics.

TRUE FALSE

48. What are three medications that can be used to treat extrapyramidal symptoms?

49. Match each of the following body function impairment with its cause:

____ 1. Tardive dyskinesia	A. This is a movement disorder characterized by an intense feeling of restlessness and a need to move. Individuals with akathisia may pace, rock back and forth, or tap their feet or fingers in an attempt to relieve the sensation
____ 2. Dystonia	B. This is characterized by a range of symptoms, including fever, muscle rigidity, tremors, and changes in consciousness
____ 3. Akathisia	C. Symptoms can include involuntary movements of the face, tongue, and limbs, as well as abnormal movements of the trunk and pelvis
____ 4. Bradykinesia	D. This includes tremors, rigidity, and bradykinesia (slowness of movement)
____ 5. Parkinsonism	E. This is a movement disorder characterized by involuntary muscle contractions that can cause twisting, repetitive movements, or abnormal postures
____ 6. Neuroleptic malignant syndrome	F. Movement disorder characterized by slowness of movement or difficulty initiating movement

50. Typical (first-generation) antipsychotics block ________________ receptors. Atypical(second-generation)antipsychoticsblock________________________ and ________________________________ receptors.

51. Complete the following table on typical, or first-generation, antipsychotics.

Medication	Potency	Adverse effects	Misc
Chlorpromazine			
Thioridazine			
Loxapine			
Thiothixene			
Molindone			
Perphenazine			
Haloperidol			
Fluphenazine			
Trifluoperazine			
Pimozide			

52. Complete the following table on atypical, or second-generation, antipsychotics.

Medication	Adverse effects	Misc
Clozapine		
Risperidone		
Quetiapine		
Olanzapine		
Ziprasidone		
Aripiprazole		
Paliperidone		
Asenapine		
Iloperidone		
Lurasidone		

53. Which labs and vitals must be monitored while a patient is taking an atypical antipsychotic?

54. Complete the following table by providing the generic or brand name for first-generation (typical) and second-generation (atypical) antipsychotic medications.

Generic	Brand
First-generation (typical) antipsychotics	
Chlorpromazine	
	Haldol
	Prolixin
Perphenazine	
Second-generation (atypical) antipsychotics	
Risperidone	
	Zyprexa
	Seroquel
	Geodon
Aripiprazole	
Paliperidone	
	Clozaril
Lurasidone	
	Saphris

55. Typical antipsychotics address ________________________ symptoms by antagonizing D2 receptors in the ________________________ pathway.

56. Atypical antipsychotics antagonize both ________________________ and ________________________ receptors. How does the mechanism of action work to benefit the patient?

57. Patients should not realistically expect full efficacy from antipsychotic medications before ____________ weeks.

58. Three dangerous adverse events associated with typical antipsychotics include: (1) ______________________________, (2) ______________________________, and (3)______________________________.

59. Second-generation antipsychotics are linked to an increased risk of ______________________. Providers should check which labs and measurements to monitor for this issue?

60. What are some high-potency antipsychotics with higher incidence risks of EPS?

61. Which group of patients is most at risk for developing tardive dyskinesia?

62. Therapy is often not recommended to patients with schizophrenia?
    TRUE FALSE

63. General spasms of the face, neck, and tongue are examples of ______________________________.

64. Extrapyramidal symptoms as sequelae of antipsychotic medication that result in resting tremor, rigidity, and bradykinesia are known as ______________________________.

65. Medications for akathisia symptom may include ______________________________ and ______________________________.

66. Dry mouth, dizziness, blurry vision, constipation, and increased body temperature are ______________________________ symptoms.

67. For a patient presenting with symptoms of tardive dyskinesia, the only step is to stop the antipsychotic medication.
    TRUE FALSE

68. A patient presents to the ED with hyperthermia, tachycardia, diaphoresis, muscle rigidity, elevated CPK, and metabolic acidosis. In addition to stopping the offending medication and starting hydration, what two medications would be expected to give? What types of medications are they?

69. Clozapine prescribers must register themselves and their patients with ______ ____ safety program required by the Food and Drug Administration (FDA) due to the drug's potential to cause ____, a life-threatening condition.

9.5 Answers and Explanations to Chapter Activities

1. Psychosis causes skewed reality and information processing problems. A person loses touch with reality, experiencing delusions, hallucinations, disorganized thinking, and strange behaviors.
2. Psychosis has three features:

   - Delusions: Unrealistic notions like believing someone is attempting to hurt you or that you have unique powers regardless of evidence to the contrary..
   - Hallucinations: Hearing voices or seeing things that are not there.
   - Unorganized Cognition and Speech: Can produce confusion, communication problems, and unorganized behavior. Jumping from topic to issue, using illogical words, or answering questions unrelatedly are examples.

3. Answers may vary, but could include: schizophrenia, mania, depression, delirium, dementia, specifically Lewy body dementia, substance use disorders, medication-induced, schizoaffective, bipolar disorder.
4. Answers may vary, but could include: neurological disorders including tumors, migraines, brain bleeds, hypoxia, syphilis, AIDS, nutritional deficiencies, adrenal, thyroid, or calcium abnormalities, MS, SLE, porphyria, dementias, encephalitis.
5.

X	Playful silliness, child-like
X	Bizarre dress, make-up, hair
X	Needs assistance with ADLs
X	Inappropriate comments or behaviors, particularly sexual
X	Misinterprets environmental stimuli, placing significance on mundane

6. To be diagnosed with brief psychotic disorder, a patient must show signs of at least two elements of psychosis for a duration of at least 1 day(s), but less than 1 month(s), with eventual full return to premorbid level of functioning.
7. 1/B, 2/D, 3/G, 4/F, 5/C, 6/A, 7/E
8. Command auditory hallucinations involve hearing nonexistent voices ordering people to perform an act.
9.

Loose association (derailment)	Jumping from one idea to another without a clear connection between them
Tangential	Going off on a tangent and talking about something unrelated to the topic at hand
Circumferential	Providing excessive and unnecessary detail when answering a question or describing a situation, without ever getting to the main point
Word salad	Using words and phrases that do not make sense or are not related to one another
Neologism	Creating new words or using words in a way that is not consistent with their usual meaning
Thought blocking	Suddenly stopping in the middle of a sentence or thought, often because of an interruption in the person's thought process
Perseveration	Repeating a particular word, phrase, or idea over and over again, even if it does not make sense in the context

10. Illusions are misinterpretations of stimuli. Illusions, unlike hallucinations, can be experienced by numerous people with the same physical stimulation.
11.

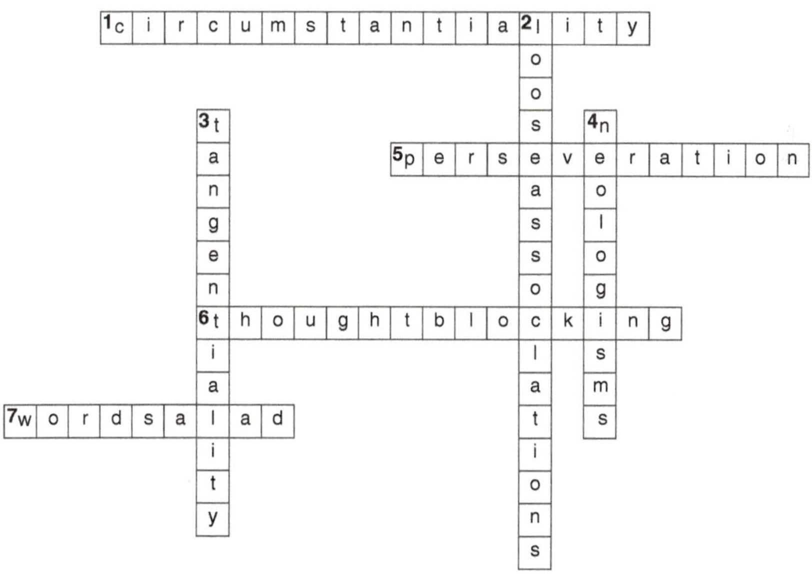

12. Delusions are false beliefs. They are often fixed and unshakable, even in the face of contradictory evidence or logical arguments.

13. Bizarre and nonbizarre delusions are two subtypes of delusions that are differentiated by the plausibility of the belief.

Bizarre delusion	Nonbizarre delusion
Bizarre delusions are those that are completely implausible and could not possibly be true. These delusions involve situations that are completely impossible or defy the laws of physics or nature	Nonbizarre delusions are those that are theoretically possible, but unlikely or improbable. These delusions typically involve situations that could occur in real life, although they may be highly unlikely
Example: A person believing that they are an alien from another planet who has been sent to earth to save humanity	Example: A person may believe that their spouse is cheating on them, even though there is no evidence to support this belief

14. To be diagnosed with delusional disorder, an individual must have nonbizarre delusions for at least 1 month and their life is not significantly impaired.
15. Delusional disorder risk rises after 40. Aging-related brain alterations may cause delusional illness. Family history, social isolation, and trauma or abuse are further risk factors for delusional condition.
16. 1/E, 2/C, 3/I, 4/F, 5/K, 6/H, 7/A, 8/G, 9/D, 10/J, 11/B
17. A uncommon mental disease called folie à deux, or shared psychotic disorder, occurs when two or more close friends share a delusional belief. One partner usually harbors a delusional or grandiose belief that the other then begins to share. People who first experience delusions are called "primary" or "inducer," while others are called "secondary" or "associated."
18. To be diagnosed with schizophrenia per the DSM, an individual must have symptoms for 6 months. Less than this period of time would qualify them for a diagnosis of schizophreniform disorder. Brief psychotic disorder lasts for 1 month or less.
19. FALSE. Schizophrenia is chronic; there is no cure.
20. TRUE. In terms of prevalence of schizophrenia among men and women, the statistics are mostly equal/similar.
21. Men tend to present with symptoms of schizophrenia from 18 to 25 years old. Women have an average onset between 25 and 35 years old.
22. Men with schizophrenia tend to have poorer outcome prognoses and negative symptoms, while women with schizophrenia experience more positive symptoms.
23.

M	Age of onset 18–25 years
W	Age of onset 25–35 years
M	More negative symptoms
W	More paranoid delusions and hallucinations
W	Fewer prodromal symptoms
M	Poorer prognosis
M	Poorer response to medications
W	Fewer neurostructural abnormalities
M	More cognitive impairment

24.

	Positive symptoms	Negative symptoms
Definition	Symptoms that are present when should not be; added to personality Respond well to antipsychotic medications	Symptoms that are missing when should be present, loss of characteristic or functioning. Atypical antipsychotics are better.
Examples	Hallucinations, delusions, disorganized behavior, thoughts, and speech, aggression, mania, paranoia, grandeur, referential thinking	Anhedonia (lack of joy, happy emotions), flat affect, poverty of speech (alogia), avolition or apathy (disinterest), poor attention, lack of insight into illness

25. Negative. These symptoms may be less obvious and unpleasant for the person experiencing them, but they can nonetheless affect daily living. Schizophrenia symptoms can start off good and negative, and some people may have a combination of both. Schizophrenia can also go into remission and recur, and symptoms might fluctuate.
26. Catatonia is characterized by motor abnormalities such as immobility, rigidity, or excessive and odd motor movements, as well as behavioral, cognitive, and emotional disorders. Agitated conduct, confrontational, unpredictable exclamations, repeated motions, unusual postures, muscle rigidity, and lack of mobility are some examples. Catatonia affects up to 30% of schizophrenia patients. Antipsychotics, benzodiazepines, and electroconvulsive treatment are used in severe cases.

27.

Aspect	Examples of findings in schizophrenia
Appearance	Disheveled clothing, poor grooming or hygiene, unusual or inappropriate dress
Speech	Rapid or pressured speech, tangential speech, loose associations or derailment, neologisms or made-up words, incoherent or unintelligible speech
Affect	Flat affect or diminished emotional expressiveness, incongruent affect, blunted affect
Mood	Dysphoric or depressed mood, anxious or fearful mood, euphoric or elated mood
Thought process	Disorganized or tangential thought process, circumstantial thought process, flight of ideas, thought blocking or thought insertion, perseveration or repetition of words or phrases
Thought content	Delusions of persecution, grandiosity, or control, paranoia or suspiciousness, ideas of reference, thought withdrawal or thought broadcasting, obsessions or compulsions
Cognition	Impaired attention or concentration, difficulty with memory or recall, disorientation to time, place, or person, poor insight or judgment
Orientation	Disorientation to time, place, or person
Memory	Impaired immediate or short-term memory, difficulty with remote or long-term memory
Concentration	Poor concentration or distractibility
Abstraction	Difficulty with abstract thinking, such as understanding proverbs or metaphors
Judgment	Poor judgment or impaired decision-making skills

28.

	Definition	Example 1	Example 2
Prodromal	Functional decline prior to first psychotic episode	Withdraw, irritable, interests in unusual groups or belief systems, mumbles to self, self-isolates, collects odd items	Decline in school/work performance, neglected hygiene/personal care
Psychosis	Hallucinations, delusions, and/or disordered thoughts	Disconnection from reality, experiencing external stimuli that are not present to others	Thoughts are unclear, choppy, and content is out of the norm, odd, and lacks coherence in topic and presentation of ideas
Residual	Post-psychosis period, similar to prodromal period in examples	Mild hallucinations or delusions	Social withdrawal and other negative symptoms

29. "Downdrift" describes schizophrenia's detrimental effects on function. Schizophrenia's cognitive and social deficiencies cause a decline in social and vocational functioning. Schizophrenia can cause attention, memory, and executive functioning issues. They may also struggle with social skills like communication and relationships. Schizophrenia patients may struggle to find work, housing, and social connections due to these deficiencies, lowering their quality of life.
30. Studies reveal that schizophrenia patients are more prone to smoke cigarettes and have worse health outcomes. Although nicotine may improve cognitive and negative symptoms in schizophrenia, smoking is more harmful.
31. The dopamine hypothesis of schizophrenia posits that overactivity of dopamine in the mesolimbic pathway may cause positive schizophrenia symptoms including delusions and hallucinations. Other neurotransmitters like glutamate and serotonin may also contribute. Schizophrenia's pathogenesis is complicated and multifactorial, and genetics, environmental stresses, and neurodevelopmental disorders may also contribute.
32. Cannabis, hallucinogens, stimulants. Hallucinogens disrupt perception, emotion, and cognitive processes and can cause odd experiences comparable to schizophrenia. LSD and psilocybin can create visual and auditory hallucinations, delusions, and disturbed thinking. Marijuana and amphetamines can potentially trigger schizophrenia-like symptoms. These substances stimulate brain dopamine.

33.

Pathway	Trek in brain	Symptoms of adverse events
Mesocortical/ prefrontal cortex	Originates in the VTA and projects to the prefrontal cortex	Blocking dopamine in this route might worsen schizophrenia symptoms such as apathy, social isolation, and cognitive impairment. Antipsychotics that block dopamine in this route can cause cognitive dulling, drowsiness, and motor slowness

Pathway	Trek in brain	Symptoms of adverse events
Mesolimbic	Originates in the VTA and projects to the limbic system	Positive schizophrenia symptoms like hallucinations and delusions can result from excessive dopamine activation in this circuit. Antipsychotics that inhibit dopamine in this route may reduce pleasant symptoms but produce sleepiness, weight gain, and metabolic abnormalities
Tuberoinfundibular	Originates in the hypothalamus and projects to the pituitary gland	Blocking dopamine in this route can produce hyperprolactinemia, which can cause gynecomastia, galactorrhea, and sexual and menstrual issues
Nigrostriatal	Originates in the substantia nigra and projects to the striatum	Dopamine blockade in this route causes pseudoparkinsonism and extrapyramidal symptoms (EPS) like tremor, stiffness, slurred speech, akathisia, and dystonia. These side effects can be especially bothersome in elderly folks and those with mobility difficulties

34. The mesolimbic dopamine pathway is linked to positive schizophrenia symptoms. This pathway's dopamine D2 receptors can be blocked by antipsychotics to diminish dopamine signaling, which is thought to cause hallucinations and delusions. Antipsychotics can also disrupt other brain dopamine pathways, however, causing mobility difficulties and cognitive impairment.
35. Schizophrenia's negative symptoms are mostly caused by mesocortical dopamine deficiency. This midbrain-to-prefrontal cortex route is thought to be important for cognitive and emotional processing. Schizophrenia symptoms including social withdrawal, apathy, and limited emotional expressiveness may be caused by dopamine signaling dysregulation in this circuit.
36. Movement-related extrapyramidal symptoms can result from nigrostriatal dopamine pathway blockade. Parkinsonism, which causes tremors, rigidity, and bradykinesia (slow movement), and dystonia, which causes involuntary muscular contractions that induce twisting, repetitive movements, or abnormal postures, might be symptoms. Akathisia, an intense feeling of restlessness and a need to move, and tardive dyskinesia, a movement disorder that can develop after prolonged use of antipsychotics, can also occur.
37. Akathisia is a subjective feeling of restlessness or discomfort and a need to move or pace. Akathisia can be treated by lowering the offending medicine, switching to a new one, or adding a symptom management medication. Behavioral therapies like relaxation and exercise may help manage akathisia.
38. Schizophrenia is linked to dopamine, GABA, glutamate, serotonin, and norepinephrine.
39. If one twin gets schizophrenia, their sibling is at 50% chance. Children of schizophrenic parents have a higher risk of developing schizophrenia than those without, but the exact risk is unknown.

40.

B	Later onset
W	Early onset
W	Poor social support
B	Positive symptoms
W	Family history
B	Few relapses
W	Gradual onset
B	Good social support
W	Male gender
W	Poor premorbid functioning
W	Many relapses
W	Negative symptoms
B	Female gender
B	Acute onset
B	Good premorbid functioning
W	Comorbid substance use
B	Mood symptoms

41. CT and MRI scans of the brains of individuals with schizophrenia are most likely to show enlargement of the ventricles and atrophy of the cortex.
42.

Speech issue	Definition	Patient example quote
Neologism	Newly invented words or phrases that have no meaning	I'm trying to find my zimmerhoodle so I can go to the store"
Echolalia	Repetition of words or phrases spoken by someone else	Interviewer: "What is your name?" patient: "Name...Name...Name."
Clang	Speech patterns based on the sound of words rather than meaning	"I'm as jumpy as a rumble-tumble, it's time to fumble"
Poverty of speech	Reduction in the amount of speech or a lack of spontaneous speech	Interviewer: "Tell me about your interests" patient: "Nothing"
Pressured speech	Increase in rate and volume of speech, often with urgency or pressure	"I need to tell you everything that's happened, and I need to tell you now"
Incoherence	Speech that is disorganized and difficult to follow	"I want to be the future and the past, the present is the present so we must stay fast"
Mutism	Complete lack of speech	No verbal response from patient
Paralogia	Illogical or tangential speech	"I need to buy some apples, but the sky is blue today"

43. Schizoaffective illness combines schizophrenia symptoms like delusions and hallucinations with mood disorder symptoms like depression or mania. Schizoaffective disorder can cause psychosis, sadness, and mania.
44. Schizophreniform illness is similar to schizophrenia but has a shorter duration of symptoms. Schizophreniform disorder is diagnosed when a person has schizophrenia-like symptoms for 1–6 months. If symptoms last longer than 6 months, schizophrenia may be diagnosed.
45. The prognoses of the following psychotic disorders range from mild to severe:

- Brief Psychotic Disorder: This usually lasts less than a month and disappears without therapy. Most people with short psychotic condition recover fully and without long-term disability.

- Schizophreniform Disorder: Like schizophrenia, but with symptoms lasting 1–6 months. Schizophreniform disorder has a better prognosis than schizophrenia, with many patients recovering fully and without long-term damage.
- Schizoaffective Disorder: This complex illness combines schizophrenia and a mood disorder like depression or mania. Schizoaffective disorder has a worse prognosis than schizophreniform disorder, with more relapses and long-term disability.
- Schizophrenia: This serious mental illness is hard to treat. Schizophrenia prognosis varies based on age of start, severity of symptoms, and treatment response. Some people with schizophrenia can control their symptoms and have productive lives, but others may have persistent symptoms and considerable daily functioning impairment.

46. None. Schizophrenia cannot be diagnosed by lab tests. Healthcare practitioners may utilize laboratory tests and imaging investigations to rule out other medical disorders or substance use that may mimic schizophrenia symptoms. The tests may include:

    - Thyroid diseases, vitamin shortages, and infections can induce symptoms similar to schizophrenia. Blood testing can rule them out.
    - Amphetamines, cocaine, and marijuana can produce psychotic symptoms; thus, this urine drug check can detect them.
    - Neuroimaging Studies: MRI or CT scans of the brain can rule out structural abnormalities or brain lesions that cause schizophrenia-like symptoms.
    - Laboratory and imaging tests can help rule out other medical conditions or substance use, but schizophrenia is usually diagnosed based on a thorough evaluation of the individual's symptoms, history, and mental status.

47. TRUE. Many antipsychotics are called neuroleptics because they cause drowsiness, motor slowness, and cognitive dulling. First-generation antipsychotics are called "typical" because they differ from later, second-generation ones, which have different mechanisms of action and fewer neurological adverse effects.
48. Antipsychotic side effects can cause extrapyramidal symptoms (EPS), a set of movement abnormalities that can be treated with different drugs. Three typical EPS medicines are:

    - Benztropine: This anticholinergic reduces EPS symptoms as tremors, rigidity, and dystonia.
    - Diphenhydramine, an antihistamine and anticholinergic, helps lessen EPS like akathisia and dystonia.
    - Amantadine, a dopamine agonist, reduces EPS symptoms like stiffness and akathisia.
    - Long-term antipsychotic usage can develop tardive dyskinesia, a movement disease that can be treated with VMAT2 inhibitors. These drugs limit brain nerve cell release of dopamine and other neurotransmitters, which can diminish involuntary movements like facial tics, tongue protrusion, and limb motions. Current tardive dyskinesia treatments include two VMAT2

inhibitors: valbenazine and deutetrabenazine. Although well-tolerated, these drugs may cause drowsiness, dry mouth, and nausea.

49. 1/C, 2/E, 3/A, 4/F, 5/D, 6/B
50. Typical (first-generation) antipsychotics block dopamine (D2) receptors. Atypical (second-generation) antipsychotics block dopamine (D2) and serotonin (5-HT2A) receptors.
51.

Medication	Potency	Adverse effects	Misc
Chlorpromazine	Low	Orthostatic hypotension Blue-gray skin discoloration Photosensitivity	Used for N/V and intractable hiccups
Thioridazine	Low	Retinitis pigmentosa	
Loxapine	Mid	Seizure risk	Metabolite is antidepressant
Thiothixene	Mid	Ocular pigment changes	
Molindone	Mid		
Perphenazine	Mid		
Haloperidol	High	Dystonia Tardive dyskinesia	Decanoate form available
Fluphenazine	High		Decanoate form available
Trifluoperazine	High		Nonpsychoatic anxiety
Pimozide	High	QTc prolongation Ventricular tachycardia	

52. Complete the following table on atypical, or second-generation, antipsychotics.

Medication	Adverse effects	Misc
Clozapine	Myocarditis Agranulocytosis Seizures Constipation Tachycardia Hypersalivation	Reduces suicide risk Used for treatment refractory schizophrenia
Risperidone	Hyperprolactinemia Gynecomastia Orthostatic hypotension	Decanoate form available
Quetiapine	Sedation Orthostatic hypotension	
Olanzapine	QTc prolongation	Less weight gain Take with 300 kcal food
Ziprasidone	Akathisia	Less weight gain
Aripiprazole		
Paliperidone		Decanoate form available
Asenapine		Orally dissolving tablet
Iloperidone		
Lurasidone		Take with 300 kcal food Used in bipolar depression

53. Labs and vitals may include:

- Weight and BMI: Atypical antipsychotics can cause weight gain and BMI changes, which can raise the risk of diabetes and cardiovascular disease.
- Fasting Blood Glucose and Lipid Levels: Atypical antipsychotics can alter glucose and lipid metabolism, increasing the risk of diabetes and cardiovascular disease.
- Blood Pressure and Heart Rate: Atypical antipsychotics can raise blood pressure and heart rate, increasing the risk of heart attack and stroke.
- Complete Blood Count (CBC) and Liver Function Tests (LFTs): Atypical antipsychotics can influence blood cell counts and liver function; therefore, doctors may monitor these labs to check for side effects.
- Electrocardiogram (ECG): Healthcare practitioners may do an ECG to check heart function and rule out cardiovascular diseases that may worsen with atypical antipsychotics.

54.

Generic	Brand
First-generation (typical) antipsychotics	
Chlorpromazine	Thorazine
Haloperidol	Haldol
Fluphenazine	Prolixin
Perphenazine	Trilafon
Second-generation (atypical) antipsychotics	
Risperidone	Risperdal
Olanzapine	Zyprexa
Quetiapine	Seroquel
Ziprasidone	Geodon
Aripiprazole	Abilify
Paliperidone	Invega
Clozapine	Clozaril
Lurasidone	Latuda
Asenapine	Saphris

55. Most antipsychotics block mesolimbic dopamine D2 receptors to treat positive schizophrenia symptoms. Dopamine signaling in this system decreases, which may cause pleasant symptoms including hallucinations and delusions. Movement difficulties, drowsiness, and cognitive deficits can result from standard antipsychotics blocking dopamine receptors in other brain circuits.
56. Atypical antipsychotics block brain dopamine and serotonin receptors. The antagonism of these receptors may help to address positive and negative symptoms of schizophrenia. Atypical antipsychotics may have a more selective and partial effect on dopamine receptor antagonism. They may be less prone to cause movement difficulties and other extrapyramidal adverse effects while still lowering mesolimbic dopamine signaling and improving positive schizophrenia symptoms. They can treat negative symptoms of schizophrenia and other mood disorders like depression and anxiety by antagonizing serotonin receptors.

57. Antipsychotics won't work fully for 4–6 weeks. However, some people may see symptom alleviation within days of treatment initiation.
58. Three hazardous side effects of conventional antipsychotics:

    - Movement disorders include dystonia, akathisia, parkinsonism, and tardive dyskinesia are extrapyramidal symptoms (EPS).
    - Neuroleptic Malignant Syndrome (NMS): Antipsychotics can cause this rare but deadly illness. Medical treatment is needed for high temperature, muscle rigidity, autonomic instability, and changed mental status.
    - Tardive Dyskinesia (TD): Long-term antipsychotic usage can cause this potentially permanent movement problem. Involuntary facial, tongue, and limb movements can be socially stigmatizing and functionally debilitating.

59. Second-generation (atypical) antipsychotics increase the risk of metabolic syndrome, which includes obesity, high blood pressure, high blood sugar, and dyslipidemia. These diseases can cause cardiovascular disease and other health issues. Healthcare practitioners should evaluate these labs and measures for metabolic syndrome:

    - Fasting glucose levels.
    - HbA1c values.
    - Cholesterol and triglycerides panel.
    - Blood pressure.
    - The BMI.
    - The waist circumference

60. High-potency antipsychotics leading to extrapyramidal symptoms (EPS) include haldol, fluphenazine, trifluoperazine (Stelazine), and thiothixene (Navane).

    - These drugs have a stronger affinity for brain dopamine D2 receptors, which may help them address positive schizophrenia symptoms. They are also more likely to cause dystonia, akathisia, parkinsonism, and tardive dyskinesia.

61. Older, female, long-term antipsychotic users are most likely to develop tardive dyskinesia. History of movement problems, higher cumulative antipsychotic doses, and high-potency antipsychotics are other risk factors. TD can affect any antipsychotic-taking patient, regardless of age, gender, or other risk factors. Involuntary facial, tongue, and limb movements can be socially stigmatizing and functionally debilitating in TD patients.
62. FALSE. Schizophrenia treatment can benefit from therapy. In addition to pharmaceutical treatment, many individuals benefit from CBT, supportive therapy, social skills training, and family therapy. Therapy can help people cope, socialize, manage stress and anxiety, and improve their quality of life. It can also provide a supportive, non-judgmental space for patients to address their problems and collaborate with their healthcare team to optimize their treatment plan.

63. Antipsychotics can cause dystonia, which causes facial, neck, and tongue spasms. Patients may struggle to take the drug because of dystonia's discomfort, agony, and functional impairment.
64. Parkinsonism is resting tremor, stiffness, and bradykinesia caused by extrapyramidal symptoms (EPS) from antipsychotics. First-generation (typical) and high-potency second-generation (atypical) antipsychotics can cause parkinsonism.
65. Medicines for akathisia may include: beta-blockers, benzodiazepines, and anticholinergics like benztropine (Cogentin) and trihexyphenidyl.
66. Anticholinergic symptoms result from acetylcholine suppression, a neurotransmitter that regulates digestion, perspiration, and body temperature.
67. FALSE. Reducing the dose or switching to a less tardive dyskinesia-prone antipsychotic are options. Tetrabenazine (Xenazine), valbenazine (Ingrezza), or deutetrabenazine (Austedo) can cure tardive dyskinesia symptoms.
68. Neuroleptic malignant syndrome (NMS), an uncommon but life-threatening antipsychotic reaction, fits the scenario. Start treating NMS by stopping the offending medicine and providing supportive care, such as hydration and vital signs and metabolic status monitoring. In addition to supportive care, several drugs can treat NMS:

    1. Dantrolene, a skeletal muscle relaxant, reduces hyperthermia and muscle rigidity. Bromocriptine, or amantadine, dopamine agonists, can relieve motor symptoms and shorten NMS.

69. Because clozapine can cause agranulocytosis, a life-threatening white blood cell count deficiency, the FDA requires prescribers and patients to register with the Clozapine REMS (Risk Evaluation and Mitigation Strategy) Program. The Clozapine REMS Program monitors patients' white blood cell counts and absolute neutrophil counts (ANCs) to detect agranulocytosis and guarantee safe clozapine treatment.

References and Resources

American Psychiatric Association, editor. Diagnostic and statistical manual of mental disorders: DSM-5-TR. 5th ed. American Psychiatric Association Publishing; 2022.

Badcock JC, Larøi F, Kamp K, Kelsall-Foreman I, Bucks RS, Weinborn M, Begemann M, Taylor JP, Collerton D, O'Brien JT, El Haj M, Ffytche D, Sommer IE. Hallucinations in older adults: a practical review. Schizophr Bull. 2020;46(6):1382–95. https://doi.org/10.1093/schbul/sbaa073.

Bhutani S, Huremovic D. Folie a deux: shared psychotic disorder in a medical unit. Case Reports in Psychiatry. 2021;2021:5520101.

Bornheimer L, Hong V, Li VJ, Fernandez L, King C. Relationships between hallucinations, delusions, depression, suicide ideation, and plan among adults presenting with psychosis in psychiatric emergency care. Psychosis. 2021;14:1–11. https://doi.org/10.1080/17522439.2021.1912815.

Johnson K, Vanderhoef D, Magrath N. Psychiatric-mental health nurse practitioner review and resource manual. American Nurses Association: American Nurses Credentialing Center; 2020.

Metzl JM. The protest psychosis: how schizophrenia became a black disease. Beacon Press; 2009.
Oh ES, Fong TG, Hshieh TT, Inouye SK. Delirium in older persons: advances in diagnosis and treatment. JAMA. 2017;318(12):1161–74. https://doi.org/10.1001/jama.2017.12067.
Pringle R. Psychosis and schizophrenia: a mental health nurse's perspective. Nurse Prescribing. 2013;11(10):505–9. https://doi.org/10.12968/npre.2013.11.10.505.
Seiler N, Nguyen T, Yung A, O'Donoghue B. Terminology and assessment tools of psychosis: a systematic narrative review. Psychiatry Clin Neurosci. 2020;74:226–46. https://doi.org/10.1111/pcn.12966.
World Health Organization. (2021). Schizophrenia. https://www.who.int/mental_health/management/schizophrenia/en/
Zakhari R. The psychiatric-mental health nurse practitioner certification review manual. Springer Publishing Company; 2021.

Notes:

Notes:

Neurocognitive Disorders and Geriatric Mental Health

10

Test your learning and check your understanding of this book's contents: use the "Springer Nature Flashcards" app to access questions using ▶ https://sn.pub/62J0Ar.

To use the app, please follow the instructions in Chap. 1.

Neurocognitive disorders, also known as cognitive disorders or brain disorders, refer to a group of conditions that affect the brain's ability to function properly. These disorders can affect a person's ability to think, remember, learn, and communicate.

One type of neurocognitive disorder is dementia, which is characterized by a decline in cognitive function. Dementia can be caused by various factors, including Alzheimer's disease, vascular dementia, and Lewy body dementia. Dementia is a significant public health concern, as it affects approximately 50 million people worldwide and is expected to affect over 131 million people by 2050 (Ferri et al. 2005). Alzheimer's disease is characterized by a decline in memory, language, and problem-solving abilities. It is the most common cause of dementia, accounting for approximately 60–80% of cases (Alzheimer's Association 2021). Frontotemporal dementia is characterized by changes in behavior, language, and decision-making abilities. It is often misdiagnosed as Alzheimer's disease due to the overlap in symptoms, but it is a distinct condition with different treatment approaches (Hudson 2014).

Another common neurocognitive disorder is traumatic brain injury (TBI), which can range from mild to severe. TBI can be caused by falls, car accidents, sports-related injuries, and other types of trauma. TBI is a leading cause of disability and death worldwide (Maas et al. 2017).

Strokes can have significant impacts on cognitive function. Strokes occur when blood flow to the brain is disrupted, which can lead to a range of symptoms, including difficulty speaking and understanding language, difficulty with memory and attention, and changes in behavior and personality. Strokes are a leading cause of

T. Stewart, *Psychiatric-Mental Health Nurse Practitioner Program Companion and Board Certification Exam Review Workbook*,
https://doi.org/10.1007/978-3-031-60894-0_10

long-term disability and are associated with a higher risk of developing cognitive decline and dementia (Wang et al. 2017).

Dementia, TBI, and strokes are just a few examples of the many types of neurocognitive disorders that PMHNPs encounter in our practice. PMHNPs may also encounter patients with other neurocognitive disorders, such as Parkinson's disease, multiple sclerosis, and brain tumors. These conditions can all have significant impacts on cognitive function and require specialized care and management. By staying up-to-date on the latest research and treatment approaches, PMHNPs can help our patients manage these conditions and improve their quality of life.

PMHNPs must also understand how neurocognitive issues affect other mental health conditions. Alzheimer's sufferers may experience anxiety and depression due to cognitive impairment. Medication, therapy, and support are possible treatments. To offer the best care for these patients, PMHNPs must typically work alongside neurologists and geriatricians.

Finally, the global elderly population is expected to approach 2 billion by 2050. Age increases the risk of mental health issues. As the older adult population grows, PMHNPs must have the skills and ability to deliver high-quality care to this vulnerable group. Age-related mental health issues include depression, anxiety, and cognitive decline. Older folks may also have persistent medical issues that affect their mental health. PMHNPs with geriatric mental health expertise can evaluate and treat older persons. Medication management, individual and group therapy, and referrals to other healthcare specialists are included. PMHNPs can also educate and support family and caregivers of older adults with mental health issues.

This chapter discusses neurocognitive illnesses like delirium, dementias (Alzheimer's, Lewy body, Pick's disease), and TBIs. Geriatric mental health is also covered. Diagnostic criteria, drugs, side effects, and treatments are provided.

10.1 Foundations of Neurocognitive Disorders

1. Define neurocognitive disorder.

2. Name the six cognitive domains that may be affected by neurocognitive disorders.
    1.
    2.
    3.
    4.
    5.
    6.

3. Neurocognitive disorders are not seen in very young patients.
   TRUE FALSE

4. Match each of the following conditions with neurocognitive impacts with their symptoms profile.

Condition	Symptoms
1. __________CVA or mass or lesion	A. Headache, altered mental status, seizures, visual and auditory deficits, and other neurological symptoms
2. __________Drug intoxication	B. Headache, confusion, altered mental status, seizures, and other neurological symptoms
3. __________Hypertensive encephalopathy	C. Cognitive impairment, memory loss, mood disturbances, and other symptoms depending on the location of the injury
4. __________Hypothyroidism	D. Altered mental status, confusion, hallucinations, delusions, agitation, and other symptoms
5.__________Lewy body disease, Parkinson's disease	E. Tremors, stiffness, gait disturbances, cognitive impairment, Kayser-Fleischer rings, and other symptoms depending on the severity and location of the injury.
6.__________Meningitis	F. Fatigue, weakness, cold intolerance, weight gain, depression, cognitive impairment, and other symptoms
7. __________Neurosyphilis	G. Headache, fever, stiff neck, nausea and vomiting, altered mental status, seizures, and other symptoms
8. __________Normal pressure hydrocephalus	H. Depending on location of injury, hemiplegia, speech disturbances, sensory loss, visual field cuts, altered mental status, and cognitive deficits
9. __________Thyrotoxicosis	I. Nervousness, irritability, tremors, weight loss, palpitations, cognitive impairment, and other symptoms
10. __________Vascular disease	J. Fatigue, weakness, tingling and numbness in the extremities, cognitive impairment, and other symptoms
11. __________Vitamin B12 deficiency	K. Gait disturbances, urinary incontinence, cognitive impairment, and other symptoms
12.__________Wilson's disease	L. Tremors, rigidity, bradykinesia, cognitive impairment, visual hallucinations, and other symptoms

5. What is the key difference between a mild and major neurocognitive disorder?

6. What would move a neurocognitive disorder from mild to major?

10.2 Delirium Foundations

7. ________________________________ presents as short-term cognitive changes, often with quick onset.

8. What are some other terms seen when referring to delirium, even though they may not be correct?

9. Describe each subtype of delirium.

Subtype	Description
Hyperactive	
Hypoactive	
Mixed	

10. Name at least 5 common risk factors for delirium.
    1.
    2.
    3.
    4.
    5.

11. Disorientation to time, place, and sometimes person are signs of ________________________________. Confusion about these changes in consciousness can cause the patient depression and anxiety.

12. Complete and memorize the following table on the mnemonic for DELIRIUM risk factors.

D	
E	
L	
I	
R	
I	
U	
M	

13. Delirium is not a serious disorder once the patient returns to baseline.
    TRUE FALSE

14. ________________________________ refers to worsening of delirium at night. Patients can become scared and combative.

15. Name 3 infections that may cause delirium or dementia signs.
    1.
    2.
    3.

10.3 Dementia Foundations

16. ______________________ often presents as memory impairment without consciousness disturbance.

17. What are 5 cognitive impairments seen commonly in dementia?
    1.
    2.
    3.
    4.
    5.

18. Dementia is often reversible, unlike delirium.

    TRUE FALSE

19. Dementia often affects ______________ hemisphere(s) of the brain, but it depends on the specific type and cause of the dementia.

20. Complete the following table on the common types of dementias. Label each as cortical (C), subcortical (S), or both cortical and subcortical (B).

Name	Description with signs and symptoms	Subtype
Dementia of Alzheimer's type		
Vascular dementia		
Lewy body disease		
Frontotemporal dementia (Pick's disease)		

Name	Description with signs and symptoms	Subtype
Dementia due to HIV disease		
Creutzfeldt-Jakob disease		
Huntington's disease		

21. Motor and affective changes are more common in the ____________________ subtype of dementia.

22. What medical conditions can cause dementia-like signs and symptoms?

23. What is the differential diagnosis if a patient has ingested substances, has personality changes and odd behaviors, but their memory and orientation are intact?

24. It is recommended that individuals 65 years of older in families at risk for dementia should receive a cognitive evaluation every __________ years. Functional motor baseline data may also prove useful.

25. There is a high correlation between dementia and depression.
    TRUE FALSE

10.4 Dementia of Alzheimer's Type

26. What is the neuropathological etiology of Alzheimer's dementia?

27. Which two neurotransmitters are decreased in patients with dementia of Alzheimer's type?

28. There is no genetic loading risk for dementia of Alzheimer's type.
    TRUE FALSE

29. Alzheimer's dementia is associated with abnormalities on chromosomes ______, ______, ______, and ______.

30. Late-onset dementia is linked to alleles for __________, which helps transport cholesterol and lipids. Its causal link to Alzheimer's is not well-understood, however.

31. A patient with dementia of Alzheimer's type may have what neuroanatomical changes visible on an MRI?

32. Which memories do dementia patients typically lose first?

33. A patient may be diagnosed with both delirium and dementia.
TRUE FALSE

10.5 Other Dementias

34. Patients with frontotemporal dementia will present with which symptoms?

35. In this frontal variant of Pick's disease, ______________________________ ______________, hypersexuality, and hyperorality are common.

36. Apraxia, emotional lability, dementia, and flu-like illness should include _____ ____ as a differential diagnosis.

37. ____________________ develops after a minor ischemic event which damages the brain, resulting in cognitive impairment.

38. Dementia with Lewy bodies should be considered if a patient presents with which symptoms?

39. Lewy body dementia is caused by an aggregation of ______________________ ____ in the basal ganglia.

40. What is the etiology of Huntington's disease?

41. In addition to delirium and dementia, the DSM includes six neurocognitive disorders (NCD). List key symptoms that build the diagnostic criteria for each.

Neurocognitive disorder	Key symptoms
Complex attention	
Executive function	
Learning and memory	
Language	
Perceptual motor	
Social cognition	

10.6 Assessment

42. Which of the following are characteristics of delirium (DL) or dementia (DM) or both (B)?
    1. _____Sudden onset
    2. _____Confusion
    3. _____Acute illness
    4. _____Slow progression
    5. _____Speech disturbances
    6. _____Psychomotor changes
    7. _____Rapid change
    8. _____Good and bad days

9. _____Recent memory loss
10. _____Irreversible
11. _____Reversible
12. _____Perceptual disturbances
13. _____Sundowning
14. _____Sleep-wake disturbances
15. _____Mute in final stages.

43. Match the following terms with their definitions. These often accompany delirium and/or dementia.

Term	Definition
_____ 1. Apraxia	A. Language disturbance.
_____ 2. Agnosis	B. Inability to recognize or identify objects.
_____ 3. Aphasia	C. Inability to carry out movements.
_____ 4. Perseveration	D. Repeating same words of phrases.
_____ 5. Asterixis	E. Repetitive uncontrolled eye movements.
_____ 6. Nystagmus	F. Involuntary muscle jerks.
_____ 7. Myoclonus	G. Flapping of wrists.

44. Why might a chest X-ray (CXR) be warranted when investigating delirium?

45. Why is it important to have documentation of an individual's baseline cognitive function?

46. Routine screening for dementia is recommended by the U.S. Preventive Services Task Force.

TRUE FALSE

47. Compare mental status exam findings for a patient with delirium to a patient with dementia.

Mental status exam findings	Delirium	Dementia
General appearance		
Speech		
Thought process		
Thought content		
Concentration		
Judgment		
Abstraction		
Affect		

Mental status exam findings	Delirium	Dementia
Mood		
Orientation		
Memory		

48. The ______________________________ is a highly sensitive and specific tool for evaluating suspected delirium. It assesses inattention, disorganized thinking, and level of consciousness. This instrument is used to assess the severity and fluctuation of delirium on 9 different measures overall.

49. Complete the following table on screening tools in geropsychiatry.

Scale	Assesses	Cut-off scores
Cornell scale for depression in dementia		
Geriatric depression scale (GDS)		
Mini-cog (word recall and clock drawing)		
Mini-mental status exam (MMSE)		
Montreal cognitive assessment (MoCA)		

50. Two cognitive tests for assessing dementia are the ______________________ ______________________________ and the ______________________ ______________________________.

51. The ____ is a screening test for major neurocognitive disorders. It assesses orientation, attention/concentration, language, constructional ability, and immediate and delayed recall. This instrument is used to screen for cognitive impairment over time, but whose score may be affected by a patient's level of education.

52. Complete the table with the score ranges for each level of the MMSE.

Cognitive function	Score
Intact	
Mild	
Moderate	
Severe	

53. A score of ____________ or above on the Montreal Cognitive Assessment (MoCA) is considered normal, or no cognitive decline.

54. The Mini-Cog tool consists of two components: (1) ______________________ ____________________________ and (2) ____________________________ ______________________.

55. What performance on the Mini-Cog would evidence cognitive impairment?

56. What screening tool may be used to determine depression in dementia patients? What score indicates depression on this scale?

57. Rapid plasma reagin (RPR) tests for __________________. Why is this an appropriate test for individuals experiencing neurocognitive changes?

58. The clinical presentation of normal pressure hydrocephalus is described as wobbly, wet, and wacky. What symptoms do these keywords capture?

59. Lewy body dementia cannot be definitively diagnosed until postmortem brain tissue is examined.
    TRUE FALSE.

10.7 Medications and Other Treatments

60. Benzodiazepines are first-line medications for treating delirium and dementia.
    TRUE FALSE

61. What is the first-line medication for treating agitation and psychosis in a patient with delirium? What medications should be avoided?

62. How can a patient's family help to address delirium in a loved one?

63. If delirium is diagnosed, what tests may be ordered to help determine etiology?

64. Medications can stop or reverse Alzheimer's dementia progression.
    TRUE FALSE

65. Most anti-dementia medications work by ______________________________ ______, resulting in increased acetylcholine in the body. Examples include donepezil and rivastigmine.

66. ______________ is a unique anti-dementia medication because it antagonizes NMDA receptors. It is recommended in ____________ cases of Alzheimer's dementia due to fewer side effects.

67. ____________________ may be prescribed to address behavior dysregulation in dementia patients, but are not considered anti-dementia agents.

68. The only SSRI to show efficacy in helping reduce agitation in dementia patients is __________________. However, EKG should be monitored for ______________________________.

69. Vitamin ______ may help to slow Alzheimer's related cognitive decline.

70. ________________________ is the best-tolerated medication among patients with Lewy body dementia, even though it is not an anti-dementia medication.

71. ____ is the preferred TCA for use with elderly patients due to its low anticholinergic side effect profile.

72. ________________________ are usually first-line treatment for frontotemporal dementia, as cholinesterase inhibitors have no effect.

73. ____ symptoms are often treated with tetrabenazine or second-generation antipsychotics.

74. ____________________________________ is the first-line treatment for Parkinson's disease, while ______________________________________ ___medications may worsen Parkinsonian symptoms.

75. Psychotropic medications should be used cautiously in patients with HIV-related dementia if they are also taking _________ or ____________. These latter medications are ___________ inhibitors.

76. What is the typical treatment for normal pressure hydrocephalus?

77. Complete the following table on use of pharmacological agents in treating different dementias.

Class	Mechanism of action	Example medication (brand name)	Target neurocognitive diseases/disorders
Acetylcholinesterase inhibitors		Donepezil (Aricept), Rivastigmine (Exelon), Galantamine (Razadyne)	
NMDA receptor antagonists			Alzheimer's disease
Second-generation antipsychotics	Block dopamine and serotonin receptors		
Antidepressants			
Psychostimulants	Increase dopamine and norepinephrine levels	Methylphenidate (Ritalin)	Cognitive dysfunction associated with multiple sclerosis and post-stroke cognitive impairment

10.8 Geriatric Mental Health

78. Elderly patients who have experienced a myocardial infarction or a stroke are more likely to develop ______________________________. These individuals are 3–4x more likely to die than their peers.

79. What is pseudodementia?

80. ________________________ is the most common mental health disorder in the elderly.

81. Electroconvulsive therapy (ECT) is not safe for use in geriatric populations.

TRUE FALSE

82. Sleep disorders increase with aging.

TRUE FALSE

83. Increased restless leg movements, or periodic leg movements (PLM), are likely due to an imbalance in the neurotransmitter ________________.

84. For elderly patients who report low appetite and sleep disturbances, ________________ is a medication to consider.

85. Elderly patients should not be prescribed stimulants.

TRUE FALSE

86. Why are older individuals more susceptible to the effects of alcohol?

87. Older female patients with cognitive decline and a lack of social support are particularly susceptible to ________________.

88. Most elder abuse is completed by family members, which goes unreported because the patient has fear of retaliation, lack of support, and guilt.

TRUE FALSE.

10.9 Traumatic Brain Injury

89. What qualifies as a traumatic brain injury (TBI)?

90. Name 3–5 examples of TBI and if each would be mild, moderate, or severe.
    1.
    2.
    3.
    4.
    5.

91. ______________________________ is the most common type of TBI.

92. What are 5 causes of traumatic brain injuries?
    1.
    2.
    3.
    4.
    5.

93. What mental health sequelae might manifest after a TBI?

94. For each location of a TBI, provide 3 potential mental health outcomes.

Location of TBI	Mental health outcomes
Frontal lobe	
Temporal lobe	
Parietal lobe	
Occipital lobe	
Brainstem	
Cerebellum	

95. What diagnostic steps might a PMHNP take in order to assess for mental health effects post-TBI?

96. How is a TBI managed?

97. What medications should be avoided or used with caution in clients with TBI?

10.10 Answers and Explanations to Chapter Activities

1. Neurocognitive disorder is a brain damage or disease-related cognitive deterioration. This decrease can impair thinking, reasoning, memory, and communication. The word "neurocognitive" stresses that brain malfunction causes cognitive impairment, not due to aging.
2. The six cognitive domains that may be affected by neurocognitive disorders are as follows:

   1. Complex attention.
   2. Executive function.
   3. Learning and memory.
   4. Language.
   5. Perceptual motor.
   6. Social cognition.
3. FALSE. Neurocognitive disorders can affect anyone, but older people are more likely to develop them. Traumatic brain damage and autism may impact younger people, for example. Children experiencing high fevers and those prescribed anticholinergic medications are vulnerable also. Genetics, environment, diseases, and trauma can create neurocognitive issues. Neurocognitive diseases should be considered in individuals of all ages who show indicators of cognitive impairment or decline and assessed to determine the cause and treatment approach.
4. 1/H, 2/D, 3/B, 4/F, 5/L, 6/G, 7/A, 8/K, 9/I, 10/C, 11/J, 12/E (Fig. 10.1)
5. Mild neurocognitive disorder (formerly mild cognitive impairment) causes cognitive impairments without daily functioning problems. Cognitive decline from major neurocognitive disorder (formerly dementia) impacts memory, language, attention, and executive function. Individuals with serious neurocognitive impairments require assistance with ADLs.

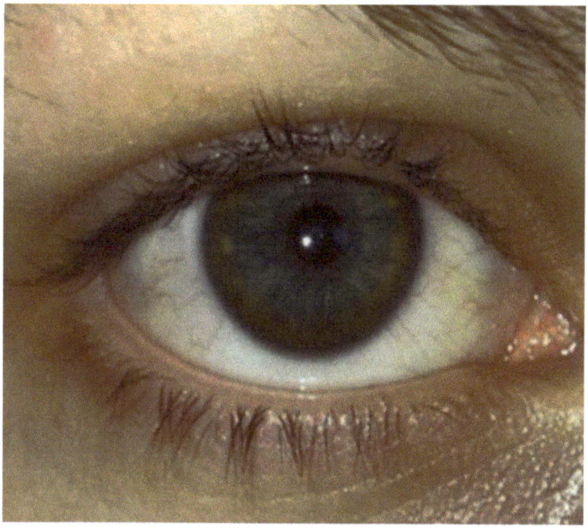

Fig. 10.1 Kayser-Fleischer Rings (From: Moraru, L.; Budianu, M.; Musteață, I.; Voidazan, T.S. Epidemiological Study on a Wilson Disease Group of Patients. Preprints 2024, 2,024,030,696. https://doi.org/10.20944/preprints202403.0696.v1. Under CC BY 4.0 DEED https://creativecommons.org/licenses/by/4.0/)

6. Disorder symptoms worsen and persist. Cognitive decline that hinders daily tasks including finances, self-care, and work is a serious neurocognitive disorder. Major neurocognitive illnesses cause memory loss, language and communication impairments, reasoning and judgment issues, and personality and behavior changes. These symptoms can impair independence and require extra care.
7. Delirium. Delirium causes confusion, disorientation, agitation, hallucinations, and sleep-wake disorders. Delirium can cause falls, hospital admissions, and death.
8. Altered mental status, encephalopathy, acute brain syndrome, acute toxic psychosis.
9.

Subtype	Description
Hyperactive	Hyperactive delirium causes agitation, restlessness, and psychomotor activity. Patients with hyperactive delirium may pace, fidget, and pull at their tubes or dressings. Delusions and hallucinations may also make it harder for them to stay in bed.
Hypoactive	Hypoactive delirium reduces arousal and activity. The hypoactive delirium patient may appear withdrawn, lethargic, or unresponsive. They may have trouble staying awake or following discussions and speak or move slowly. Patients may not show the same agitation or behavioral abnormalities as in hyperactive delirium, making it difficult to diagnose.
Mixed	Hyperactive and hypoactive signs characterize mixed delirium. Mixed delirium patients may have moments of agitation and lethargy. Their symptoms may include disorientation, confusion, and sleep-wake abnormalities.

10. Common delirium risk factors are as follows:

    - Delirium is more common in older people, especially over 65 years.
    - People with dementia or mild cognitive impairment are more prone to have delirium.
    - Chronic diseases: Heart disease, diabetes, and COPD increase delirium risk.
    - Long-term hospitalization raises delirium risk.
    - Major surgery, especially in the elderly, can produce delirium.
    - Drugs like sedatives and painkillers can produce delirium.
    - Victims of alcohol or benzodiazepine addiction are more likely to develop delirium.
    - Sleep deprivation, sensory impairment, stress, and trauma can cause delirium. These risk variables must be minimized by healthcare practitioners to reduce delirium risk in sensitive individuals.

11. Cognitive impairment, including delirium, dementia, or stroke.
12.

D	Drugs
E	Electrolytes/emotional disturbances
L	Low O_2/lack of medication
I	Infection
R	Reduced sensory input/retention
I	Intracranial/ictal/infection
U	Undernutrition
M	Myocardial/metabolic

13. FALSE. Delirium treatment may cause cognitive impairment or other issues. Within a year, delirium nearly doubles injury or nosocomial infection mortality, such as pneumonia or hunger.
14. Dementia and other cognitive issues worsen delirium at night, called sundowning. Patients may become confused, worried, fearful, or combative and have difficulties sleeping or wandering. Patients and caregivers may struggle due to circadian rhythm disturbances, sensory overload, and other difficulties. Sundowning can be managed by treating medical issues, creating a tranquil and predictable environment, limiting sensory input, and encouraging relaxation and sleep hygiene. Medications can treat symptoms and regulate sleep-wake cycles.
15. Examples include the following:

    - UTIs.
    - Pneumonia.
    - Sepsis.
    - HIV/AIDS.
    - Meningitis.
    - Encephalitis.
    - Lyme disease.
    - Syphilis.

16. Memory loss without consciousness disturbance is dementia. There is no cure for dementia, but therapies and interventions can help patients and family manage symptoms and enhance quality of life.
17. In dementia, cognitive abnormalities might arise, such as:

- Memory loss is a frequent early dementia sign. Patients may recall past events but not recent ones.
- Patients may struggle with words, a debate, or written or spoken language.
- Poor judgment and decision-making: Patients may struggle to solve problems, estimate risks, and make decisions.
- Patients may struggle with depth perception, distance measurement, and face recognition.
- Patients may struggle to focus or follow directions.
- Impaired executive function: Patients may have trouble planning, organizing, starting, and monitoring their activity and adapting to changes.
- Psychological symptoms: Agitation, apathy, anger, and depression may occur.
- Disorientation: Patients may lose track of time, place, or identity.

18. FALSE. Delirium is often reversible, while dementia is not.
19. 2 (both) hemispheres
20.

Name	Description with signs and symptoms	Subtype
Dementia of Alzheimer's type	Memory loss, progressive, amyloid deposits, neurofibrillary tangles	C
Vascular dementia	Can see changes in mood, due to infarcts in cerebral vessels from cardiovascular disease and HTN	B
Lewy body disease	Visual hallucinations coupled with parkinsonian-like psychomotor signs, fast onset, cortical inclusions, antipsychotics not effective	B
Frontotemporal dementia (Pick's disease)	Sexual inappropriateness, odd social behavior, aphasia, often not affecting memory, see loss of neurons, seen more in men	C
Dementia due to HIV disease	Combination of cognitive, motor, affective, and behavioral decline, vascular abnormalities, death within 6 months, may manifest in seizures, hallucinations, OCD, bipolar depression symptoms	S
Creutzfeldt-Jakob disease	Fatal <6 months after initial symptoms, presents as influenza with cognitive impairment, neurological deficits, and psychiatric symptoms	C
Huntington's disease	Genetic disorder, progressive jerky motor movements in shoulders, arms, face, high incidence of suicide, retains memory and language abilities	S

21. Motor and affective changes are more common in the subcortical subtype of dementia.
22. Several medical conditions can cause dementia-like symptoms:

- Hypo- or hyperthyroid.
- B1, B12, or folate deficiencies.

- Brain tumors, infections.
- Parkinson's, Huntington's, multiple sclerosis.
- Normal pressure hydrocephalus.
- Brain injury.
- Chronic alcoholism with HIV/AIDS.
- Cancers.
- Metabolic issues.
- Infections.
- Ketoacidosis.

23. The differential diagnosis is acute intoxication, substance-induced mood illness, psychosis, or delusional disorder. To assess symptoms, PMHNPs must obtain a comprehensive substance use history, physical exam, and lab tests.
24. 3 years
25. TRUE. Half of dementia sufferers are depressed.
26. Neuronal **β**-amyloid plaques and neurofibrillary tangles (i.e., **τ**-protein accumulations) in neurons cause Alzheimer's dementia. Due to these two abnormal structures obstructing communication, neurons misfire and die. Presenilin-1 or presenilin-2 may contribute. Apolipoprotein gene polymorphism promotes early-onset Alzheimer's. Lifestyle, genetics, and environment can cause Alzheimer's.
27. Alzheimer's lowers acetylcholine and norepinephrine.
28. FALSE. Dementia risk threatens first-order relatives. Early detection and intervention are needed for at-risk households.
29. Chromosomes 1, 14, 19, 21.
30. Late-onset dementia is linked to cholesterol-transporting APOE alleles. The ε4 allele of APOE is associated with an increased risk of Alzheimer's disease, although the mechanism remains unknown.
31. Alzheimer's patients' MRIs may show neuroanatomical changes like:

    - Shrinkage of the hippocampus: Memory development requires it. MRI shows the hippocampus shrinking first in Alzheimer's disease.
    - The fluid-filled brain ventricles enlarge to cushion and protect the brain. Alzheimer's disease shrinks brain tissue, making ventricles appear larger on MRIs.
    - Decreased cortical brain tissue: The cortex governs thought, language, and perception. MRIs may show a thinner cortex in Alzheimer's disease, indicating brain tissue loss.
    - Alzheimer's disease produces brain protein buildup and amyloid plaques and neurofibrillary tangles. Brain tissue can show these deposits after death or with other imaging modalities, but not on an MRI.

32. Dementia patients lose recent memories first.
33. TRUE. If an acute illness or drug change induces delirium, a dementia patient may be diagnosed with both.

34. Symptoms of FTD include psychological changes such as:

 - Indifference, disinhibition, inappropriate social behavior, and lack of empathy.
 - Language and communication difficulties such as wordlessness, stuttering, and misspeaking.
 - Poor planning, problem-solving, and decision-making.
 - Lack of interest in hobbies.
 - Hoarding, excessive eating, and later-stage motor symptoms such as muscle weakness, stiffness, and tremors may indicate the condition.
 - Lack of impulse control, hyperorality (sweets), hypersexuality (touching, propositioning), aphasia

35. Kluver-Bucy syndrome.
36. Creutzfeldt-Jakob disease.
37. Vascular dementia.
38. Dementia with Lewy bodies (DLB) should be considered if a patient presents with the following symptoms:

 - Fluctuating cognition.
 - Visual hallucinations.
 - Parkinsonism (e.g., tremors, stiffness, slow movement).
 - REM sleep behavior disorder (e.g., acting out dreams during sleep).
 - Severe sensitivity to antipsychotic medications.

39. α-synuclein
40. HTT protein trinucleotide (CAG) repeats in the Huntingtin gene on chromosome 4 causing Huntington's disease. The mutation creates huntingtin, a defective protein that causes neurodegeneration in brain neurons. The mechanism is unknown, but mitochondrial function, transcriptional regulation, and axonal transport may be affected. Huntington's disease usually affects the cortex and basal ganglia, which control cognition and perception and coordinate movement. Cognitive decline, mobility limitations, and mental concerns develop in midlife. Therapy can manage symptoms and enhance quality of life, but Huntington's disease has no cure.
41.

Neurocognitive disorder	Key symptoms
Complex attention	Change in ability to sustain attention and speed to process information
Executive function	Decline in planning, decision-making, working memory, and inhibitions
Learning and memory	Decline in memory and recall
Language	Notable changes in fluency, reception, expression, word use, labeling
Perceptual motor	Visual and tactile perception decreases, motor praxis manipulation less fine-tuned
Social cognition	Emotional dysregulation

42. __DL____Sudden onset
__B____Confusion.
__DL____Acute illness.
__DM____Slow progression.
__B___Speech disturbances.
__DL___Psychomotor changes.
__DL___Rapid change.
__DM___Good and bad days.
__DM___Recent memory loss.
__DM___Irreversible.
__DL___Reversible.
__DL___Perceptual disturbances.
__DL___Sundowning.
__B___Sleep-wake disturbances.
__DM___Mute in final stages
43. 1/C, 2/B, 3/A, 4/D, 5/G, 6/E, 7/F
44. Pneumonia can produce delirium, requiring a chest X-ray. Occasionally, a chest X-ray may detect respiratory disorders causing delirium. COPD and other chronic lung illnesses may increase the likelihood of delirium during an acute exacerbation.
45. Baseline cognitive function aids cognitive disease progression analysis. Baseline information may include cognitive capacity, memory, language, and other cognitive functions.
46. FALSE. Routine cognitive impairment or dementia screening is not recommended by recent USPSTF guidelines. They recommend screening for cognitive impairment in persons with symptoms and considering the risks and benefits individually.
47.

Mental status exam findings	Delirium	Dementia
General appearance	May appear agitated, restless, or lethargic. Example: May pace back and forth, or appear drowsy or unresponsive.	May appear alert, but with gradual decline in grooming, hygiene, and self-care. Example: May wear soiled clothing or forget to bathe or groom.
Speech	May be rapid or slow, with slurred or nonsensical speech. Example. May speak incoherently or use words that do not make sense.	May be slow, with difficulty finding the right words or expressing themselves. Example: May have a limited vocabulary or use repetitive phrases.
Thought process	Disorganized, with rapid or tangential thoughts, or disorientation to time, place, or person. Example: May jump between unrelated topics or make nonsensical statements.	Disorganized, with gradual loss of ability to plan, organize, or problem-solve. Example: May have difficulty making decisions or solving simple problems.

Mental status exam findings	Delirium	Dementia
Thought content	May have delusions or hallucinations, or be preoccupied with fear or paranoia. Example: May believe that they are being followed or that someone is trying to harm them.	May have difficulty distinguishing reality from fantasy, but typically do not have delusions or hallucinations. Example: May have difficulty recognizing familiar people or places, or may be confused about time or location.
Concentration	Impaired, with difficulty focusing and sustaining attention. Example: May have a short attention span or be easily distracted.	Impaired, with difficulty following complex instructions or completing multi-step tasks. Example: May forget what they were doing or lose track of their thoughts.
Judgment	Impaired, with difficulty making decisions or solving problems. Example: May make poor decisions or engage in risky behavior.	Impaired, with difficulty planning or organizing daily activities. Example: May forget to take medication or engage in other self-care activities.
Abstraction	Impaired, with difficulty understanding abstract concepts or making associations. Example: May be unable to recognize similarities between objects or understand metaphors.	Impaired, with difficulty with higher-level thinking or reasoning. Example: May have difficulty with simple arithmetic or following directions.
Affect	May have a labile or flat affect. Example: May exhibit inappropriate or exaggerated emotional responses, or may have a blunted emotional response.	May have a blunted or flattened affect. Example: May appear indifferent or apathetic, or may have a reduced range of emotional expression.
Mood	May have a dysphoric or anxious mood. Example: May exhibit signs of depression or anxiety, or may appear restless or agitated.	May have a flat or apathetic mood. Example: May appear indifferent or disinterested in their environment.
Orientation	Disoriented to time, place, or person. Example: May not know their name, where they are, or what day it is.	Gradual loss of orientation, starting with time and progressing to place and person. Example: May forget the date or time, then become confused about their location, and eventually forget familiar people.
Memory	Impaired, with difficulty forming new memories or recalling recent events. Example: May forget conversations or events that occurred a few hours or days ago.	Impaired, with difficulty forming new memories and recalling past events. Example: May forget important life events or personal details from their past.

48. The Confusion Assessment Method (CAM) detects probable delirium with high sensitivity and specificity. It evaluates awareness, inattention, and disorder.

49.

Scale	Assesses	Cut-off scores
Cornell scale for depression in dementia	Depression in elderly adults with dementia	>12 possible depression
Geriatric depression scale (GDS)	Depression	>10 needs follow-up
Mini-cog (word recall and clock drawing)	Cognitive impairment	0–2 word recall and abnormal clock = impairment 1–2 word recall and normal clock = none 3 words = no dementia
Mini-mental status exam (MMSE)	Cognitive impairment	<24 mild, <20 moderate, <9 severe
Montreal cognitive assessment (MoCA)	Cognitive decline	>26 normal

50. Two cognitive tests for assessing dementia are the Mini-Mental State Examination (MMSE) and the Montreal Cognitive Assessment (MoCA).
51. Mini-Mental State Examination (MMSE) detects severe neurocognitive deficits. MMSE tests are often given to older persons and those suspected of cognitive impairment. Easy to administer, the exam takes 10 minutes. Cognitive domains are tested with questions and tasks. These include time and place orientation, attention, focus, language, visuospatial ability, and immediate and delayed memory. The MMSE can diagnose Alzheimer's, vascular dementia, and other neurocognitive disorders with excellent sensitivity and specificity.
52.

Cognitive function	Score
Intact	25–30
Mild	21–24
Moderate	10–20
Severe	<9

53. 26 out of 30
54. The Mini-Cog comprises three-item recall and clock-drawing tests. The three-item memory test requires recalling and repeating three unrelated words after a pause. Sketching a clock face and arranging the hands is the clock-drawing test. The Mini-Cog cognitive impairment testing takes around five minutes. The Mini-Cog reliably and correctly detects cognitive impairment, including dementia, in primary care offices, clinics, and hospitals.
55. Missing 0/3 words on recall, or missing 1–2 words on recall and an abnormal clock-drawing test.

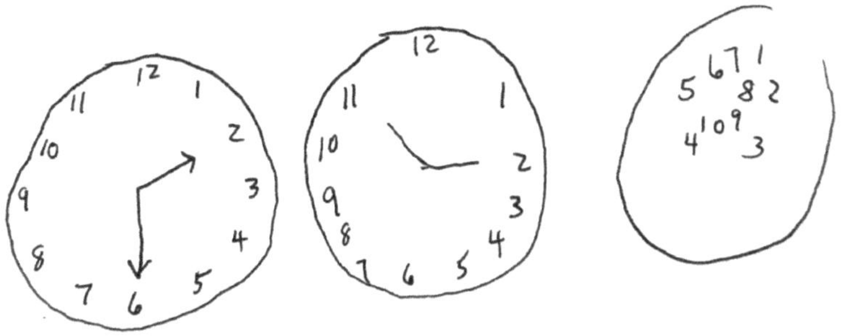

Normal Early Alzheimer's Dementia Late Alzheimer's Dementia

56. The Cornell Scale for Depression in Dementia is a screening tool used to determine depression in dementia patients. A score of 12 or higher on this scale indicates depression in dementia patients.
57. RPR tests for Treponema pallidum-caused syphilis. The blood RPR test reveals bacterium-induced antibodies. Syphilis can affect the brain and neurological system. Confusion, behavioral abnormalities, and coordination and balance difficulties may emerge as the infection progresses.
58. "Wobbly" refers to gait instability, "wet" to urinary incontinence, and "wacky" to cognitive impairment such as dementia, memory loss, and psychiatric issues like hallucinations or delusions.
59. TRUE. Postmortem brain tissue testing confirms Lewy body dementia diagnosis.
60. FALSE. Benzodiazepines tend to worsen disorientation and cognitive impairment; hence, they are rarely used to treat delirium and dementia.
61. Haloperidol is the first-line treatment for delirium-related agitation and psychosis. Avoid anticholinergics and benzodiazepines, which might worsen delirium.
62. To assist loved ones with delirium, family members should:

    - Report symptoms to hospital workers.
    - Reassuring delirium patients: They may feel scared, nervous, and bewildered. Family members can comfort patients.
    - Bring home comforts: Family photos, blankets, and other items might help orient and comfort the patient.
    - Reorientation: Talking, playing games, or physical treatment may minimize delirium symptoms.
    - Best sleep habits: Reduce noise and light, adopt a sleep regimen, and relax to promote sleep and prevent delirium.
    - Family involvement in discharge planning can help ensure that their loved one's care plan includes follow-up appointments, medication monitoring, and environmental adjustments to prevent delirium.
    - Visit often, talk to patient, post time and date, help with meals and water, stimulate patient, add personal touches.

63. Blood glucose, O_2 saturation, arterial blood gases, ECG, CMP, CBC, UA and culture, drug screen, therapeutic medication levels, thyroid hormone, liver function tests, head CT and/or lumbar puncture if neurological deficit.
64. FALSE. Alzheimer's disease has no cure; however, drugs can slow its course and alleviate symptoms.
65. Inhibiting cholinesterase.
66. Memantine; severe.
67. Use antipsychotics with caution in dementia patients due to an increased risk of stroke and mortality. For dementia behavioral and psychological symptoms, nonpharmacological therapies should be explored first, and antipsychotics should only be used if they fail and the benefits outweigh the dangers.
68. Citalopram; QTC prolongation.
69. Vitamin E.
70. Quetiapine.
71. Nortriptyline.
72. SSRIs or other serotonergic medications.
73. Huntington's disease.
74. Carbidopa-Levodopa; antipsychotic (dopamine antagonist).
75. HIV patients with dementia using protease inhibitors or NNRTIs should use psychotropic medicines cautiously. Some medications inhibit CYP3A4.
76. A ventriculoperitoneal shunt drains CSF from the brain to the abdomen to treat normal pressure hydrocephalus. The shunt may need to be replaced over time to work properly.
77.

Class	Mechanism of action	Example medication (brand name)	Target neurocognitive diseases/disorders
Acetylcholinesterase inhibitors	Inhibit acetylcholinesterase which breaks down acetylcholine	Donepezil (Aricept), Rivastigmine (Exelon), Galantamine (Razadyne)	Alzheimer's disease and dementia-associated with Parkinson's disease
NMDA receptor antagonists	Blocks NMDA receptors and inhibits glutamate action	Memantine (Namenda)	Alzheimer's disease
Second-generation antipsychotics	Block dopamine and serotonin receptors	Quetiapine (Seroquel)	Behavioral and psychological symptoms of dementia (BPSD)
Antidepressants	Increase monoamine neurotransmitter levels	Sertraline (Zoloft)	Dementia-related depression and anxiety
Psychostimulants	Increase dopamine and norepinephrine levels	Methylphenidate (Ritalin)	Cognitive dysfunction associated with multiple sclerosis and post-stroke cognitive impairment

78. Depression; they are also at increased risk of vascular dementia.
79. Pseudodementia is a disorder in which depression causes dementia symptoms including memory loss and cognitive deterioration. Since "pseudo" implies false, pseudodementia is false dementia. Depression medication can alleviate cognitive symptoms in pseudodementia. Because of treatment differences, pseudodementia and dementia must be distinguished. Depression requires psychotherapy, medicine, or both, while dementia may require medication and supportive care.
80. Major depressive disorder.
81. FALSE. ECT can be safe and effective in senior patients, but medical and psychological comorbidities must be considered. However, it is contraindicated in patients with dementia as it can induce short-term memory loss.
82. TRUE. Sleep disorders include insomnia, decreased REM, daytime napping, sleep apnea, and restless leg syndrome are more common in older persons.
83. Dopamine.
84. Mirtazapine (Remeron),
85. FALSE. If needed, older people can be given stimulants. Consider the risks and advantages and start the treatment at a modest dose. Recent research reveals stimulants do not worsen cardiac incidents.
86. Body composition, water content, and liver function make older persons more alcohol-sensitive. Increasing body fat and decreasing body water content as people age raises their blood alcohol concentration after drinking the same amount. Alcohol metabolism slows and stays in the blood when liver function declines with age. Long-term alcohol usage can cause cognitive impairment, falls, and other health difficulties.
87. Elder abuse.
88. TRUE.
89. TBIs are brain injuries caused by bumps, blows, or jolts to the head or penetrating head injuries that affect brain function. Its symptoms can range from modest (short changes in consciousness or mental status) to severe (long unconsciousness or memory loss).
90.
    - Concussion—mild.
    - Contusion—moderate to severe.
    - Diffuse axonal injury—severe.
    - Penetration injury—severe.
    - Coup-contrecoup injury—severe.
    - Shaken baby syndrome—severe.
    - Anoxic brain injury—severe.
    - Toxic brain injury—mild to severe.
    - Hypoxic brain injury—mild to severe.
    - Secondary impact syndrome—severe.
91. Concussion.

92. Traumatic brain injuries (TBIs) can be caused by a variety of factors, including:

- Falls (the most common cause of TBIs).
- Motor vehicle accidents.
- Sports-related injuries.
- Violence (such as gunshot wounds or physical assaults).
- Explosive blasts (such as those experienced by military personnel).
- Shaken baby syndrome.
- Penetrating injuries (such as from a sharp object).
- Medical procedures (such as surgeries).
- Drug overdoses.
- Electric shock or lightning strikes.

93. A TBI can result in a range of mental health sequelae. These can include:

- Cognitive impairment, such as difficulty with attention, memory, and executive functioning.
- Mood disorders, including depression and anxiety.
- Behavioral changes, such as irritability, impulsivity, and aggression.
- Post-traumatic stress disorder (PTSD).
- Substance use disorders, particularly alcohol and other drugs used to cope with TBI symptoms.
- Personality changes, including decreased empathy and increased self-centeredness.
- Insomnia and other sleep disturbances.

94.

Location of TBI	Mental health outcomes
Frontal lobe	Impulsivity, poor judgment, mood lability, decreased initiation and motivation, difficulty with executive functioning (planning, organizing, problem-solving)
Temporal lobe	Aggression, impulsivity, irritability, memory difficulties (both short- and long-term), difficulty recognizing faces or objects, difficulty with language comprehension and expression
Parietal lobe	Difficulty with sensory processing, difficulty with spatial orientation, difficulty with reading and writing, difficulty with math calculations
Occipital lobe	Visual disturbances, difficulty with reading and writing, difficulty with color identification and contrast sensitivity, difficulty with depth perception
Brainstem	Difficulty with arousal, vegetative functions (e.g., breathing, heart rate), cranial nerve deficits
Cerebellum	Difficulty with balance, coordination, fine motor movements

95. A PMHNP may diagnose post-TBI mental health problems using the following steps:

- Reviewing medical history: If the patient has a history of brain injury, the PMHNP will look for risk factors for TBI-related mental health issues.
- A physical exam will assess for neurological impairments, balance, coordination, and other TBI symptoms.
- Image studies: CT scans and MRIs may be ordered to assess brain injury and structural abnormalities.
- Neuropsychological testing provides a complete examination of cognitive, behavioral, and emotional functioning. It measures brain damage and cognitive deficiencies.
- Mental health assessment: A mental health assessment evaluates TBI-related emotional or behavioral issues such as depression, anxiety, and PTSD. Clinical interviews, screening questionnaires, and patient behavior observation may be used.
- Refer to specialist: PMHNPs may refer TBI patients to specialists for examination and therapy. A neuropsychologist, neurologist, or rehabilitation specialist may be needed, depending on the patient's symptoms.

96. TBI severity may affect treatment. Patient stabilization, oxygenation, blood flow, and damage prevention are the main goals of first care. Surgery may lessen brain edema and pressure if the injury is severe. A TBI recovery team may include a neurologist, physical therapist, occupational therapist, speech therapist, and neuropsychologist. Rehabilitation may include physical activity, cognitive treatment, and emotional support to assist the patient adjust to life changes. Depending on symptoms, the PMHNP may employ psychotherapy and antidepressants, anxiolytics, or antipsychotics for mental health impacts. The PMHNP may also assess TBI-related cognitive deficits and mood swings.
97. Certain drugs can worsen symptoms or cause complications in people with traumatic brain injuries (TBIs). These drugs include:

- A benzodiazepine, used to treat anxiety and agitation, can increase the risk of disorientation, cognitive impairment, and falls in TBI patients.
- Anticholinergic medications treat allergies, Parkinson's disease, and urine incontinence. They may cause cognitive impairment, confusion, and delirium in older persons and TBI patients.
- Opioids, often recommended for pain management, can induce cognitive impairment, dizziness, and falls, which are especially risky for TBI patients.
- Tricyclic antidepressants: Used to treat depression, anxiety, and chronic pain, these medicines can cause confusion, cognitive impairment, and falls in TBI patients.
- Antipsychotics: Used to treat agitation and violence in TBI patients, these medicines can produce cognitive impairment, drowsiness, and other adverse effects that worsen symptoms.

References and Resources

Alzheimer's Association. (2021). Alzheimer's disease facts and figures. https://www.alz.org/alzheimers-dementia/facts-figures.

American Psychiatric Association, editor. Diagnostic and statistical manual of mental disorders: DSM-5-TR. 5th ed. American Psychiatric Association Publishing; 2022.

Cerveira CCT, Pupo CC, Dos Santos SDS, Santos JEM. Delirium in the elderly: a systematic review of pharmacological and non-pharmacological treatments. Dement Neuropsychol. 2017;11(3):270–5. https://doi.org/10.1590/1980-57642016dn11-030009.

Downing LJ, Caprio TV, Lyness JM. Geriatric psychiatry review: differential diagnosis and treatment of the 3 D's - delirium, dementia, and depression. Curr Psychiatry Rep. 2013;15(6):365. https://doi.org/10.1007/s11920-013-0365-4.

Ferri CP, Prince M, Brayne C, Brodaty H, Fratiglioni L, Ganguli M, Guerchet M. Global prevalence of dementia: a Delphi consensus study. Lancet. 2005;366(9503):2112–7. https://doi.org/10.1016/S0140-6736(05)67889-0.

Hudson B. Understanding Alzheimer's disease: A comprehensive review. J Geriatr Psychiatry Neurol. 2014;27(3):128–39. https://doi.org/10.1177/0891988714524622.

Johnson K, Vanderhoef D, Magrath N. Psychiatric-mental health nurse practitioner review and resource manual. American Nurses Association: American Nurses Credentialing Center; 2020.

Kuźma E, Lourida I, Moore SF, Levine DA, Ukoumunne OC, Llewellyn DJ. Stroke and dementia risk: a systematic review and meta-analysis. Alzheimers Dement. 2018;14(11):1416–26. https://doi.org/10.1016/j.jalz.2018.06.3061.

Maas AI, Menon DK, Adelson PD, Andelic N, Bell MJ, Belli A, Wu T. Traumatic brain injury: integrated approaches to improve prevention, clinical care, and research. Lancet Neurol. 2017;16(4):455–516. https://doi.org/10.1016/S1474-4422(17)30371-X.

Mohandas E, Rajmohan V. Frontotemporal dementia: an updated overview. Indian J Psychiatry. 2009;51 Suppl 1(Suppl1):S65–9.

Nash M, Foidel S, editors. Neurocognitive behavioral disorders: an interdisciplinary approach to patient-centered care. Springer Nature; 2019.

Piscopo P, Crestini A, Carbone E, Rivabene R, Ancidoni A, Lo Giudice M, Corbo M, Vanacore N, Lacorte E. A systematic review on drugs for synaptic plasticity in the treatment of dementia. Ageing Res Rev. 2022;81(101726):101726. https://doi.org/10.1016/j.arr.2022.101726.

Prendergast NT, Tiberio PJ, Girard TD. Treatment of delirium during critical illness. Annu Rev Med. 2022;73(1):407–21. https://doi.org/10.1146/annurev-med-042220-013015.

Simoes E, Justino JD. HIV-associated neurocognitive disorders: a review for NPs. Nurse Pract. 2015;40(7):1–7. https://doi.org/10.1097/01.NPR.0000466501.42049.99.

Wang H, Peng Y, Wang Y, Xu Y, Zhang Y, Zhao J, et al. Stroke and its relationship with disability and cognitive decline in older adults. Stroke. 2017;48(1):102–8. https://doi.org/10.1161/STROKEAHA.116.014909.

Zakhari R. The psychiatric-mental health nurse practitioner certification review manual. Springer Publishing Company; 2021.

Notes:

Notes:

Substance-Related and Addictive Disorders 11

Test your learning and check your understanding of this book's contents: use the "Springer Nature Flashcards" app to access questions using ▶ https://sn.pub/62J0Ar.

To use the app, please follow the instructions in Chap. 1.

Substance-related disorders are characterized by a pattern of impaired control over substance use, leading to significant negative physical, emotional, and social consequences for individuals and their families (American Psychiatric Association 2022). Further, substance-related disorders and addictions are significant public health issues. According to data from the National Highway Traffic Safety Administration (NHTSA), in 2020, there were 10,265 deaths in alcohol-impaired-driving crashes in the United States. This accounted for 28% of all traffic fatalities that year. Drug overdose deaths in the United States have been on the rise in recent years as well. In 2020, the CDC reported that there were almost 67,500 drug overdose deaths in the United States. The majority of these deaths were caused by opioids, including prescription painkillers and illicit drugs like heroin and fentanyl.

These disorders can include substance abuse, substance dependence, and substance-induced disorders. Substance abuse refers to the use of a substance in a manner that is harmful to oneself or others, such as driving under the influence or engaging in risky sexual behavior. Substance dependence refers to a more severe form of substance abuse, characterized by a strong craving for the substance and the inability to control use even when it causes negative consequences. Substance-induced disorders are conditions that are caused or exacerbated by substance use, such as substance-induced mood disorder or substance-induced anxiety disorder. Substance use disorder (SUD) is often comorbid with other psychiatric disorders.

T. Stewart, *Psychiatric-Mental Health Nurse Practitioner Program Companion and Board Certification Exam Review Workbook*,
https://doi.org/10.1007/978-3-031-60894-0_11

The challenges that individuals with substance-related disorders may face can include stigma, lack of access to treatment resources, and financial barriers. Also, the increasing legalization and decriminalization of some substances complicate diagnosis and treatment. As of 2021, cannabis has been legalized for recreational use in 15 states and the District of Columbia, and it has been legalized for medical use in 36 states and the District of Columbia. Some states have also passed laws to decriminalize the possession of small amounts of cannabis, meaning that possession of the drug is punishable by a fine rather than jail time (National Conference of State Legislatures 2023).

Psilocybin, on the other hand, is currently classified as a Schedule I controlled substance in the United States, meaning that it is illegal to manufacture, distribute, or possess the drug (Drug Enforcement Administration 2021). However, there have been efforts in recent years to legalize or decriminalize the use of psilocybin for medicinal or therapeutic purposes. In 2021, Oregon became the first state to legalize the therapeutic use of psilocybin (OHA 2021). Colorado has decriminalized the possession of psilocybin. Other states are considering similar measures (Klee 2023).

PMHNPs must have a thorough understanding of these disorders and their treatment in order to provide the best possible care for patients. Further, they need advanced understanding of the different substances that can be abused and their specific effects on the body and brain. PMHNPs should also be familiar with the signs and symptoms of substance abuse and dependence, as well as the potential co-occurring mental health disorders that may be present. According to the National Institute on Drug Abuse (NIDA), people with psychiatric disorders, particularly schizophrenia and bipolar disorder, are at increased risk for developing SUD (NIDA 2021). Through a combination of pharmacotherapy and psychotherapy, PMHNPs can help individuals with substance-related disorders achieve lasting recovery and improve their overall quality of life.

This chapter covers substance-related disorders and addictions. Content focuses on substance-specific symptoms and overdose, including pharmacological interventions. Diagnostic criteria, pertinent medications, along with side effects, and therapies are presented.

11.1 Foundations

1. Define substance use disorder.

2. To be diagnosed with a substance use disorder (SUD) according to the Diagnostic and Statistical Manual of Mental Disorders (DSM-5), symptoms must be present for at least _______ months.
3. What are some symptoms that may be met in order to diagnose a patient with substance use disorder?

4. Explain the neurobiological foundation to addiction.

5. What protein has been found to be involved in all addictions? It stimulates dopamine-producing neurons.

6. Match each term below with its definition on the right.

Term	Definition
______1. Dependence	A. Multi-substance dependence, usually simultaneous. PSD complicates treatment and worsens withdrawal and health.
______ 2. Tolerance	B. A pattern of substance use that impairs or distresses the ability to meet employment, school, family, legal, financial, or social commitments. Drug abuse can lead to addiction.
______ 3. Withdrawal	C. When drug use compromises judgment, conduct, and health. Some intoxicants produce slurred speech, coordination difficulties, and altered perception.
______4. Substance abuse	D. When the body needs more chemical to get the same effect. Tolerance to prescription and illegal drugs can cause addiction.
______5. Intoxication	E. The use of a substance in a manner that is inconsistent with medical or legal guidelines, such as taking a medication in a way that is not prescribed or using an illicit substance. Misuse can lead to negative consequences and can increase the risk of dependence and addiction.
______ 6. Polysubstance dependence (PSD)	F. A set of symptoms that occur when a person stops using a substance after becoming dependent on it. Depending on the substance, withdrawal symptoms include nausea, tremors, anxiety, and depression.
__________ 7. Addiction	G. Where the body has acclimated to a substance and needs it to function. H. Chronic drug addiction with recurrent usage despite undesirable effects. After quitting, physical, psychological, or both dependencies cause withdrawal symptoms.
__________ 8. Misuse	H. A chronic and relapsing disorder characterized by compulsive drug-seeking behavior and the continued use of a substance despite negative consequences. Addiction is thought to involve changes in the brain's reward system and other brain regions involved in motivation, decision-making, and impulse control.

7. What mental illnesses most often have substance use as a co-occurring disorder?

8. Most substance use disorders have their roots during the ____________________ years, when many individuals experiment with substances for the first time.

9. List common signs of abuse and dependence for each drug.

Drug	Signs
Opiates	
Alcohol	
Stimulants	
Cannabis	
Sedatives/hypnotics	
Tobacco	

10. For each of the substances in the left column, identify those drugs/substances for which they may produce a FALSE positive laboratory result. LSD and PCP do not have any common causes of FALSE positive results.

Amantadine	
Bupropion	
Chlorpromazine	
Dextromethorphan	
Diphenhydramine	
Efavirenz (HIV medication)	
Mouthwash	
NSAIDs	
Phentermine	
Poppy seeds	
Promethazine	
Proton pump inhibitors	
Pseudoephedrine	
Quetiapine	
Quinolone antibiotics (e.g., rifampin)	

Sertraline	
Trazodone	
Venlafaxine	
Verapamil	
Weight loss pills	

11.2 Caffeine

11. Caffeine is a xanthine-type drug which binds to ________________ receptors, causing the release of the neurotransmitter ____________________.

12. What are common symptoms of caffeine withdrawal? What treatment is provided?

13. It is recommended that an individual stop consuming caffeine at least __________ hours before bedtime.

11.3 Nicotine

14. Nicotine is an alkaloid that binds to the __________________ receptors in the CNS. It affects practically every neurotransmitter.

15. In addition to cancer, what are 3–5 other adverse effects linked to nicotine?

    1.
    2.
    3.
    4.
    5.

16. How do the mechanisms of action of bupropion and varenicline support smoking cessation?

11.4 Alcohol

17. Which 3 neurotransmitters are increased with the acute consumption of alcohol?
    1.
    2.
    3.
18. What are 3-5 medical adverse effects linked to chronic alcohol consumption?
    1.
    2.
    3.
    4.
    5.
19. Name 3–5 signs of fetal alcohol syndrome.
    1.
    2.
    3.
    4.
    5.
20. What is the legal blood alcohol concentration (BAC) in the United States?

21. What is Wernicke-Korsakoff syndrome? What are its etiology, symptoms, and treatment?

22. Thiamine should be administered to a patient who is a chronic alcohol drinker prior to giving ________________, or Wernicke-Korsakoff symptoms may worsen.

23. On the arrow below, list symptoms associated with each level of alcohol withdrawal.

Mild	Moderate	Severe
→	→	→

24. What is delirium tremens, its signs and symptoms, and development timeline?

25. ________________________________ are used to prevent delirium tremens in individuals who recently stopped drinking alcohol.

26. Chronic alcohol use may be tested by comparing the ratio of liver enzymes aspartate transaminase (AST) to alanine transaminase (ALT). If AST is _______ times that of ALT, then it is a sign that the patient is a chronic user of alcohol. Elevated gamma-glutamyl (GGT) is also a common test. ______________ is

often elevated, showing macrocytic anemia, as well as increased amylase/lipase levels due to ________________.

27. What are three medications that can be prescribed to help treat alcohol abuse? Provide the mechanism of action and outcome of use of each as well.

    1.
    2.
    3.

28. A client with a history of alcohol dependence, who has not had an alcoholic drink within ______________ week(s), is typically out of danger for complicated withdrawal. It is still smart to monitor the individual regardless.

11.5 Cannabis

29. ________________________ is the primary psychoactive substance in cannabis. After metabolism by the liver, this substance becomes ______________ ________________, which are fat-soluble molecules that attach to endocannabinoid receptors (CB1, CB2).

30. Early marijuana use can increase later risk of psychiatric disorders.
    TRUE FALSE

31. What are 5–7 effects associated with cannabis intoxication?

    1.
    2.
    3.
    4.
    5.
    6.
    7.

32. What are common cannabis withdrawal symptoms?

11.6 Stimulants

33. Cocaine increases dopaminergic activity in ____________________________, ____________________________, and ______________________ areas/structures of the brain. It also blocks norepinephrine reuptake.

34. For patients on a ________________________________, simultaneous cocaine use may lead to a hypertensive crisis due to adrenergic stimulation.

35. What is formication?

36. What visual hallucinations may cocaine users report?

37. Indicate if each psychological and physiological sign and symptom is increased (↑) or decreased (↓) with cocaine use. Place an X in the correct box.

Sign/symptom	↑	↓
Mood		
Energy		
Sex drive		
Concentration		
Sleep		
Anxiety		
Irritability		
Judgment		
Heart rate		
Blood pressure		
Body temperature		
Sweating		
Blood vessel diameter		
Pupil size		
Seizure risk		

38. What symptoms can a chronic user of cocaine experience during withdrawals from the drug?

39. Patients who overdose on cocaine may present with hyperthermia, seizures, malignant hypertension, and agitation. What medications may be used to treat each of these symptoms?

40. Although used off-label, which medications have been shown to reduce the amount and frequency of cocaine use?

41. What neurotransmitters are affected by amphetamines?

42. What effects do amphetamine users often report? What adverse effects may be seen with amphetamine use?

43. A woman presents to the emergency department with low respiratory rate and miosis (pinpoint pupils). The physician thinks she has taken stimulants.
TRUE FALSE

44. Stimulants Are Physiologically Mediated by the ________________________ ________________ Nervous System

11.7 Opioids

45. Identify each drug as a natural opioid, semisynthetic opioid, or synthetic opioid.

Drug	Natural	Semisynthetic	Synthetic
Morphine			
Heroin			
Hydrocodone			
Oxycodone			
Methadone			
Propoxyphene			
Fentanyl			

46. The three major opioid receptors are ______________, ________________, and ______________.

47. Buprenorphine is a partial agonist at the _____________ opiate receptor.

48. What opioid antagonists block all opiate receptor sites?

49. Which opiate is used in gastrointestinal procedures to dilate the sphincter of Oddi? If a patient is on this medication, a PMHNP may avoid prescribing what common psychotherapeutics?

50. A patient who is receiving methadone for opiate dependence cannot overdose if they use other opiates simultaneously.

TRUE FALSE

51. ______________________________ is the primary cause of death due to opiate overdose.

52. A patient experiencing withdrawal from opiates will be very uncomfortable. Name 3–5 symptoms that the patient may experience.

1.
2.
3.
4.
5.

53. To address opiate withdrawal symptoms, what medications are commonly used?

54. What is the Drug Addiction Treatment Act of 2000 (DATA) waiver?

55. Is an individual withdrawing from opioids in danger? Why/why not?

11.8 Hallucinogens

56. LSD is an abbreviation for ______________________________ ____________.

57. The chemical LSD is akin to the neurotransmitter ____________________. Psilocybin (mushrooms) and mescaline (peyote) also act on this neurotransmitter.

58. Dissociative hallucinogens, which cause alterations in one's perception of self and reality, include these three drugs:

    1.
    2.
    3.

59. There are no known withdrawal symptoms with LSD.

    TRUE FALSE

60. LSD may cause users to have flashbacks, engage in dangerous behaviors, and other adverse reactions. In addition to placing the patient in a soothing environment, what medication may be used?

11.9 Psychedelics

61. The psychoactive chemical in "magic mushrooms" is ______________________.

62. 3,4-Methylenedioxymethamphetamine (MDMA) is better known as ______________________ and is chemically structured like methamphetamine yet stimulates serotonin more than dopamine.

63. MDMA may have various physiological effects. Name 3–5 harmful effects.
MDMA can have various physiological effects, including:

    1.
    2.
    3.
    4.
    5.

64. A patient who is dissociating, presents with vertical nystagmus, and has increased deep tendon reflexes, is likely on the hallucinogen ______________________________.

65. "Robo-tripping" is the consumption of over-the-counter cough medicines with the hallucinogen ____________________________. This chemical blocks NMDA receptors and increases dopamine, resulting in heightened perceptions and visual hallucinations.

11.10 Inhalants

66. The use of inhalants, like glue, gasoline, degreasers, and spray paints, is known as "huffing." While high, an individual will feel happy, dizzy, and disinhibited. Afterwards, an individual may have headaches, nystagmus, and GI distress. What are possible adverse effects from chronic use?

11.11 Diagnosis and Treatment

67. In addition to a comprehensive medical history and physical examination, what are the diagnostic and laboratory findings that can aid in the diagnosis and management of substance use disorders?

68. On average, illicit substances will be identifiable via a urine drug screen for ____ to ____ days, except marijuana which may show positive results for up to _____ weeks.

69. For each of the screening instruments/scales below, provide its full name and a brief description of the instrument/scale as used in substance use disorders.

Acronym	Full name	Description
AUDIT		

Acronym	Full name	Description
CAGE		
CIWA		
CINA		
COWS		
CRAFFT		
S-MAST		

70. What is MAT vis-a-vis the treatment of opioid addiction?

71. What are examples of 12-step programs? What is their purpose and how do they differ from more formal therapy?

72. Explain the relapse prevention model.

73. For each medication below, place an X under the corresponding substance for which it is used to combat withdrawal symptoms or addictions to the substance.

Medication	Alcohol	Opioid	Cannabis	Nicotine	Sedatives	Stimulants
Acamprosate						
Baclofen						
Benzodiazepines						
Buprenorphine						
Bupropion						
Disulfiram						
Dronabinol						
Flumazenil						
Methadone						
Naltrexone						
Topiramate						
Varenicline						

11.12 Answers and Explanations to Chapter Activities

1. SUD is the development of tolerance to the substance, withdrawal symptoms when not using, using more than intended, unsuccessful attempts to quit or cut down, and spending a lot of time obtaining or using it, according to the DSM-5. They might be mild or severe and affect social and professional functioning. Constellation of disorders with cognitive, behavioral, and physiological signs that suggest substance use despite major difficulties.
2. SUD symptoms must endure 12 months, but intensity and frequency vary. SUD may also be diagnosed if the person shows significant impairment or distress.
3. The DSM-5 requires at least two of the following symptoms within a 12-month period to diagnose substance use disorder (SUD). Mild SUD has two or three symptoms, moderate four or five, and severe six or more.

   - Trying or failing to cut back on drugs.
   - Slow to recover.
   - Strong desire to use.

- Substance use causing missed job, school, or household duties.
- Using despite ongoing social or interpersonal challenges caused by the substance.
- Avoiding important social, occupational, and leisure activities owing to substance use.
- Finds self in dangerous scenarios like driving or operating machines.
- Use despite knowing you have a persistent physical or mental ailment caused by it.
- Tolerance occurs when you need more or less of a substance to achieve the desired effect.
- Avoiding withdrawal by using the drug.

4. Neuropeptides release dopamine in the ventral tegmental area and nucleus accumbens, resulting in feelings of happiness after drug reinforcement. The hippocampus is involved in emotional memory, while the amygdala is responsible for sensing and processing emotions. The prefrontal cortex assists in planning and decision-making. Chronic substance use leads to neuroadaptation, making quitting challenging. Repeated drug use decreases dopamine receptor availability, reducing pleasure from natural rewards and increasing the need for medication to stimulate the reward system.
5. All addictions include **δ**FosB-stimulated dopamine neurons. **δ**FosB regulates neuron gene expression via transcription. It builds up in specific brain regions after persistent drug use and irreversibly alters neuron function. **δ**FosB may cause addiction by increasing drug cravings. Dopamine-producing neurons in the brain's reward system become more sensitive to drug-related stimuli and use. These changes might encourage addicts to crave drugs obsessively and make treatment difficult.
6. 1/G, 2/D, 3/F, 4/B, 5/C, 6/A, 7/H, 8/E.
7. Mental illnesses that often accompany SUD include:

   - MDD causes persistent melancholy, pessimism, and a loss of interest in activities. MDD individuals may self-medicate for stress or symptoms.
   - Mental disorders that induce excessive dread or worry are anxiety disorders. Examples: panic, social, and generalized anxiety. Drugs may help anxiety sufferers manage stress.
   - PTSD sufferers may use medicines for flashbacks, nightmares, and hyperarousal.
   - Depression and mania characterize bipolar disorder. Drugs may alleviate depression or promote mania in bipolar individuals.
   - Schizophrenia causes hallucinations, delusions, and disordered thinking. Drugs may help schizophrenia patients manage symptoms or antipsychotic side effects.
   - Antisocial personality disorder involves chronic disrespect and rights violations. Substance abuse can worsen ASPD symptoms including impulsivity and aggression and increase criminal risk.

8. Adolescent drug and alcohol use can damage brain structure and function. Adolescent drug and alcohol usage can cause dependence, addiction, cognitive impairment, mental health concerns, and social and legal issues.
9.

Drug	Signs
Opiates	• Needle marks, old scars • Pupillary miosis (with intoxication) • Pruritus (itching) • Constipation • Hepatitis C infection
Alcohol	• Enlarged or shrunken liver • Alcohol on breath • Spider angioma (spider-like blood vessels on the skin) • Palmar erythema (redness on the palms of the hands) • Elevated liver function tests • Elevated prothrombin time/international normalized ratio (INR)
Stimulants	• Burn marks on dominant finger and lips (if smoking) • Dilated pupils • Rapid speech • Elevated blood pressure • Tachycardia (rapid heart rate) • Nasal problems (when snorted) • Needle marks (if injecting)
Cannabis	• Bloodshot eyes • Hunger • Tachycardia (rapid heart rate)
Sedatives/hypnotics	• Sleepiness • Poor coordination
Tobacco	• Smells of cigarettes • Nicotine stains on fingers or teeth • Elevated carboxylated hemoglobin (a marker of tobacco use)

10.

Amantadine	Amphetamine
Bupropion	Amphetamine
Chlorpromazine	Amphetamine
Dextromethorphan	PCP
Diphenhydramine	Opioids (methadone), PCP
Efavirenz (HIV medication)	THC
Mouthwash	Alcohol
NSAIDs	THC, barbiturates
Phentermine	Amphetamine
Poppy seeds	Opioids
Promethazine	Amphetamine
Proton pump inhibitors	THC
Pseudoephedrine	Amphetamine
Quetiapine	Opioids (methadone)
Quinolone antibiotics (e.g., rifampin)	Opioids
Sertraline	Benzodiazepines, LSD
Trazodone	Amphetamine
Venlafaxine	Opioid (tramadol), PCP
Verapamil	Opioid, LSD
Weight loss pills	Amphetamine

11. Caffeine suppresses adenosine, a neurotransmitter that promotes sleep and lowers wakefulness, in the central nervous system. Caffeine increases brain activity and releases dopamine and norepinephrine by blocking adenosine receptors. In the brain's reward system, dopamine produces pleasure and motivation. Caffeine may boost mood, cognition, and alertness through dopamine release. Norepinephrine increases heart rate, blood pressure, and breathing in "fight or flight" reactions. Norepinephrine release from caffeine raises heart rate, blood pressure, and energy.
12.

    Common caffeine withdrawal symptoms:

    - Headache.
    - Fatigue.
    - Depression or agitation.
    - Concentration issues.
    - Nausea, vomiting, and muscle pain are flu-like symptoms.

    Treatment options include:

    - Consider tapering caffeine instead of discontinuing it for effective withdrawal tactics.
    - Keep hydrated with water.
    - Getting enough sleep.
    - Exercise improves mood and reduces symptoms.
    - Taking OTC medications like acetaminophen or ibuprofen for headaches and other symptoms.

13. Stop consuming caffeine at least 6 h before bedtime to avoid sleep disruption. Caffeine boosts alertness, delays sleep, and reduces sleep quality and length. The effects of caffeine vary on metabolism, sensitivity, dosage, and timing. Caffeine-sensitive people or those who have trouble sleeping should limit or avoid caffeine, especially at night.
14. Nicotine stimulates nicotinic acetylcholine receptors in the CNS (central nervous system). Nicotine regulates central nervous system dopamine, norepinephrine, and serotonin release. Nicotine attaches to these receptors, releasing neurotransmitters that boost mood, arousal, and cognition. Along with neurotransmitters, nicotine triggers the brain's reward system and may create addiction. Regular nicotine use changes brain reward pathways, making quitting smoking or other tobacco products difficult.
15. Nicotine use carries health hazards beyond cancer:

    - Nicotine elevates blood pressure, heart rate, and heart attack and stroke risk.
    - Nicotine promotes lung inflammation and damage, increasing the risk of chronic bronchitis and emphysema.
    - Nicotine can cause fertility loss, erectile dysfunction, and menstrual irregularities.
    - Nicotine can cause gum disease, tooth damage, and oral cancer.
    - Nicotine may impair night vision and increase cataract risk.

- Nicotine can cause depression, anxiety, and schizophrenia.
- Nicotine is highly addictive and causes withdrawal symptoms. Nicotine addiction may require professional help.

16. Bupropion and varenicline are FDA-approved smoking cessation medications. Both limit nicotine's pleasure by targeting the brain's reward system, making quitting smoking simpler. The antidepressant bupropion boosts brain dopamine and norepinephrine. Bupropion boosts neurotransmitters to lessen nicotine withdrawal, cravings, and smoking enjoyment. Bupropion tablets are used once or twice a day for 7–12 weeks. Varenicline partially binds brain nicotinic acetylcholine receptors. Varenicline partially stimulates these receptors to reduce nicotine withdrawal, cravings, and smoking enjoyment. For 12–24 weeks, varenicline is taken twice daily as a pill.
17. Alcohol enhances GABA's tendency to "calm" neuronal activity. Alcohol calms, tires, and suppresses anxiety. Alcohol increases dopamine release from the reward system's nucleus accumbens. Pleasure, euphoria, and reinforcement can foster alcohol and addiction. Alcohol influences serotonin release and reuptake, which controls mood, hunger, and other functions. Due to serotonin changes, alcohol can promote mood swings, impulsivity, and behavioral disinhibition.
18. Chronic alcohol usage can cause many ailments such as:

    - Fatty liver, hepatitis, and cirrhosis.
    - Increased blood pressure, heart attack, and stroke risk.
    - Painful pancreatitis.
    - Malignancies are linked to alcohol use.
    - Memory loss, cognitive deterioration, and peripheral neuropathy.
    - Ulcers, gastritis, and reflux.
    - Libido loss, erectile dysfunction, and infertility.
    - Lowers immunity, increasing infection.
    - Depression, anxiety, and alcoholism.
    - Damage relationships, careers, and laws.

19. Newborns with fetal alcohol syndrome (FAS) often exhibit physical characteristics such as smooth philtrum, thin upper lips, and small eye apertures, alongside potential health complications. FAS can result in lower birth weight, stunted growth, and reduced head circumference. Furthermore, it may lead to central nervous system abnormalities, contributing to intellectual challenges, developmental delays, and attention or memory issues in affected children. Additionally, FAS can impact hearing, potentially causing strabismus and visual problems. Long-term cardiac and kidney issues are also associated with FAS. Skeletal abnormalities may manifest as joint problems, irregular spine curvature, and shortened fingers or limbs. In terms of social interactions, children with FAS might encounter difficulties in connecting with others, interpreting social cues, and exercising impulse control, often displaying hyperactivity and impulsivity.
20. The legal BAC limit for driving or other alert and coordinated activities is BAC. US drivers can drive with 0.08% BAC. A driver with a BAC of 0.08% or more may be charged with DUI or DWI. Alcohol can impair cognitive and

motor function, increase accident and injury risk, and affect health and well-being at lower BAC levels.

21. Wernicke-Korsakoff syndrome (WKS) is a neurological disorder caused by severe thiamine deficiency from chronic alcohol consumption and inadequate diet and vitamin absorption. Thiamine deficiency and WKS can also result from malnutrition, gastrointestinal issues, and bariatric surgery. Disorientation, ataxia, ophthalmoplegia, nystagmus, anisocoria, and mental state can result from Wernicke's encephalopathy (Figs. 11.1 and 11.2). Korsakoff's condition involves severe memory loss, confabulation, and cognitive problems. Not treating WKS symptoms quickly can be disastrous. WKS is treated with fast intravenous thiamine and long-term nutrition.

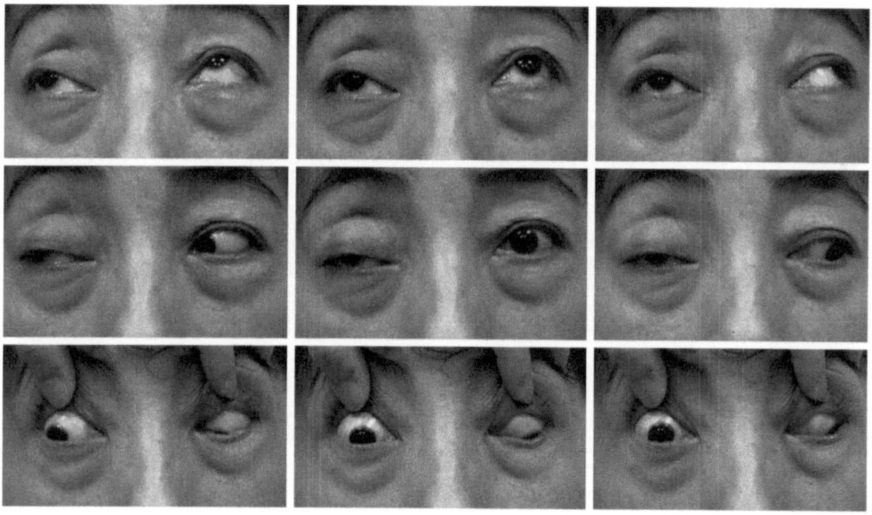

Fig. 11.1 Ophthalmoplegia (With permission from: Wang, AG. (2018). Tolosa-Hunt Syndrome. In: Emergency Neuro-ophthalmology . Springer, Singapore. https://doi.org/10.1007/978-981-10-7668-8_27)

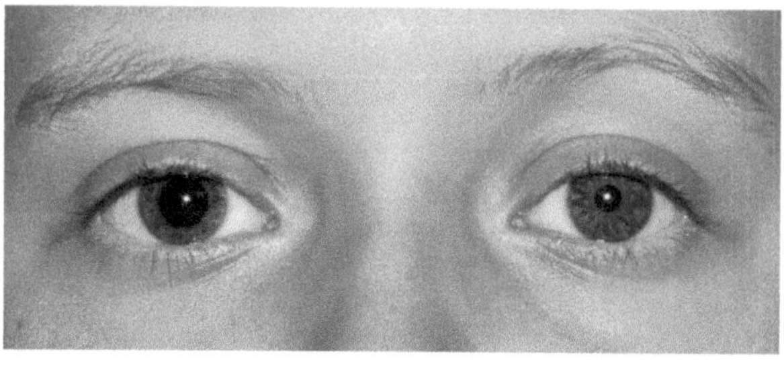

Fig. 11.2 Anisocoria (From: Macchiaiolo, M., Vignati, E., Gonfiantini, M.V. et al. An unusual case of anisocoria by vegetal intoxication: a case report. *Ital J Pediatr* 36, 50 (2010). https://doi.org/10.1186/1824-7288-36-50. Published under the terms of the Creative Commons Attribution License (http://creativecommons.org/licenses/by/2.0))

22. Chronic alcohol drinkers should be administered thiamine before glucose. Since glucose rapidly depletes thiamine levels in thiamine-deficient patients, it may aggravate neurological symptoms such as disorientation, ataxia, and ophthalmoplegia.
23.

    Mild alcohol withdrawal:

    - Anxiety, nervousness, or restlessness.
    - Insomnia or difficulty sleeping.
    - Tremors or shaking, especially in the hands.
    - Sweating, especially at night.
    - Headache.
    - Gastrointestinal symptoms, such as nausea, vomiting, or diarrhea.
    - Loss of appetite.
    - Mild increase in heart rate or blood pressure.

    Moderate alcohol withdrawal:

    - Increased intensity of mild symptoms.
    - Agitation or irritability.
    - Confusion or disorientation.
    - Hallucinations (seeing or hearing things that are not there).
    - Seizures.
    - Increased heart rate or blood pressure.
    - Fever.
    - Rapid breathing or shortness of breath.

    Severe alcohol withdrawal:

    - Increased intensity of moderate symptoms.
    - Delirium tremens (DTs), which is a severe and potentially life-threatening form of alcohol withdrawal that can include:
      - Severe confusion or disorientation.
      - Agitation, restlessness, or irritability.
      - Hallucinations (seeing or hearing things that are not there).
      - Seizures.
      - High fever.
      - Rapid heart rate or irregular heartbeat.
      - Profuse sweating.
      - Severe dehydration.
      - Respiratory distress or failure.

24. Long-term alcohol use can cause life-threatening delirium tremens (DTs). DT normally occurs 2–3 days after the previous drink but can occur up to 10 days later.

    Tremens delirium symptoms:

    - Extreme confusion.

- Restlessness, agitation.
- Unreal sights or sounds.
- Seizures.
- High fever.
- Fast or erratic pulse.
- Lots of sweat.
- Extreme thirst.
- Respiratory issues.

25. Benzodiazepines.
26. The liver enzyme ratio of AST to ALT can indicate persistent alcohol use. A twofold increase in AST over ALT implies chronic alcohol use. Gamma-glutamyl is increased in many chronic alcohol testing. Other lab tests can detect the health impacts of chronic alcohol use besides liver enzyme tests. Chronic alcoholism can cause macrocytic anemia, enlarged red blood cells. Measure MCV, a red blood cell size indicator, to detect it. Pancreatitis, which elevates amylase and lipase levels, can result from chronic alcohol usage. Chronic alcohol use raises AST/ALT over ALT. Remember the larger AST increase from drinking and becoming wasted. Another liver enzyme that shows chronic alcohol use is gamma-glutamyl transferase (GGT). High AST/ALT suggests chronic alcohol usage. You may imagine GGT with alcohol in Gonna Get Trashed.
27. Naltrexone blocks opioids, including alcohol-released endorphins. Naltrexone blocks alcohol-GABA binding, preventing alcohol effects. Acamprosate decreases alcohol cravings via NMDA receptors and calcium channels. It repairs brain neurotransmitters destroyed by alcohol. Acamprosate may reduce alcohol cravings, withdrawal anxiety, and depression. It lowers relapse risk with behavioral therapy. Disulfiram blocks acetaldehyde dehydrogenase. Alcohol intake while on disulfiram causes flushing, nausea, and vomiting due to acetaldehyde buildup. Disulfiram may restrict drinking by connecting alcohol with these unpleasant feelings. Disulfiram reduces drinking frequency, intensity, and relapse risk in a comprehensive treatment. Avoid if taking warfarin, metronidazole, phenytoin, or isoniazid.
28. A client with a history of alcohol dependence who consumed no alcohol in a week is unlikely to develop difficult withdrawal. Alcohol withdrawal intensity and duration depend on alcohol intake, metabolism and sensitivity, age, gender, and health. Relapse is common in early recovery, so persons with a history of alcohol dependence should undergo ongoing monitoring and therapy to prevent relapse and address any medical or mental health difficulties.
29. **δ**-9-tetrahydrocannabinol (THC) is the primary psychoactive substance in cannabis. After metabolism by the liver, this substance becomes active metabolites known as 11-hydroxy-THC and 11-nor-9-carboxy-THC, which are fat-soluble molecules that attach to endocannabinoid receptors (CB1, CB2).
30. TRUE. Early marijuana use raises the risk of anxiety, depression, psychotic disorders like schizophrenia, and substance use problems later in life. Early marijuana usage may harm brain development but this is unknown. Genetics and environment also cause psychiatric illnesses; therefore, not all marijuana users get them.

31. Euphoria, giddiness, time perception disturbance, appetite stimulation, perceptual enhancement, paranoia, consciousness, short-term memory, and cognition. Negative effects include dry mouth, minor tremor, incoordination, slurred speech, bloodshot eyes, nausea, headache, and muscle tension. MI risk rises.
32. Cannabis withdrawal symptoms (within 7–10 days) may include:

    - Mood changes and daily life disruption.
    - Sleeplessness.
    - Lower appetite and food intake, weight loss or nutritional deficiencies.
    - Anxiety, especially in anxious persons.
    - Depression.
    - Headaches.
    - Nighttime sweating.
    - Nausea or vomiting.

33. Mesolimbic, mesocortical, striatum.
34. Cocaine can cause hypertension in individuals taking an MAOI. MAOIs enhance brain neurotransmitters like dopamine, norepinephrine, and serotonin. Cocaine stimulates neurotransmitter release, which raises blood pressure and heart rate, especially in MAOI users.
35. Formication is itching, burning, or tingling, or the sensation of bugs crawling on or under the skin. Cocaine, amphetamines, and methamphetamine usage are frequently associated with it, but delirium tremens, menopause, and peripheral neuropathy can also cause it. Black, "insect-like" spots may appear on cocaine users and their surroundings. They are known as "coke bugs."
36. Cocaine users may see:

    - Users may see a spinning item or a person's face melt or shift.
    - Distortions: Users may see brighter or darker colors or larger or smaller objects.
    - Paranoia or terror may result from seeing invisible people or objects.
    - Flashbacks or visual disturbances like patterns or geometric shapes may occur without the drug.
    - Shadow people.
    - Coke bugs, darting objects, and lights.

37.

Sign/symptom	↑	↓
Mood	X	
Energy	X	
Sex drive	X	
Concentration	X	
Sleep		X
Anxiety	X	
Irritability	X	
Judgment		X
Heart rate	X	
Blood pressure	X	

Sign/symptom	↑	↓
Body temperature	X	
Sweating	X	
Blood vessel diameter		X
Pupil size	X	
Seizure risk	X	

38. Chronic Cocaine Users in Withdrawal May Experience

- Days or weeks of fatigue.
- Depression.
- Increased appetite.
- Vivid, sleep-interrupting dreams.
- Irritability and ruin relationships.
- Anxiety or paranoia.
- Restlessness and fidgeting, which can be difficult to manage.
- Loneliness and social disengagement.

39. Cocaine overdose can cause hyperthermia, requiring immediate medical intervention. Benzodiazepines and cold packs or blankets can calm the patient and reduce muscle activity. Bromocriptine and dantrolene may lower body temperature and muscle activity.

- Cocaine overdose can cause seizures, requiring medical attention. Benzodiazepines like lorazepam and diazepam and anticonvulsants like phenytoin and valproate can control seizures.
- Malignant hypertension from cocaine overdose can induce stroke or other cardiovascular issues. Nitroprusside, labetalol, or nicardipine lower blood pressure and prevent complications.
- Lorazepam or diazepam can alleviate agitation after cocaine overdose. Haloperidol or olanzapine may treat psychosis or severe agitation.

40. In addition to treating alcohol use disorder, disulfiram has been used off-label for cocaine use disorder. Disulfiram blocks the cocaine-degrading enzyme, raising blood levels and possibly exacerbating negative effects. Modafinil helps narcolepsy and other sleep disorders but has been used off-label for cocaine use disorder. Modafinil promotes alertness and lowers cocaine cravings by increasing brain dopamine. Topiramate treats cocaine use disorder off-label in addition to epilepsy and migraines. Topiramate boosts brain GABA, lowering cocaine cravings and enhancing mood and anxiety. Off-label, baclofen treats muscle spasms and cocaine use disorder. Baclofen boosts brain GABA, lowering cocaine cravings and improving mood and anxiety.
41. Amphetamines stimulate the brain with dopamine, causing pleasure and motivation. Amphetamines induce cerebral norepinephrine release, which boosts heart rate, blood pressure, respiration, alertness, and focus. Amphetamines increase brain serotonin, providing happiness and well-being.
42. The range of effects includes elevated mood, enhanced focus, mental clarity, and increased energy. Conversely, negative effects encompass anxiety, paranoia, insomnia, anorexia, excessive sweating, hypersexuality, elevated blood

pressure, heart rate, dilated pupils, and tremors. Psychosis is a common and serious side effect, characterized by persecution delusions, ideas of reference, as well as visual and auditory hallucinations.

43. FALSE. A woman with low respiratory rate and miosis (pinpoint pupils) is more likely to have used heroin or opioid prescription drugs rather than stimulants. Most stimulants increase respiration and pupil size. Stimulants produce tachycardia, mydriasis, hypertension, rapid breathing, hyperthermia, and psychosis at high doses.
44. Sympathetic nerves control stimulants. The "fight or flight" response—increased heart rate, blood pressure, respiration, dilated pupils, perspiration, and decreased hunger—is caused by the sympathetic nervous energy, alertness, and exhilaration resulting from sympathetic nervous system stimulation.
45.

Drug	Natural	Semisynthetic	Synthetic
Morphine	X		
Heroin		X	
Hydrocodone		X	
Oxycodone		X	
Methadone			X
Propoxyphene			X
Fentanyl			X

46. Mu (μ), delta (δ), and kappa (κ) are the primary opioid receptors.
47. Mu opioid receptors are affected by buprenorphine, but it activates μ-opioid receptors less than heroin or oxycodone. Buprenorphine reduces opioid withdrawal symptoms without euphoria or overdose.
48. Naltrexone blocks all opioid receptors. Once opioids leave receptors, these drugs quickly restore breathing and other functions following overdose. Nasal spray and injections last less than oral naltrexone.
49. The opiate used in gastrointestinal procedures to dilate the sphincter of Oddi is called Meperidine (also known by its brand name, Demerol). When a patient is on Meperidine, a psychiatric-mental health nurse practitioner (PMHNP) may avoid prescribing certain common psychotherapeutic medications, particularly those that are classified as monoamine oxidase inhibitors (MAOIs). When these two drugs are taken together, there is a risk of a severe and potentially life-threatening condition called serotonin syndrome. Serotonin syndrome can cause symptoms such as confusion, agitation, rapid heartbeat, high blood pressure, fever, muscle stiffness, and even coma.
50. FALSE. Methadone binds plasma proteins and has a long liver half-life. Overdose and respiratory depression can result if an individual uses other opiates or CNS depressants simultaneously.
51. Respiratory depression kills most opiate overdose victims. Opioids reduce brainstem respiratory centers, limiting breathing.
52. Rhinorrhea.

    - Bone pain.
    - Exhaustion.
    - Spasticity.

- Diarrhea, nausea, vomiting.
- Chills, sweat.
- Low-quality sleep.
- Agitated and concerned.
- Depressed, moody, anxious.
- Drug cravings.

53. Drugs for opioid withdrawal include methadone, which reduces cravings and withdrawal without causing euphoria or overdose. Under medical supervision, methadone is used daily.

    - Buprenorphine reduces cravings and withdrawal without increasing bliss. Daily or long-term buprenorphine injections are available.
    - Clonidine lowers opioid withdrawal symptoms like anxiety and agitation by influencing the autonomic nervous system.
    - NSAIDs like ibuprofen and naproxen can relieve opiate withdrawal muscle pain.
    - Treatment for opioid withdrawal diarrhea includes loperamide, diphenoxylate/atrop, and tramadol.

54. Under the federal Drug Addiction Treatment Act of 2000 (DATA) waiver, competent prescribers can prescribe and administer buprenorphine for opioid use disorder. DATA waivers allow qualified clinicians to prescribe buprenorphine for opioid use disorder without DEA registration. Under the DATA waiver, doctors must undergo 8 h of opioid use disorder treatment training to stay licensed. Once licensed, doctors can prescribe and administer buprenorphine to 30 outpatients or 100 with training. Buprenorphine prescribers no longer need this waiver as of 2023.
55. Individuals withdrawing from opioids can indeed be in danger due to the potential severity of withdrawal symptoms and the associated risks. Opioid withdrawal can lead to complications such as dehydration, electrolyte imbalances, fluctuations in blood pressure and heart rate, and severe psychological distress, including anxiety and depression. There is also a risk of relapse, which could result in overdose, and in some cases, individuals might experience increased sensitivity to opioids, leading to respiratory depression if they relapse. Moreover, coexisting medical conditions can be exacerbated during withdrawal, adding to the danger.
56. Lysergic acid diethylamide (LSD).
57. Serotonin.
58. Dextromethorphan (DXM), ketamine, phencyclidine (PCP).
59. TRUE. There are typically no known withdrawal symptoms associated with LSD (lysergic acid diethylamide). Unlike some other substances, such as opioids or alcohol, LSD does not typically lead to physical dependence, and individuals who use LSD do not experience withdrawal symptoms when they stop using the drug. However, it is important to note that LSD can have psychological effects, and some individuals may experience psychological discomfort or

"flashbacks" in the days or weeks following LSD use, but this is not considered withdrawal in the same sense as with physically addictive substances.

60. LSD use can lead to distressing experiences like flashbacks, where users re-experience aspects of previous hallucinogenic trips, sometimes resulting in dangerous behaviors or adverse reactions. To manage acute distress during these episodes, healthcare providers may administer medications like benzodiazepines, such as diazepam or lorazepam, to alleviate anxiety and agitation. However, it is crucial to use these medications under medical supervision, as they should be administered judiciously to prevent further complications. In addition to medication, a soothing environment and supportive therapy are often necessary to address adverse reactions associated with LSD use effectively.
61. "Magic mushrooms" contain psilocybin. Psilocybin binds 5-HT2A brain serotonin receptors. The binding alters brain activity and transmission, causing awareness, sensory distortions, deep emotion, perception, and cognition. Psilocybin, traditionally spiritual and therapeutic, is being researched for depression, anxiety, and addiction.
62. "Ecstasy" or "molly," which contains MDMA (3,4-methylenedioxymethamphe tamine), is a synthetic amphetamine-like substance that primarily releases serotonin rather than dopamine, leading to feelings of pleasure, openness, and empathy.
63. Tachycardia, fever, diaphoresis, dehydration, liver failure, anxiety, panic, muscle rigidity, and thirst mechanism antagonism.
64. "Angel dust" phencyclidine (PCP) can produce dissociation, vertical nystagmus, and increased deep tendon reflexes. PCP can produce dissociation, distortions, disorientation, numbness, and coordination issues. Chronic hallucinations, delusions, and psychosis can result. Convulsions, respiratory depression, and coma can ensue with PCP.
65. "Robo-tripping" involves dextromethorphan-containing OTC cough medications. DXM causes dissociation, visual and auditory hallucinations, and other psychedelic effects by inhibiting NMDA receptors and increasing dopamine.
66. Brain damage, hearing loss, respiratory suppression, cardiovascular issues, cognitive impairment, blood dyscrasias, liver and kidney failure, and neuron demyelination.
67. In addition to a comprehensive medical history and physical examination, various diagnostic and laboratory findings play a crucial role in the diagnosis and management of substance use disorders. These include chemical profiles, thy roid function tests, CBCs, and B12 levels to rule out underlying metabolic or medical conditions that may contribute to substance use disorders. Pharmaceutical toxicity screening, guided by the patient's history, can help identify specific substances contributing to symptoms. Elevated blood alcohol levels, especially exceeding 100 mg/dL in outpatients, 150 with symptoms, or 300 anytime, can indicate alcohol abuse. Assessments like the AST/ALT ratio can measure liver function, with a ratio exceeding 2.0 suggesting alcohol-induced liver damage. Additionally, markers such as glutamyl transferase, MCV, prothrombin time, uric acid, total cholesterol, and triglycerides can

increase with alcohol use, reflecting liver damage, while decreased levels of magnesium, calcium, potassium, BUN, hemoglobin, hematocrit, platelet count, and albumin may signal other underlying medical issues associated with alcohol consumption.

68. Urine drug testing detects illegal narcotics in 2–4 days, whereas marijuana takes 4–6 weeks.

69.

Acronym	Full name	Description
AUDIT	Alcohol use disorders identification test	A 10-item questionnaire used to screen for hazardous or harmful alcohol consumption.
CAGE	Screening tool for alcohol abuse	A 4-item questionnaire used to identify alcohol dependence. Clients scoring 2 or greater are at mild to moderate risk for alcohol dependency, while clients scoring 3 to 4 are considered at high risk.
CIWA	Clinical institute withdrawal assessment for alcohol	An 8-item scale used to assess and monitor the severity of alcohol withdrawal symptoms.
CINA	Clinical institute withdrawal assessment for narcotics	A 5-item scale used to assess and monitor the severity of opioid withdrawal symptoms.
COWS	Clinical opioid withdrawal scale	A 11-item scale used to assess and monitor the severity of opioid withdrawal symptoms.
CRAFFT	Car, relax, alone, forget, friends, trouble	A 6-item questionnaire used to screen for substance use disorders in children and adolescents under 21 years of age.
S-MAST	Short Michigan alcoholism screening test	A 22-item questionnaire used to screen for alcohol dependence.

70. Medication-assisted treatment (MAT) uses behavioral therapy and drugs to treat opioid addiction. For opioid addiction, methadone, buprenorphine, or naltrexone addresses withdrawal symptoms and cravings so the addict may focus on recovery and sobriety.
71. Alcoholics Anonymous, Narcotics Anonymous, Cocaine Anonymous, and Marijuana Anonymous are examples of 12-step groups. To support recovery and personal growth, members discuss their strengths, hopes, and experiences and follow a set of principles and standards. Key differences distinguish 12-step meetings from professional therapy. Traditional therapy is led by mental health professionals and may be court-ordered. Peer-directed therapy is voluntary. The 12-step groups emphasize spirituality, whereas formal therapy may emphasize tailored and evidence-based treatments. The 12-step groups are free and widely available, unlike formal therapy, which has waitlists. Finally, whereas official therapy is time-limited, 12-step groups are open-ended and may need ongoing attendance.
72. Cognitive-behavioral relapse prevention is an approach focused on addressing addiction and preventing relapse by targeting both cognitive and behavioral factors. It views addiction as a chronic condition requiring ongoing treatment and management. This method emphasizes the replacement of maladaptive coping

strategies with healthier ones, particularly in response to triggers and high-risk situations. The process involves stages such as initial assessment, education on addiction, relapse, triggers, and high-risk management, stress and problem-solving skills, cognitive restructuring, relapse avoidance planning, and the availability of counseling, support groups, and medical support to help individuals manage their addiction and reduce the risk of relapse. This approach recognizes that addiction treatment should be tailored to the individual's specific needs and circumstances.

73.

Medication	Alcohol	Opioid	Cannabis	Nicotine	Sedatives	Stimulants
Acamprosate	X					
Baclofen						X
Benzodiazepines	X				X	
Buprenorphine		X				
Bupropion				X		
Disulfiram	X					
Dronabinol			X			
Flumazenil						
Methadone		X				
Naltrexone	X	X	X			
Topiramate						X
Varenicline				X		

References and Resources

American Psychiatric Association, editor. Diagnostic and statistical manual of mental disorders: DSM-5-TR. 5th ed. American Psychiatric Association Publishing; 2022.

Brewerton TD, Dennis AB, editors. Eating disorders, addictions and substance use disorders: research, clinical and treatment perspectives. Springer; 2016.

Drug Enforcement Administration. (2021). Controlled Substances - Alphabetical Order. https://www.deadiversion.usdoj.gov/schedules/orangebook/c_cs_alpha.pdf.

Enoch MA, Goldman D. Problem drinking and alcoholism: diagnosis and treatment. Am Fam Physician. 2002;65(3):441–50.

Johnson K, Vanderhoef D, Magrath N. Psychiatric-mental health nurse practitioner review and resource manual. American Nurses Credentialing Center, American Nurses Association; 2020.

Larimer ME, Palmer RS, Marlatt GA. (1999). Relapse prevention: an overview of Marlatt's cognitive-behavioral model. Alcohol Res Health. 1999;23(2):151–60. https://pubs.niaaa.nih.gov/publications/arh23-2/151-160.pdf

Moberg CA, Bradford DE, Kaye JT, Curtin JJ. Increased startle potentiation to unpredictable stressors in alcohol dependence: possible stress neuroadaptation in humans. J Abnorm Psychol. 2017;126(4):441–53. https://doi.org/10.1037/abn0000265.

Moore DJ. A nurse practitioner's perspective on prescribing suboxone for opioid use disorder. J Addict Nurs. 2018;29(3):226–9. https://doi.org/10.1097/JAN.0000000000000242.

Morgen KJ. Substance use disorders and addictions. SAGE Publications; 2017.

National Conference of State Legislatures. (2023). State Medical Cannabis Laws. https://www.ncsl.org/research/health/state-medical-marijuana-laws.aspx.

National Institute on Drug Abuse (NIDA). Psychiatric disorders and increased risk of substance use disorders. 2021. Available from: https://www.drugabuse.gov/publications/research-reports/psychiatric-disorders-and-substance-abuse.

Oregon Health Authority (OHA). Oregon Psilocybin Services Act: Overview and regulations. 2021. Available from: https://www.oregon.gov/oha/PH/PREVENTIONWELLNESS/Documents/psilocybin.pdf.

Klee M. The Battle for the future of psychedelics. Rolling Stone; 2023. https://www.rollingstone.com/culture/culture-features/fight-legalize-psychadelics-mdma-psilocybin-ketamine-1234778259/

SAMHSA (Substance Abuse and Mental Health Services Administration). Telehealth for the treatment of serious mental illness and substance use disorders. SAMHSA; 2021. https://store.samhsa.gov/sites/default/files/pep21-06-02-001.pdf

Soltis-Jarrett V. Integrating behavioral health and substance use models for advanced PMHN practice in primary care: Progress made in the 21st century. Arch Psychiatr Nurs. 2020;34(5):363–9. https://doi.org/10.1016/j.apnu.2020.07.026.

Song J, Park JH, Han DH, Roh S, Son JH, Choi TY, Lee YS. Comparative study of the effects of bupropion and escitalopram on internet gaming disorder. Psychiatry Clin Neurosci. 2016;70(11):527–35. https://doi.org/10.1111/pcn.12429.

Swift RM, Aston ER. Pharmacotherapy for alcohol use disorder: current and emerging therapies. Harv Rev Psychiatry. 2015;23(2):122–33. https://doi.org/10.1097/HRP.0000000000000079.

Tompkins DA, Bigelow GE, Harrison JA, Johnson RE, Fudala PJ, Strain EC. Concurrent validation of the clinical opiate withdrawal scale (COWS) and single-item indices against the clinical institute narcotic assessment (CINA) opioid withdrawal instrument. Drug Alcohol Depend. 2009;105(1–2):154–9. https://doi.org/10.1016/j.drugalcdep.2009.07.001.

Vashi P, Edwin P, Popiel B, Lammersfeld C, Gupta D. Methylmalonic acid and homocysteine as indicators of vitamin B12 deficiency in cancer. PLoS One. 2016;11(1):e0147843. https://doi.org/10.1371/journal.pone.0147843.

Wesson DR, Ling W. The clinical opiate withdrawal scale (COWS). J Psychoactive Drugs. 2003;35(2):253–9. https://doi.org/10.1080/02791072.2003.10400007.

Winslow BT, Onysko M, Hebert M. Medications for alcohol use disorder. Am Fam Physician. 2016;93:457–65.

Yuodelis-Flores C, Ries RK. Addiction and suicide: a review. Am J Addict. 2015;24(2):98–104. https://doi.org/10.1111/ajad.12185.

Zakhari R. The psychiatric-mental health nurse practitioner certification review manual. Springer Publishing Company; 2021.

Notes:

Notes:

12 Personality Disorders

Test your learning and check your understanding of this book's contents: use the "Springer Nature Flashcards" app to access questions using ▶ https://sn.pub/62J0Ar.
To use the app, please follow the instructions in Chap. 1.

Personality disorders are defined by long-standing patterns of thinking, feeling, and behaving that deviate significantly from cultural norms and cause significant distress or impairment in an individual's life. Personality disorders are important for psychiatric-mental health nurse practitioners (PMHNPs) to understand because they are relatively common and frequently co-occur with other mental health conditions such as depression, anxiety, and substance use disorders (SUDs). Approximately 9% of the general population has a personality disorder, with borderline personality disorder being the most common (APA, 2022). They frequently manifest in adolescence, affect men and women fairly equally (with some variations among individual disorders), and are long-lasting.

Personality disorders are among the most intriguing and difficult mental health diagnoses. They are fascinating because we can spot signs of personality disorders in many of our clients, friends and family, and even ourselves. They are difficult because personality is not a static factor. We all have a variety of personality traits that change depending on the situation. Experiences, culture, nurture, genetics, and other mental and medical illnesses all have a strong influence on personality. Further, personality disorders are sensationalized and popularized in the entertainment industry because they make for dramatic, mysterious, and even criminal characters. However, depictions are frequently skewed for ratings, leading to misunderstandings of personality disorders. When they do not resemble the extreme examples depicted on television and in movies, some people may downplay their

T. Stewart, *Psychiatric-Mental Health Nurse Practitioner Program Companion and Board Certification Exam Review Workbook*,
https://doi.org/10.1007/978-3-031-60894-0_12

disorders. Because of the stigma associated with personality disorders, some clinicians will also avoid making the diagnosis.

Personality disorders can be difficult to treat due to the entrenched nature of the associated patterns of thinking and behavior. As a society, we accept that there are various personality types that can change over time as we mature and gain new experiences. Individuals with a personality disorder face additional challenges because they frequently lack insight into their condition, and they may accept who they are because they can function in society, maintaining a job and relationships if desired. We might label them as strange, eccentric, self-serving, or introverted. However, the person may be distressed.

Psychopharmacological treatments are also limited. Even some personality disorders are resistant to treatment. While therapy is still the first line of treatment for most personality disorders, it is difficult to keep people on track due to the time, expense, and difficulties in looking inward. Dialectical behavior therapy (DBT), which was specifically developed for the treatment of borderline personality disorder, has been found to be effective in reducing self-harm behaviors and improving overall functioning when used. DBT combines individual therapy, group skills training, and phone coaching to help people learn new ways to cope with stress and regulate their emotions (Linehan, 1993).

PMHNPs can assist individuals with personality disorders in managing their condition and improving their overall functioning and quality of life by using evidence-based approaches such as DBT and providing education and support to patients and their families. This chapter discusses the three DSM-5 personality disorder clusters. Diagnostic criteria, relevant medications, side effects, and therapies are all presented.

12.1 Foundations

1. Define personality.

2. An individual's personality is fixed in early life, and cannot be altered.

   TRUE FALSE

3. What makes a personality trait become a personality disorder?

4. Behavioral manifestations of an individual (e.g., interpersonal relations, coping skills, situational beliefs) are known as ______________________________. They can be either ego-syntonic or ego-dystonic.

5. ______________________________ patterns of behavior are consistent with an individual's personality and cause little discomfort to the individual.

6. ______________________________ patterns of behavior are uncomfortable, cause discomfort, and are so inconsistent with an individual's personality that they seek help.

7. An individual can be diagnosed with more than one personality disorder simultaneously.

   TRUE FALSE

8. According to ____ theory, an individual who fails to develop a distinct identity of self-representation from their mother may be at risk of developing a personality disorder. Family enmeshment and social isolation complicate separation and individuation efforts.

9. Using an X, identify if each of the following is increased and decreased in personality disorders.

_____dopamine regulation.
_____gray matter in prefrontal cortex.
_____limbic regulation.
_____serotonin.
_____norepinephrine

10. Maladaptive traits are universal, making it easy to diagnose personality disorders across culturally diverse populations.

    TRUE FALSE

11. According to "Object Relations," the ability to maintain a relationship is known as object ______________________________.

12. With regard to treatment for patients with personality disorders, what are key elements to avoid relapse and severity?

13. During which developmental periods do personality disorders usually become most apparent?

14. A diagnosis of antisocial personality disorder is not given until ________ years old.

15. Complete the following table on the "Big Five" personality traits using the acronym OCEAN. Provide the name of each trait and a brief description of the characteristics of an individual who has high or low levels of each particular trait.

	Trait	High level of trait	Low level of trait
O			
C			
E			
A			
N			

16. ________________________ tend to be diagnosed with personality disorders in the clinical setting. ________________________ with personality disorders are most often seen in court settings.

17. Individuals with personality disorders have ________________________ rates of morbidity and mortality. Why?

18. Treatment of personality disorders should focus on curative outcomes.
TRUE FALSE

19. Personality disorders are often (under or over) diagnosed. Why?

20. Personality disorders can be diagnosed if the individual's behavior does not align with cultural expectations and affects at least two of the following. This can be remembered through the mnemonic CAPRI.

C	
A	
P	
R	
I	

21. What are 3–5 medical conditions that may cause changes in personality?

    1.
    2.
    3.
    4.
    5.

22. Match the personality disorder on the left with the best description or example on the right.

1. Paranoid______	A. Breaks law, manipulates others to do work, thinks rules are made to be broken
2. Schizoid______	B.Has same set of friends as partner, falls into abusive relationships easily
3. Schizotypal______	C.Thinks hidden meaning behind benign remarks, perceives unintentional insults; unforgiving
4. Narcissistic______	D. Will let you know he is an expert in his field, your work tarnished his reputation, you should be luck to work with him
5. Borderline______	E.Loner, does not seem to have emotional range
6. Histrionic______	F.Individual eats lunch alone at desk even though invited by co-workers and wants to go, cried during evaluation due to one area of "needs improvement"
7. Antisocial______	G. Constantly bounces between relationships because she thinks their partner is cheating or will leave her anyway, picks arguments because assumes individual was talking about them, either love or hate you
8. Obsessive-compulsive______	H. Slams door when leaving during class, talks loudly to person sitting next to her, best friends with everyone
9. Avoidant______	I. Rewrites notes, turns in work late because always editing, setting up study area just right takes up most study time
10. Dependent______	J. Believes in clairvoyance, telepathy, magic; speaks, dresses, and acts bizarrely

12.2 Cluster A—Weird (Odd/Eccentric)

23. Complete the following table on personality disorders within cluster A. Then, in the middle column, provide a description of each disorder. Lastly, in the right column, identify if the personality disorder is more commonly diagnosed in males (M), females (F), or both equally (B).

Personality disorders	Description of disorder	Gender

Personality disorders	Description of disorder	Gender

24. Cluster A of personality disorders may be incorrectly diagnosed as a psychotic disorder.

    TRUE FALSE

25. What is a key difference between paranoid personality disorder and schizophrenia?

26. What types of therapy should be avoided with those with paranoid personality disorder?

27. ______________________ personality disorder is considered premorbid for individuals with schizophrenia.

12.3 Cluster B—Wild (Dramatic/Erratic)

28. Complete the following table on personality disorders within cluster B. Then, in the middle column, provide a description of each disorder. Lastly, in the right column, identify if the personality disorder is more commonly diagnosed in males (M), females (F), or both equally (B).

Personality disorders	Description of disorder	Gender

Personality disorders	Description of disorder	Gender

29. ______________________ personality disorder is rarely given as a primary diagnosis.
30. What makes histrionic personality disorder unique among cluster B personality disorders?
31. Borderline personality disorder symptoms can overlap with what other mental illnesses?
32. What is the difference between psychopathic and non-psychopathic antisocial personality disorders?

33. Individuals diagnosed with antisocial personality disorder often were previously diagnosed in childhood with ________________________________ ________________or ________________________________ __________.

34. Why is antisocial personality disorder difficult to treat?

35. Individuals diagnosed with ______________________ personality disorder often grew up with parents with a substance use disorder.

36. ____________ years old is the minimum age required per the DSM-5 for someone to be diagnosed with antisocial personality disorder

37. The symptoms of antisocial personality disorder can be remembered using the mnemonic CONDUCT. What are the symptoms?

C	
O	
N	
D	
U	
C	
T	

38. The mnemonic IMPULSIVE can be used to remember the symptoms of borderline personality disorder. List the symptoms below.

I	
M	
P	
U	

L	
S	
I	
V	
E	

39. Explain the defense mechanism "splitting."

40. "Borderline" in borderline personality disorder captures how these clients are between ____________________________ and ____________________________.

41. ____________________________ personality disorder has the highest risk of suicide.

42. ____________________________ is an immature defense mechanism, often found in borderline personality disorder, in which the patient cannot deal with their conflicting emotions and, therefore, treats others as either "good" or "bad." The view of the same individual can change from interaction to interaction.

43. ____________________________________ is the most common defense mechanism used by individuals with histrionic personality disorder. However, this behavior may lessen with maturation.

44. How can a PMHNP distinguish antisocial personality disorder from histrionic personality disorder in terms of the patient's goals?

12.4 Cluster C—Worried (Anxious/Inhibited)

45. Complete the following table on personality disorders within cluster C. Then, in the middle column, provide a description of each disorder. Lastly, in the right column, identify if the personality disorder is more commonly diagnosed in males (M), females (F), or both equally (B).

Personality disorders	Description of disorder	Gender

46. Patients with anorexia nervosa have behaviors similar to ______________________ personality disorder.

47. Avoidant personality disorder may be best conceptualized as ______________________ disorder, albeit more severe and chronic.

48. Social anxiety disorder overlaps with ______________________ personality disorder due to their shared symptoms of fear of rejection and avoidance of social interaction.

49. The symptoms of avoidant personality disorder can be remembered through the mnemonic AFRAID. What are the symptoms for each letter?

A	
F	
R	
A	
I	
D	

50. The mnemonic OBEDIENT is useful for remembering the symptoms of dependent personality disorder. List the symptoms for each letter below.

O	
B	
E	
D	

I	
E	
N	
T	

51. Clients with borderline, histrionic, and dependent personality disorders all endorse dependence on a significant other in a relationship. What are the distinctions among the three?

52. What are the key differences between obsessive-compulsive disorder (OCD) and obsessive-compulsive personality disorder (OCPD)?

12.5 Treatments

53. Pharmacotherapy is the most common form of treatment for personality disorders.

    TRUE FALSE

54. What are common forms of therapy for personality disorders?

55. Name 5 goals of psychotherapy for clients with personality disorders.

    1.
    2.
    3.
    4.
    5.

56. Cluster _____ personality disorders are most likely to lead to hospitalization during an acute episode.

57. Which anxiolytic is usually avoided when treating patients with personality disorders? Why?

58. What are two neurocognitive disorders that may present as personality changes/ disorders?

59. Hospitalized patients are susceptible to developing _______________ ___________________, which may manifest as alterations in their personality, even across a single day.

60. Developed by Marsha Linehan, _________________________________ __________is an evidence-based behavior therapy used to help patients to control their outbursts and to reduce their sensitivity to criticism. Therapists set clear limits and take a firm approach with clients under this model. It is most widely used with clients with ________________________ personality disorder.

61. Complete the crossword puzzle by deciding which personality disorder is described in each clue.

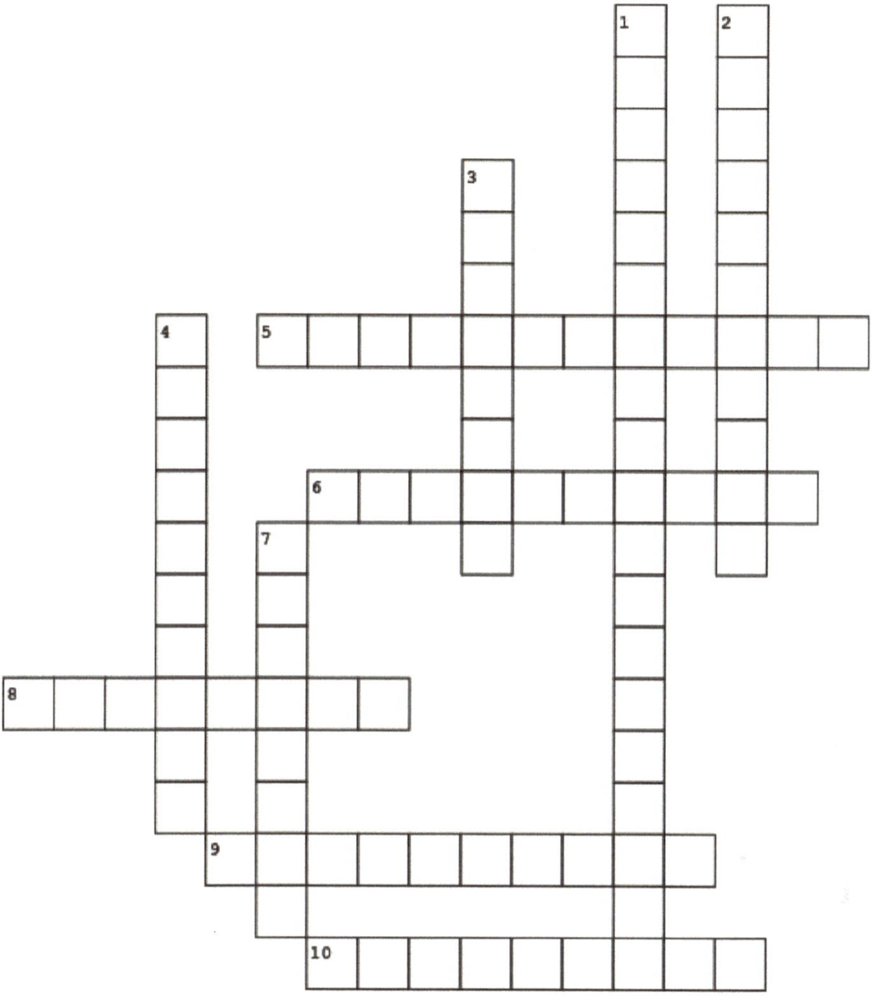

Across		Down	
5.	Hakeem will not applaud his first-place classmate. Later, he complains that his project was more inventive and investigated. He counts his awards. Classmate hears Hakeem. No sympathy from Hakeem.	1.	Patrick has always been a scheduler. Lists, order, and cleanliness please him. Before starting a career, he anticipates and avoids problems. He avoids commencing the project due to worry. Despite skipping leisure activities for work, he routinely misses deadlines due to his substandard output.

Across		Down	
6.	Frederick was often arrested for violence. He is under investigation for theft and arson. Parents told cops Frederick bullied others and tried to kick their pet. Fred shrugs when questioned about his activities.	2.	Harmony marches to the beat of her own drum. Her unique dress draws attention. Her accents vary. Working from home, harmony plays video games. She primarily connects with LARPers at weekend cosplay battles.
8.	Sonia has a close group of friends that she is known since college. At work, she shows up, finishes her tasks, and goes home. Although she likes trivia, she never attends the after-work trivia contest at the local bar because she is afraid that she might make an embarrassing comment.	3.	Tobias is a software coder. He likes being alone and having few friends. Tobias codes well but refuses compliments. Usually regarded as stoic and sex-averse.
9.	Tamara talks on her phone in class and then stomps out, slamming the door. Classmates talk TV at lunch. Boredom makes Tamara loosely connect her phone conversation to the TV plot. She often touches her male classmate and speaks sexually.	4.	Katherine has had several turbulent relationships. She cheats and cries to her partner. She claims victimhood and requests second chances. Katherine enters psychiatric hospital after suicidal threat. She befriends two male nurses and critiques females.
10.	Raquel has been with her girlfriend for 10 years. Raquel calls her multiple times a day to ask what to wear, make for supper, or buy at the grocery store while her beloved is at a conference.	7.	Jack is shopping. He is accidentally bumped by another patron. Jack believes the action was meant to harm him on purpose even though the other customer apologized profusely. Jack refuses the apology, asking "who sent you?"

12.6 Answers and Explanations to Chapter Activities

1. Personality refers to the unique and relatively enduring pattern of thoughts, feelings, behaviors, and characteristics that define an individual and distinguish them from others. It encompasses a person's consistent traits, tendencies, and ways of interacting with the world and others. Personality traits can encompass a wide range of dimensions, including but not limited to extraversion, introversion, openness, conscientiousness, agreeableness, and neuroticism. These traits influence an individual's reactions to various situations, their interpersonal relationships, and their overall behavior, contributing to the stability and consistency of their identity over time. Personality is shaped by a combination of genetic, environmental, and developmental factors and plays a fundamental role in understanding and predicting how individuals perceive and engage with the world around them.
2. FALSE. Personality can change. Life events, the environment, and other factors can change personality traits.
3. Personality traits are normal cognitive, feeling, and behavior differences. Their personality is healthy and adaptive. However, rigid, maladaptive personality

traits that produce serious anxiety or functional difficulties may suggest a personality disorder.

4. Personality attributes include social skills, coping, and situational beliefs. They may be ego-syntonic or ego-dystonic. Ego-syntonic qualities are healthy and adaptive and fit self-image. However, personality traits that contradict with self-image may cause unhappiness or hinder functioning. In personality disorders, rigid and persistent ego-dystonic traits can cause considerable distress or limit daily functioning.
5. Ego-syntonic activity suits a person and is comfortable. These activities are usually healthy, adaptable, and in line with individual values, beliefs, and self-image.
6. Contrary to personality, ego-dystonic behavior can be stressful. These limiting behaviors can seriously impair daily life.
7. TRUE. Coexisting personality disorders are possible.
8. Object relations theory studies how relationships shape personalities. According to this concept, a child who does not differentiate from their mother may have a personality disorder. Family and social seclusion, which are essential to self-development, may hamper detachment and individuation. According to object relations theory, people form their identities through relationships, and issues in these relationships can impact personality. Identity-based personality disorders like borderline personality disorder are better understood and treated with this notion.
9. All decrease except norepinephrine. Studies suggest borderline personality disorder patients may have dopamine and serotonin modulation issues, which affect mood and emotion, for example.
10. FALSE. Personality and diseases vary widely among cultures, contrary to popular notion. Values, beliefs, and norms can influence how people express their thoughts, feelings, and actions and what is typical or aberrant in a culture.
11. Object constancy is the ability to maintain a relationship with someone or something when absent. Healthy relationships include the ability to think and feel about someone or something when they are away.
12. Reducing relapse and managing symptoms in individuals with personality disorders can be achieved through several key factors. Early diagnosis and regular consultations with therapists and PHMNPs provide the necessary support and guidance to control symptoms and prevent recurrence. Medication may be prescribed to address mood or anxiety-related aspects of personality disorders, and collaboration among mental health specialists is essential to create an effective treatment plan. Psychotherapy, including cognitive behavioral therapy (CBT) and dialectical behavior therapy (DBT), is valuable for identifying and changing detrimental thought and behavior patterns while enhancing coping skills. Supportive relationships with family, friends, and others play a crucial role in reducing symptoms and preventing relapse, offering emotional and practical assistance. Prioritizing self-care through exercise, a healthy diet, and adequate rest can aid in symptom management and relapse prevention by promoting overall mental and physical well-being.

13. Personality issues peak in youth and early adulthood. Consistent and ego-dystonic behavioral patterns may become more obvious or tougher to maintain during stressful or changeful phases like adolescence or early adulthood.
14. Antisocial personality disorder (ASPD) is usually diagnosed around 18, but symptoms may occur younger. ASPD is characterized by remorselessness and disregard for others' rights. ASPD sufferers may lie, steal, or attack and break the law. A long-term pattern of behavior is used to diagnose ASPD.
15.

	Trait	High level of trait	Low level of trait
O	Openness to experience	Imaginative, interested in new experiences	Conventional and traditional
C	Conscientiousness	Align with personal and social expectations, rules, order, planners, associated with depression and OCD conduct issues and addiction	Spontaneous, free-spirited, disorganized, associated with
E	Extroversion	Engage with environment, gain energy interacting with others	Introverted, focused on own inner mental state, need to "recharge" after socializing
A	Agreeableness	Gets along with others, puts others' interests first, helpful, trustworthy, may be prone to social pressure, associated with anxiety	Less willing to help others, skeptical, suspicious, associated with conduct disorders
N	Neuroticism	Negative emotions, anger, sad, anxiety, present-oriented, worry about future, stress	Positive emotions, happiness, joy, content, less reactive and stressed, does not equate with positive mood

16. Women; men.
17. The general population has lower morbidity and mortality than individuals with personality disorders. Mental health issues including depression and anxiety and a higher risk of substance addiction may explain this. Personality disorders can increase morbidity and mortality due to self-harm and suicide. Personality problems can make managing emotions, stress, and relationships difficult, causing physical and mental health issues.
18. FALSE. Treatment should address thoughts/behaviors for a happier life and relationships, focusing on the most distressing and dysfunctional symptoms.
19. Underdiagnosed. Those with personality disorders may not know their thoughts, feelings, and actions are damaging and may not seek help. Due to their complexity and overlap with other mental health issues, personality disorders are often underdiagnosed.
20. Cognition, affect, personal relations, impulse control.
21. TBI, TIA, seizures, infections, cancer, Huntington's, MS, thyroid conditions, HIV, SLE, hypercortisolism, and many others.
22. 1/C, 2/E, 3/J, 4/D, 5/G, 6H/, 7/A, 8/I, 9/F, 10/B

23.

Personality disorders	Description of disorder	Gender
1. Paranoid	Persistent pattern of fear, mistrust, and suspicion directed at most people, multiple paranoid ideas, low agreeableness, socially isolated	M
2. Schizoid	Avoids social relationships, introversion, solitary, aloof, detached, but not bothered by this isolation, do not get lonely, can be seen as cold/flat affect, apathetic, fond of fantasy and imaginative worlds, little interest in sex	M
3. Schizotypal	Odd beliefs, magical thinking, difficulty relating to others, lonely and isolated because they fear ostracism for their beliefs and behaviors, clear link to schizophrenia (1/3 progress), socially anxious	M

24. TRUE. Paranoid, schizoid, and schizotypal personality disorders are often misdiagnosed as psychotic. Delusions and aberrant thinking may be signs in some personality disorders.
25. Schizophrenia and paranoid personality disorder have different symptom durations and intensity. Paranoid personality disorder involves constant mistrust and suspicion of others, yet it does not affect reality or daily life. However, schizophrenia causes hallucinations, delusions, and other abnormal thought processes that disrupt reality and daily living.
26. Those with paranoid personality disorder may struggle with trust and vulnerability in group therapy. Misinterpretation of group treatment statements might cause mistrust. CBT, which modifies negative thought and behavior patterns, may be difficult for paranoid personality disorder sufferers also. Paranoid personality disorder sufferers may struggle with confronting ideas and actions in this therapy.
27. Schizotypal.
28.

Personality disorders	Description of disorder	Gender
1. Narcissistic	Exaggerated behaviors for attention, sense of superiority to others although they often are insecure and fear being unloved, lack of empathy, continuous boasting of accomplishments and importance, arrogant	M
2. Borderline	Chronic instability, dysregulation of emotion, relationship insecurity, low self-worth, impulsive, tendency toward anger, shame, and depression and anxiety, seeks approval, history of abuse/neglect common	F
3. Histrionic	Exaggerated behavior, attention seeking, dramatic, often flirtatious and sexual, unstable self-image, seen as obnoxious, shifting, and shallow emotions	F
4. Antisocial	Infringes on others' rights, deceptive, aggressive, manipulative, lacks conscientiousness and remorse, comorbid substance abuse common, impulsive	M

29. Histrionic personality disorder entails intense attention seeking, exaggerated moods and behaviors, and demanding attention. Though common, histrionic personality disorder is generally diagnosed secondary. This may be because mood or anxiety issues typically accompany histrionic personality disorder. Primary diagnoses are mental health problems that cause the most suffering or damage, while secondary diagnoses are additional conditions that may be causing symptoms.
30. Histrionic personality disorder is distinguished from other cluster B personality disorders by its intense need for attention, exaggerated emotions and behaviors, and urge to be the center of attention. In contrast to cluster B personality disorders, which behave differently. Histrionic folks are rarely violent.
31. Fluctuating mood, poor self-image, relationship instability, impulsivity, and self-destruction characterize BPD. BPD is difficult to diagnose and treat due to its complex symptoms and overlap with mood, anxiety, and addiction disorders.
32. Antisocial personality disorder entails ignoring others' rights and not feeling remorseful. ASPD is sociopathy/psychopathy. Because of the debate over psychopathic and non-psychopathic ASPD, both terms are commonly used interchangeably. Some experts believe ASPD's psychopathic and non-psychopathic forms are distinct disorders. Psychotic ASPD lacks empathy, regret, guilt, and is more likely to harm others. Non-psychopathic persons are too emotional when rejected or humiliated, externalize negative sentiments, have mood dysregulation, and can be aggressive but usually respond premeditatedly.
33. Oppositional defiant disorder; conduct disorder.
34. People with ASPD may resist treatment or not view their behavior as inappropriate, making treatment difficult. They may not comprehend how their actions damage others and refuse to change. ASPD patients may often fail to create and sustain relationships, making therapy and therapeutic alliances challenging. ASPD in conjunction with mood or substance addiction disorders makes therapy challenging.
35. Antisocial personality disorder.
36. 18 years old
37. Capriciousness, oppressive, no empathy or responsibility, deceitful, unlawful, carefree, temper.
38. Impulsive, moody, paranoid, unstable self-image, labile relationships, suicidal, inappropriate anger, vulnerable to abandonment, emptiness.
39. The defense mechanism called "splitting" is the inability to mix positive and negative features of oneself or others. This can create a black-and-white worldview where people and things are either good or bad. BPD sufferers may split by idealizing and disparaging others. Borderline personality disorder patients may initially idealize their romantic partners as perfect. If the connection disappoints or irritates the person, they may suddenly devalue their spouse as unworthy of loyalty. Further, these individuals may feel confident and self-important one minute and depressed and worthless the next. Splitting is a personality disorder protective strategy and may suggest emotional instability. Splitting patients need psychotherapy to improve emotional regulation and coping.

40. Neurosis; psychosis.
41. Borderline personality disorder (>10%).
42. Splitting.
43. "Acting out" is a prevalent HPD coping mechanism. Acting out is expressing unconscious thoughts or feelings via actions rather than words or analysis. Histrionic personality disorder sufferers may act out to escape bad emotions or attention. Examples include impulsivity, attention seeking, and outbursts. Better coping and self-awareness may reduce histrionic personality disorder symptoms. Psychotherapy can help histrionic personality disorder patients overcome underlying issues and improve coping skills.
44. Histrionic personality disorder entails intense attention seeking, exaggerated moods and behaviors, and demanding attention. People with histrionic personality disorder think they deserve special treatment. Their reputation is inflated. When unappreciated, they show dread and depression. Borderline individuals crave power and possessions. Antisocial personality disorder entails ignoring others' rights and not feeling remorseful. PMHNPs can distinguish these two personality disorders based on patient intentions and actions in several ways. The patient's behavior goals separate ASPD from histrionic personality disorder. ASPD sufferers may exploit people without regard for their rights or feelings. Histrionic personality disorder sufferers may want attention to fit in. Another way to distinguish these diseases is via patient relationships. ASPD sufferers may struggle with authority and relationships. However, histrionic personality disorder sufferers may seek connections and over-rely on others for affirmation.
45.

Personality disorders	Description of disorder	Gender
1. Obsessive-compulsive	Rigid emotions and behaviors, seek control and structure, inflexible, "perfectionist" qualities, procrastination	M
2. Avoidant	Avoid others, but desire companionship, sense of inadequacy, sensitive to rejection	B
3. Dependent	Over-reliance on others, highly agreeable in relationships to avoid abandonment, can become subservient to and abused by others	F

46. Idealization, control, and inflexibility characterize obsessive-compulsive personality disorder (OCPD). Due to their obsession with order, efficiency, and perfection, OCPD clients may struggle to make decisions and delegate work. Those with anorexia nervosa may share OCPD symptoms such as compulsive weight concerns and body image, diet and exercise management, and change issues. They may also struggle with perfectionism, judgment, and chore delegation.
47. Social anxiety disorder.
48. Avoidant personality disorder.

49. Avoid social occupations, fear of embarrassment, reserved behavior, always concerned about rejection, isolates from relationships (platonic and romantic), distances from others due to shyness.
50. Obsessed with approval, bound by others' decisions, enterprises rarely initiated, decisions difficult, invalidating feelings when alone, engrossed with fears of self-reliance, needs relationship, tentative decision-maker.
51. In BPD, mood, self-image, relationship instability, impulsivity, and self-destruction are present. Borderline personality disorder sufferers may cling due to abandonment fears. Histrionic personality disorder involves an insatiable demand for attention, exaggerated emotions and behaviors, and a drive to be noticed. People with histrionic personality disorder may crave attention and validation from others. Dependent personality disorder causes separation anxiety and excessive caregiving. Dependent personality disorder patients may have trouble making decisions and taking care of themselves.
52. OCD and OCPD are often conflated mental health disorders. Personality disorder OCPD is different from anxiety disorder OCD. While personality problems create rigidity and inappropriate conduct, worry disorders cause excessive fear and worry. Obsessions and compulsions are symptoms of OCD. Distressing obsessions and compulsions can disrupt life. Perfectionism, control, and change issues define OCPD. Due to their obsession with order, efficiency, and perfection, OCPD sufferers may struggle to make decisions and delegate work. Their symptoms are ego-syntonic and they reject obsessions and compulsions. OCD individuals consider their symptoms pathological and want them gone.
53. FALSE. Nonpharmacological, psychotherapy is the most common form.
54. Dialectical behavior therapy, milieu therapy, CBT, behavioral therapy, interpersonal therapy, psychodynamic therapy.
55. Coping skills, limit-setting, avoiding self-harm, interpersonal skills, expectation formation, healthy self-appraisal, environmental structuring.
56. Cluster B.
57. Benzodiazepines. SSRIs and mood stabilizers are first-line medications. Due to dependence and abuse, benzodiazepines are rarely prescribed to patients with personality disorders. Impulsive, dangerous borderline or narcissistic personality disorder patients are significantly affected. Sedation from benzodiazepines may impede personality disorder therapy and rehabilitation. Antisocial personality disorder sufferers may abuse benzodiazepines.
58. Cerebrovascular accidents, TBI, and dementia can cause agitation, irritability, apathy, disinhibition, aggression, and impulsivity.
59. Delirium.
60. Dialectical behavioral therapy (DBT); borderline personality disorder.

61.

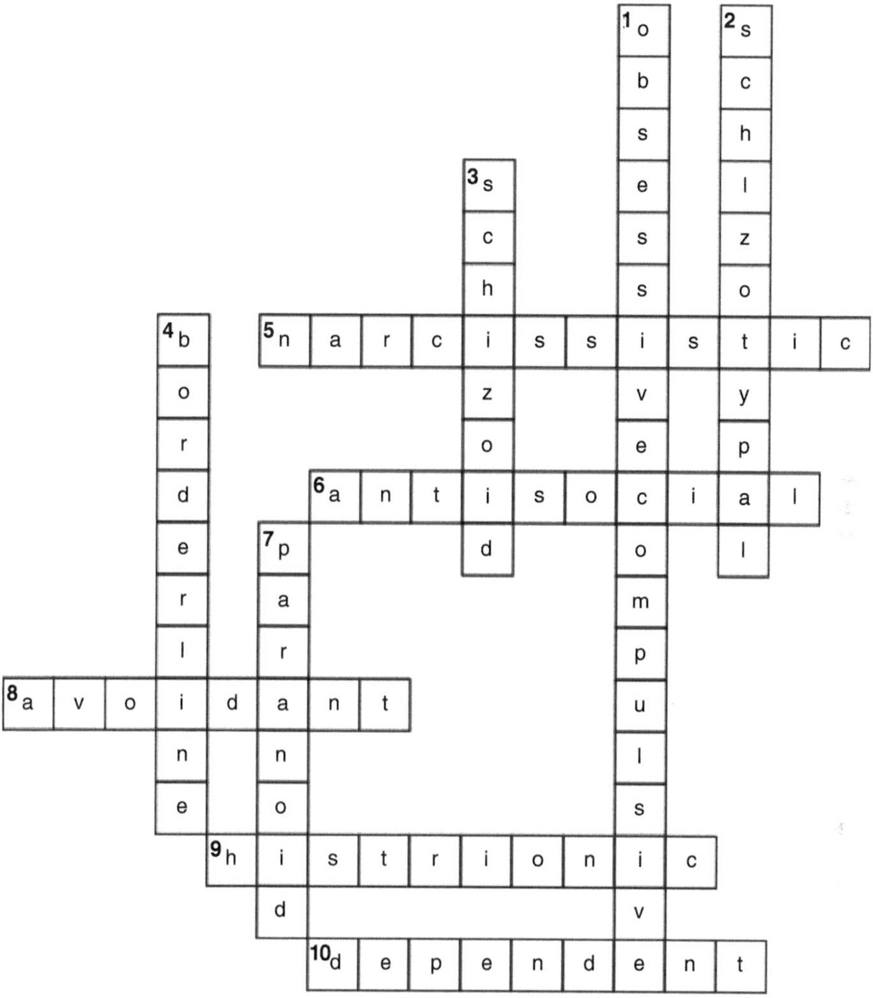
1 obsessivecompulsive
2 schizotypal
3 schizoid
4 borderline
5 narcissistic
6 antisocial
7 paranoid
8 avoidant
9 histrionic
10 dependent

References and Resources

American Psychiatric Association, editor. Diagnostic and statistical manual of mental disorders:DSM-5-TR. 5th ed. American Psychiatric Association Publishing; 2022.

Anderson JL, Kelley SE. Antisocial personality disorder and psychopathy: the AMPD in review. Personal Disord. 2022;13(4):397–401. https://doi.org/10.1037/per0000525.

Bateman A, Fonagy P. Psychotherapy for borderline personality disorder: Mentalization-based treatment. Oxford University Press; 2004.

Bhola P, Devi KD. Personality disorders in women: an overview. In: Chandra PS, Herrman H, Fisher J, Riecher-Rössler A, editors. Mental health and illness of women. Springer Nature Singapore Pte Ltd.; 2020. p. 379–402. https://doi.org/10.1007/978-981-10-2369-9_27.

Clemente MJ, Martins Silva AS, Pozzolo Pedro MO, Paiva HS, de Azevedo Marques Périco, C., Torales, J., Ventriglio, A., & Castaldelli-Maia, J.M. A meta-analysis and meta-regression analysis of the global prevalence of obsessive-compulsive personality disorder. Heliyon. 2022;8(7):e09912. https://doi.org/10.1016/j.heliyon.2022.e09912.

Daros AR, Williams GE. A meta-analysis and systematic review of emotion-regulation strategies in borderline personality disorder. Harv Rev Psychiatry. 2019;27(4):217–32. https://doi.org/10.1097/HRP.0000000000000212.

de Reus RJM, Emmelkamp PMG. Obsessive-compulsive personality disorder: A review of current empirical findings. Personal Ment Health. 2012;6(1):1–21. https://doi.org/10.1002/pmh.144.

Emmelkamp PMG, Meyerbröker K. Personality disorders. 2nd ed. Psychology Press; 2019. https://doi.org/10.4324/9781351055901.

Esterberg ML, Goulding SM, Walker EF. Cluster A personality disorders: schizotypal, schizoid and paranoid personality disorders in childhood and adolescence. J Psychopathol Behav Assess. 2010;32(4):515–28. https://doi.org/10.1007/s10862-010-9183-8.

Gibbon S, Khalifa NR, Cheung NH-Y, Völlm BA, McCarthy L. Psychological interventions for antisocial personality disorder. Cochrane Database Syst Rev. 2020;9(9):CD007668. https://doi.org/10.1002/14651858.CD007668.pub3.

Harned MS, Korslund KE, Linehan MM. A pilot randomized controlled trial of dialectical behavior therapy with and without the dialectical behavior therapy prolonged exposure protocol for suicidal and self-injuring women with borderline personality disorder and PTSD. Behav Res Ther. 2014;55:7–17. https://doi.org/10.1016/j.brat.2014.01.008.

Johnson K, Vanderhoef D, Magrath N. Psychiatric-mental health nurse practitioner review and resource manual. American Nurses Association: American Nurses Credentialing Center; 2020.

Johnson SC, Elbogen EB. Personality disorders at the interface of psychiatry and the law: legal use and clinical classification. Dialogues Clin Neurosci. 2013;15(2):203–11. https://doi.org/10.31887/DCNS.2013.15.2/sjohnson.

Klein P, Fairweather AK, Lawn S. Structural stigma and its impact on healthcare for borderline personality disorder: A scoping review. Int J Ment Health Syst. 2022;16(1):48. https://doi.org/10.1186/s13033-022-00558-3.

Leichsenring F, Fonagy P, Heim N, Kernberg OF, Leweke F, Luyten P, Salzer S, Spitzer C, Steinert C. Borderline personality disorder: A comprehensive review of diagnosis and clinical presentation, etiology, treatment, and current controversies. World Psychiatry. 2024;1:4–25. https://doi.org/10.1002/wps.21156.

Linehan MM. Cognitive-behavioral treatment of borderline personality disorder. Guilford Press; 1993.

Magid M, Fox I. Histrionic personality disorder. In: Feinstein RE, editor. Personality disorders. Oxford University Press; 2021. p. 501–22.

Marincowitz C, Lochner C, Stein DJ. The neurobiology of obsessive-compulsive personality disorder: A systematic review. CNS Spectr. 2021;27:664–75. https://doi.org/10.1017/S1092852921000754.

Masland SR, Victor SE, Peters JR, Fitzpatrick S, Dixon-Gordon KL, Bettis AH, Navarre KM, Rizvi SL. Destigmatizing borderline personality disorder: A call to action for psychological science. Perspect Psychol Sci. 2023;18(2):445–60. https://doi.org/10.1177/17456916221100464.

Muir O, Weinfeld JN, Ruiz D, Ostrovsky D, Fiolhais M, MacMillan C. Mental health clinicians' attitudes toward narcissistic personality disorder. Personal Disord. 2021;12(5):389–99. https://doi.org/10.1037/per0000510.

Mulay AL, Thurnauer H, Cain NM. Schizoid personality disorder. In: Encyclopedia of personality and individual differences. Springer International Publishing; 2020. p. 4567–75.

Paris J. Personality disorders over time: precursors, course, and outcome. American Psychiatric Pub; 2003.

Perrotta G. Histrionic personality disorder: definition, clinical profiles, differential diagnosis and therapeutic framework. Arch Public Health Community Med. 2021;7:001–5. https://doi.org/10.17352/2455-5479.000123.

Ronningstam E. Introduction to the special issue on narcissistic personality disorder. J Personal Disord. 2020;34(Suppl):1–5. https://doi.org/10.1521/pedi.2020.34.supp.1.

Ryder AG, Sunohara M, Kirmayer LJ. Culture and personality disorder: from a fragmented literature to a contextually-grounded alternative. Curr Opin Psychiatry. 2015;29(1):40–5. https://doi.org/10.1097/YCO.0000000000000120.

Skabeikyte G, Barkauskiene R. A systematic review of the factors associated with the course of borderline personality disorder symptoms in adolescence. Borderline Personal Disord Emot Dysregul. 2021;8(1):12. https://doi.org/10.1186/s40479-021-00151-z.

Volkert J, Gablonski TC, Rabung S. Prevalence of personality disorders in the general adult population in Western countries: systematic review and meta-analysis. Br J Psychiatry. 2018;213(6):709–15. https://doi.org/10.1192/bjp.2018.202.

Weinberg I, Ronningstam E. Dos and don'ts in treatments of patients with narcissistic personality disorder. J Personal Disord. 2020;34(Suppl):122–42. https://doi.org/10.1521/pedi.2020.34.supp.122.

Weinbrecht A, Schulze L, Boettcher J, Renneberg B. Avoidant personality disorder: A current review. Curr Psychiatry Rep. 2016;18(3):29. https://doi.org/10.1007/s11920-016-0665-6.

Yu R, Geddes JR, Fazel S. Personality disorders, violence, and antisocial behavior: A systematic review and meta-regression analysis. J Personal Disord. 2012;26(5):775–92. https://doi.org/10.1521/pedi.2012.26.5.775.

Zakhari R. The psychiatric-mental health nurse practitioner certification review manual. Springer Publishing Company; 2021.

Notes:

Notes:

Child/Adolescent Neurodevelopmental, Psychiatric, and Eating/Feeding Disorders

13

Test your learning and check your understanding of this book's contents: use the "Springer Nature Flashcards" app to access questions using ▶ https://sn.pub/62J0Ar.
To use the app, please follow the instructions in Chap. 1.

Understanding child and adolescent psychiatric illnesses and eating disorders is crucial for psychiatric-mental health nurse practitioners (PMHNPs). According to the World Health Organization (WHO), mental disorders are the leading cause of disability among children and adolescents, affecting up to 10% of this population (WHO 2021). PMHNPs are well-positioned to identify and assess these conditions early on, as they often have the opportunity to interact with children and adolescents in various settings, including primary care, schools, and community mental health centers.

One common psychiatric illness in children and adolescents is attention-deficit hyperactivity disorder (ADHD). ADHD is a neurodevelopmental disorder characterized by inattention, hyperactivity, and impulsivity (American Psychiatric Association 2022). It is one of the most prevalent psychiatric disorders in children, affecting around 9% of children worldwide (Polanczyk et al. 2007). Early identification and treatment of ADHD are crucial as they can have significant impacts on a child's academic and social development (Barkley et al. 2015).

Depression also can have significant impacts on a child's functioning and well-being. The prevalence of depression in children and adolescents ranges from 2% to 8% (Kessler et al. 2005). Early identification and treatment of depression are essential as they can lead to improved outcomes and prevent the development of more severe and chronic forms of the disorder (Kovacs 1985).

T. Stewart, *Psychiatric-Mental Health Nurse Practitioner Program Companion and Board Certification Exam Review Workbook*,
https://doi.org/10.1007/978-3-031-60894-0_13

Eating disorders are an area of concern for PMHNPs working with children and adolescents. Eating disorders are serious mental illnesses characterized by abnormal eating behaviors and distorted body image. They include conditions such as anorexia nervosa, bulimia nervosa, and binge-eating disorder. Eating disorders have significant impacts on physical and mental health and can have serious consequences if left untreated (Steinhausen 2002). The prevalence of eating disorders in children and adolescents ranges from 0.5% to 3% (Hudson et al. 2007).

This chapter presents these and other neurodevelopmental and psychiatric disorders common among children and adolescents. Topics will cover disruptive and mood dysregulation disorders (e.g., oppositional defiant disorder, conduct disorder, impulse control disorder), ADHD, autism spectrum disorder, and Rett syndrome. Feeding and eating disorders and elimination disorders will be discussed in this chapter as these disorders tend to start during the younger years. Diagnostic criteria, pertinent medications, along with side effects, and therapies are presented.

13.1 Child and Adolescent Development

1. For each age range, list example behavioral and developmental milestones. Try to include language, motor, social, cognitive, sexual, and affective development as warranted.

2 months	4–6 months	6–8 months	9–12 months	18 months–3 years	4–5 years	6–12 years	13–21 years

2. The ____
__ is a standardized test for assessing the development of infants and young children. It is typically administered by a healthcare provider, while the Ages and Stages Questionnaire (ASQ) is completed by parents.

3. The HEADDS screening tool examines the psychosocial factors that influence the physical and emotional health of adolescents. Complete the HEADDS mnemonic below, and provide sample questions for each category.

	Question 1	Question 2	Question 3
Home			
Education			
Activities			
Drugs/drinking			
Sex/sexuality			
Suicidality/mental health			

4. Complete the following table on Erikson's development Theory for children and adolescents.

Age range	Stage	Tasks
0–1½ years		

Age range	Stage	Tasks
1½–3 years		
3–5 years		
6–12 years		
12–20 years		

5. Continuous exposure to ______________________________ stress overtime is more likely to lead to psychopathologies in children. In contrast, a(n) ______________________________ trauma typically does not, although families may react and treat the child(ren) as if there is a psychopathology.

6. Children who speak only in the home or to a limited number of individuals may have anxiety manifesting as ______________________________. It is not commonly caused by developmental delay, as their speech comprehension and production abilities are intact.

7. Assessment and care for pediatric populations take less time than adults.

   TRUE FALSE

8. What period of development is key when conducting a history on a child's growth and developmental milestones?

9. Previously known as mental retardation, a(n) ______________________________ ______________ refers to severely impaired cognitive and social functioning.

10. For each area of functioning below, provide several examples of deficits that one might see in an individual with an intellectual disability. Both assessments are essential for diagnosing intellectual and developmental disabilities and tailoring support and interventions accordingly.

Area of functioning	Deficits
Intellectual functioning An individual's cognitive abilities, including reasoning, problem-solving, and memory, often measured using standardized IQ tests to assess their intellectual capacity relative to their age and developmental stage	
Adaptive functioning A person's practical, everyday skills required for independent living and social functioning, encompassing areas like communication, self-care, and socialization, reflecting their ability to navigate and adapt to their environment effectively	

11. Fragile X syndrome is caused by a mutation to the ____________________ gene. It affects males more than females.

12. ____ is caused by several mutations on chromosome 15. Typical signs include learning difficulties, myotonia, small stature, and chronic feeling of hunger. Metabolic orders can be severe in these children without caretaker education.

13. ____ is a monosomic 5p-mutation causing high-pitched cries, intellectual disabilities, microcephaly, and a flat nose bridge.

14. What are noted causes of intellectual disabilities?

15. ______________________________ accounts for approximately 80% of intellectual disability cases.

16. Down syndrome is caused by a(n) ____________________ of chromosome __________.

17. The average IQ is ________________.

18. ____ describes individuals with an IQ range of 71–84. They require academic accommodations and assistance with the development of social skills.

19. An aberration on the X-linked gene coding for FMR-1 results in ____________________________________.

20. Tay-Sachs disease is a hereditary ____________________________ disorder. These individuals have intellectual disabilities.

21. Complete the table on the levels of intellectual disability.

Level	IQ	Independence	School level	Work
Mild				
Moderate				
Severe				
Profound				

22. What are the most common features of fetal alcohol syndrome?

23. Name three to five mental status exam findings that may be noted for a child with an intellectual disability.
    1.
    2.
    3.
    4.
    5.

24. To receive a diagnosis of global developmental delay, a patient must be no older than ________________ years old. Documentation of their failure to meet developmental milestones in several areas of intellectual functioning is required.

25. Name several risk factors for the development of a specific learning disorder.

26. Children that struggle with the social use of verbal and nonverbal communication may receive a diagnosis of social or pragmatic communication disorder. However, if restrictive and repetitive behaviors, activities, or interests are also present, the child may receive a diagnosis of ____________________________ ______________________.

13.2 Psychiatric Assessment and Diagnosis

27. Psychiatric diagnoses in pediatric populations must take into account what factors?

28. The provider should interview the child or adolescent separately from their adult guardians because the adults will steer the conversation.
    TRUE FALSE

29. The same approach to the mental status examination is used for pediatric populations as adults.
    TRUE FALSE

30. What are three to five ways in which the mental status examination may need to be modified when working with children?
    1.
    2.
    3.
    4.
    5.

31. Match each diagnosis with its description or set of symptoms.

Diagnosis	Description
_____1. Oppositional defiant disorder	A. Persistent, violation of rules and laws (truancy, theft, arson, lacks empathy for others or animals), distractible, symptoms present for 12 months
_____2. Conduct disorder	B. Repetitive movements, atypical communication and interaction behaviors, like routines, broad phenotypic presentation and level of disability, including agitation, self-harm, reduced interpersonal reciprocity
_____3. Attention-deficit hyperactivity disorder	C. Restrict calories, fear of weight gain even what would be considered "normal" BMI, distorted body image
_____4. Autism spectrum disorder	D. Irritable, argues and refuses to follow rules, blames others, vindictive, impaired concentration; >6 months
_____5. Rett syndrome	E. Persistent, impulsive, trouble focusing, disorganized, fidgets, interrupts or difficulty waiting; seen in at least two different settings
_____6. Anorexia nervosa	F. Lack of control when eating at least 2 days/week for 6 months, no purging behaviors
_____7. Bulimia nervosa	G. Excessive eating at times then purging to control weight, normal or slightly elevated BMI
_____8. Binge-eating disorder	H. Hand movements, social withdrawal, poor coordination, language impairment; develops after a period of normal development
_____9. Intellectual disability	I. Diagnosed <18 years, irritable mood with explosive temper
_____10. Disruptive mood dysregulation disorder	J. Diagnosed <18 years, can affect intellectual and adaptive functioning, genetic, toxins, infections, or issues in utero can be caused
_____11. Enuresis	K. >4 years old, defecates in culturally unacceptably places (bed, floors, clothes), linked to constipation
_____12. Encopresis	L. Self-wetting although can control bladder

32. Oppositional defiant disorder is less common in (males/females).

33. A child diagnosed with oppositional defiant disorder should be monitored for future development of ______________________________, another pediatric psychiatric disorder.

34. Which of the following are common psychiatric diagnoses of parents of children later diagnosed with oppositional defiant disorder? Select all that apply.
    __________Conduct disorder
    __________Dissociative identity disorder
    __________Schizoid personality disorder
    __________ADHD
    __________Substance use disorders
    __________Antisocial personality disorder
    __________Bipolar I/II disorders
    __________Kluver-Bucy syndrome
    __________Paraphilias

35. What behavior by parents is most linked to children's development of ODD?

36. The ingestion of ________________________, an environmental toxin found in many houses built before the 1980s, may be linked to ODD. Laboratory tests should screen for levels.

37. Parents of children with ODD should seek therapy and education, particularly related to ____________________________________ skills.

38. Name two psychiatric disorders common in parents of children diagnosed with conduct disorder.
    1.
    2.
    3.
    4.
    5.

39. Conduct disorder occurs in both boys and girls. Boys have a higher incidence, but its onset is early for girls.
    TRUE FALSE

40. What classes of medications may be used to address aggression and agitation in youth with conduct disorder?

41. A diagnosis of conduct disorder can only be given to those <18 years old. If 18 years old or older, a diagnosis of antisocial personality disorder is used.
    TRUE FALSE

42. Disruptive mood dysregulation disorder (DMDD) occurs more often in which age group and biological sex?

43. To be diagnosed with DMDD, a child must have temper outbursts disproportionate to the provoking circumstance at least ______________ times a week for ______________ months.

44. Name at least three comorbid disorders to be assessed before a diagnosis of DMDD.
    1.
    2.
    3.
    4.
    5.

45. One environmental issue that the PMHNP must consider when assessing a child's negative behavior or developmental delay is ______________ ______________. A survey is often given to parents to ascertain the child's early life experiences.

46. PMHNPs are mandated reporters, meaning if they even suspect child abuse is occurring then they must report it. What are some agencies/organizations to which the PMHNP may report?

47. ______________________________ enuresis is when a child loses bladder control after at least one year of bladder control.

48. During which sleep stages does nocturnal enuresis usually occur?

49. Nocturnal enuresis is an elimination disorder and a sleep disorder known as a(n) ______________________________.

50. What is diurnal enuresis? What is its important distinction from nocturnal enuresis?

51. The etiology of enuresis can be varied. Complete the mnemonic CAP'IM in the table below for some causes.

C	
A	
P	
I	
M	

52. ______________________ is when a child involuntarily defecates in an inappropriate place. It is associated with constipation.

53. Enuresis affects girls more than boys.
TRUE FALSE

54. As the PMHNP to a 7-year-old boy with enuresis, what advice and/or medications would you provide to his parents?

55. What is the mechanism of action of desmopressin (DDAVP)?

56. A common characteristic of ______________________________ is that the child constantly worries about potential harm to their caregivers when they are apart from one another.

57. Permission from a guardian to treat is always required.
TRUE FALSE

58. In all states, adolescents need guardian consent for birth control, STI assessment and treatment, and substance abuse treatment.
TRUE FALSE

59. ______________________________ and ______________________________ are the FDA-approved antidepressants for treating major depressive disorder in adolescents.

60. Which SNRI has strong evidence for treating pediatric anxiety?

61. Children often need lower doses of psychotropic medications due to their lower body weights.
TRUE FALSE

62. Identify each of the following statements about the psychopharmacological management of pediatric patients with ADHD as TRUE (T) or FALSE (F)

	Medications with adverse effects should never be used with pediatric populations
	Assessment of therapeutic response should include behavior and academic achievement
	Reassessment should occur every 2 weeks for the first year
	If the patient's height and weight cross two percentiles, a drug holiday may be warranted
	During low-stress periods, such as vacation, a drug holiday should be considered
	Medication can be stopped if the patient exhibits no symptoms after 2 years or reaches age 18
	If the medication is not working, the first step should be to switch to another medication
	Behavioral therapy and psychoeducational interventions should be assessed and offered as needed

63. A child with ____ gravitates away from their caregiver, perhaps due to abuse or neglect at an early age. They have inhibited emotional range. Often, they do not seek comfort during negative, threatening interactions.

64. ____
_____ is characterized by a child who lacks boundaries. They are friendly with strangers, including accompanying a stranger without informing their caregiver. However, forming emotional bonds is difficult for these children.

65. To receive a diagnosis of Tourette's disorder, a patient must have ________________ motor tics and ________________ vocal tic lasting for at least ______________ before the age of ________________.

66. Tic disorders do not need to cause distress in order to receive a diagnosis.
TRUE FALSE

67. Rett syndrome disproportionately affects (boys/girls) more.

68. Rett syndrome is linked to a mutation in the ___________________________
___________________________ gene.

69. Match each stage of Rett syndrome with its associated clinical findings.

_____Stage 1 (6–18 months)	A. EPS, seizures, teeth grinding, involuntary movements, cachexia
_____Stage 2 (1–4 years)	B. Holds breath, reduction in eye contact, does not meet developmental milestones
_____Stage 3 (2–10 years)	C. Hand movements, parasomnias, irritable, absence seizures
_____Stage 4 (>10 years)	D. Seizures decrease, loss of gross motor skills (ataxia), increased involuntary movements

13.3 Attention-Deficit/Hyperactivity Disorder (ADHD)

70. ADHD can be either ________________ type or ________________ type, or combined type.

71. It is expected by most providers that a diagnosis of ADHD is predicated on symptoms being present before the age of ____________.

72. Abnormalities in the neurotransmitters ________________ and ________________ are most often associated with ADHD.

73. Why might abnormalities in the reticular activating system (RAS), a collection of neurons located in the brain stem, be linked to ADHD?

74. The ________________ and ________________ are additional neuroanatomical structures associated with ADHD symptoms.

75. (Boys/girls) are twice as likely to be diagnosed with ADHD.

76. Which symptoms of ADHD persist most often into adulthood? Circle all that apply.

    Inattention Hyperactivity Impulsivity

77. Symptoms of ADHD must be observed in at least ____________ different settings to qualify for a diagnosis.

78. Name three to five symptoms of ADHD.

79. Name five medical conditions that mimic ADHD symptoms.
    1.
    2.
    3.
    4.
    5.

80. Attention-deficit/hyperactivity disorder has a typical onset prior to ____________ years old. Symptoms must be present for at least ____________ months and in at least ____________ different settings.

81. ADHD has two symptom domains—inattentiveness and hyperactivity/impulsivity. Under each domain, list as many symptoms as possible.

Inattentive	Hyperactivity/impulsivity

82. Children with ____ Disorder tend to have more injuries caused by accidents.

83. What are five side effects of stimulants that the PMHNP should share with parents and patients?
    1.
    2.
    3.
    4.
    5.

84. Complete the table of ADHD agents with generic medication and name brand, and if the medication is controlled substance. Note sustained- and extended-release options with a *.

Generic	Brand(s)	Controlled	Duration (h)	Key info
Methylphenidate	Ritalin* Metadate* Concerta Methylin* Daytrana			>6 years First-line stimulant Short duration associated with rebound irritability and hyperactivity Long duration may affect sleep Avoid if cardiac issues
	Dexedrine Adderall*	Yes (Schedule II)		
Dexmethylphenidate	Focalin*			
	Vyvanse			
Atomoxetine	Strattera		24	
Guanfacine	Intuniv		24	
	Catapres	No		
Bupropion	Wellbutrin*			Lowers seizure threshold
	Tofranil			
Nortriptyline	Pamelor			

85. Which of the above are not first-line medications if hyperactivity is a symptom?

86. Candy, sodas with high fructose corn syrup, and sweetened breakfast cereals are leading causes of ADHD.
    TRUE FALSE

87. Name at least two standardized rating instruments for ADHD.

13.4 Autism Spectrum Disorder (ASD)

88. According to the DSM-5, what two areas of impairments characterize autism spectrum disorder (ASD)?
    1.
    2.
    3.
    4.
    5.

89. What neurostructural abnormalities are implicated in ASD?

90. Imbalances in what three neurotransmitters are linked to ASD?

91. Males are ________________ times more likely to be diagnosed with ASD.

92. ______________________________ refers to an individual repeating exactly what they hear. This is common in ASD and also seen in psychotic disorders such as schizophrenia. It is associated with a desire to maintain equilibrium and sameness in their environment.

93. Before ___________ years old, the onset of symptoms of ASD is notable.

94. Name at least two screening tools for ASD.

95. Patients with ASD may be prescribed ______________________________ to address aggression and tantrums.

96. Antidepressants may be used to reduce ______________________________ behaviors in patients with ASD. Other potential medications include naltrexone and clonidine.

97. ____ therapy is recommended for patients with ASD who need assistance with impulsive or aggressive behavior.

13.5 Eating/Feeding Disorders

98. What two neurotransmitters are often decreased in patients with eating disorders?

99. Eating disorders are most common among girls between ages _________ and _________ years old.

100. Providers should consider admitting patients with anorexia nervosa for acute care when their BMI is _______ or less.

101. What are the two subtypes of anorexia nervosa?

102. Name at least three behaviors in which patients with bulimia nervosa may compensate for weight gain. Identify which behaviors are purging vs. non-purging.

Purging	Non-purging

103. What is Russell's sign?

104. Explain refeeding syndrome and why it is dangerous.

105. Muscular weakness among patients with eating disorders is often due to hypo-_______________.

106. Name three hobbies/activities with higher than average prevalence of eating disorders. Make sure to include at least one activity in which males typically participate more.

107. The antidepressant _______________ should not be prescribed to patients with eating disorders as it lowers the seizure threshold.

108. What oral pathologies may be seen in a patient who purges by vomiting?

109. Circle the sign/characteristic among each pair that is most associated with anorexia nervosa.

BMI	High	Low
Menstrual cycle	More frequent	Less frequent
Heart rate	Tachycardia	Bradycardia
Blood pressure	Hypertension	Hypotension
ECG	Elevated T-waves	Inverted T-waves
	Elevated ST segment	Depressed ST segment
	Shortened QT interval	Prolonged QT interval
Body temperature	Hyperthermia	Hypothermia
Skin	Moist	Dry

110. ________________________ refers to the fine, downy body hair that individuals with anorexia may grow.

111. What laboratory changes may be expected in patients with anorexia nervosa and bulimia nervosa?

112. The antidepressant ________________________ is FDA-approved for bulimia nervosa.

113. Patients with anorexia nervosa and bulimia nervosa both have dysfunctional beliefs about body image and maladaptive behaviors to cope with these beliefs, specifically pertaining to food.
TRUE FALSE

114. Patients with anorexia nervosa see themselves as overweight/underweight, but tend to be (overweight/underweight).

115. What behavioral habits do patients with anorexia nervosa engage in to control weight?

116. Once individuals with anorexia nervosa reach their goal weight, they end their maladaptive behaviors.
TRUE FALSE

117. Anorexia is considered ego-syntonic/ego-dystonic. Why?

118. To which personality disorder may anorexia nervosa be linked?

119. Individuals with anorexia nervosa unconsciously restrict and control food/eating behaviors.
TRUE FALSE

120. The most deadly mental illness is ____, primarily due to the severe physical health complications.

121. Name five medical issues experienced by individuals with anorexia nervosa.
    1.
    2.
    3.
    4.
    5.

122. Men do not experience anorexia nervosa.
    TRUE FALSE

123. What is the typical treatment plan for anorexia nervosa? What medications show the most efficacy?

124. Patients with anorexia nervosa with a BMI <__________ are recommended for hospitalization.

125. In addition to a low BMI, what other criteria should be considered when considering hospitalization for patients with anorexia nervosa?

126. When an individual eats a large amount of food in a short period of time, to the point where they are physically uncomfortable, it is known as ____________________________.

127. When an individual engages in some behavior to stop the digestion or absorption of food, this is called ____________________________.

128. What are some binging behaviors characteristics and behaviors seen in patients with bulimia nervosa?

129. ____, a personality disorder, has high comorbidity with bulimia nervosa, as they share interpersonal rejection sensitivity.

130. Bulimia nervosa is more/less common than anorexia nervosa.

131. What are at least three common signs on physical exam evidence purging behavior?

132. ____ is when the esophagus is damaged over time by frequent vomiting, so that it ultimately ruptures. Other health problems associated with bulimia nervosa include dehydration, ulcers, metabolic alkalosis, and electrolyte imbalances.

133. ____ are first-line pharmacotherapy for bulimia nervosa, along with cognitive behavioral therapy and interpersonal therapy.

134. Why should a PMHNP avoid the prescription of the antidepressant bupropion for patients with bulimia nervosa, and what alternative treatments are typically recommended for individuals with this eating disorder who also have co-occurring mood disorders?

135. Binge-eating disorder is similar to bulimia nervosa except there is no ______ __________________________________ behaviors by binge eaters.

136. Label each sign or symptom as being most associated with anorexia nervosa (AN), bulimia nervosa (BN), or binge-eating disorder (BE).

__________Distorted body image
__________Food avoidance
__________Severe medical complications
__________ Amenorrhea
__________ Purges through vomiting, excessive exercise, laxatives, or strict diets
__________Excessive caloric intake in a short period of time
__________Underweight
_________ Normal weight
__________Overweight
__________Strong association with cluster B personality disorders
__________Extremely sensitive to interpersonal rejection
__________Most deadly mental illness

137. The only eating disorder with equal prevalence between men and women is ____.

138. What are key elements to ask about when assessing a patient for an eating disorder?

13.6 Answers and Explanations to Chapter Activities

1.

2 months	4–6 months	6–8 months	9–12 months	18 months–3 years	4–5 years	6–12 years	13–21 years
Responds to loud sounds	Symmetrical eye movement	Explores	Sits on own	Walks, kicks	Jumps	Friendly, social interaction	Sexual development
Visual tracking	Shows affection	Babbles	Babbles two syllable words (mama, dada)	Copies others	Scribbles, draw pictures	Emotional range	Fine and gross motor maturity
Smiles	Pushes down with legs	Attempts to grab	Responds to name	Responds to absence/ presence of people	Social interest, speech understood by strangers	Fantasy play	Sense of morality
Hands to mouth	Rolls over	Rock on hands, knees	Recognizes faces	Simple toy play	Two-part commands	Dresses/ undresses on own	Abstract thinking
Holds up head when prone	Laughs		Gestures, points	Poor communication	Differentiates real from imaginary	Seeks approval, attention	Sense of self
			Stranger danger		Full name	Adapts to environment	
			Crawls		Dress, wash hand by self		

2. The Denver Developmental Screening Test evaluates a child's linguistic, social, gross, and fine motor skills. A healthcare provider or skilled expert administers the 10–15-min test. Standardized tests like the Ages and Stages Questionnaires (ASQ) examine newborn and young child development. This screening tests children's communication, gross motor, fine motor, problem-solving, and personal-social abilities. Parents can complete the ASQ at home or in a hospital environment.
3. The HEADDS screening tool examines the psychosocial factors that influence the physical and emotional health of adolescents. The categories and some example questions are:
   1. Home
      - Do you live with both parents?
      - Is there tension or fighting at home?
      - Do you feel safe at home?
      - Do you have a quiet place to do homework?
   2. Education
      - How are your grades?
      - Are you having any problems with your teachers or classmates?
      - Are you involved in any extracurricular activities?
      - Do you plan on attending college?
   3. Activities
      - What activities do you enjoy doing?
      - How often do you participate in physical activity?
      - Do you have any hobbies?
      - Are you involved in any community service?
   4. Drugs/drinking
      - Have you ever tried alcohol or drugs?
      - Do you know anyone who uses drugs or alcohol?
      - Do you feel pressure to drink or use drugs?
      - Do you know the risks associated with drug or alcohol use?
   5. Sex/sexuality
      - Are you sexually active?
      - Have you ever had unprotected sex?
      - Do you feel comfortable talking to your partner about sex?
      - Do you know about safe sex practices?
   6. Suicidality/mental health
      - Have you ever felt sad or hopeless for a long period of time?
      - Have you ever had thoughts of hurting yourself or ending your life?
      - Do you have a support system in place if you are feeling down or stressed?
      - Have you ever been diagnosed with a mental health condition such as depression or anxiety?

4.

Age range	Stage	Tasks
0–1½ years	Trust vs. mistrust	Child learns to believe that the world will provide consistent and predictable care. Building confidence in the world enhances a child's sense of self from their mother
1½–3 years	Autonomy versus shame and doubt	Child gains independence, self-control, and self-esteem. Through autonomy, children learn self-expression and cooperation
3–5 years	Initiative versus guilt	The child is active and testing what may be accomplished and the associated outcomes
6–12 years	Industry versus inferiority and inadequacy	The child learns to be productive, work, and compete
12–20 years	Identity versus role confusion	The adolescent develops personal, and occupational identity from their parents

5. Continuous exposure to chronic stress over time is more likely to lead to psychopathologies in children. In contrast, an acute, isolated trauma typically does not.
6. Selective mutism.
7. FALSE. Assessment and care for pediatric populations often take more time and require a sensitive and developmentally appropriate approach to build trust.
8. The period of development from birth to 5 years old is key when conducting a history on a child's growth and developmental milestones. Birth to 2 years is arguably the most important period during this range.
9. Intellectual disability
10.

Area of functioning	Deficits
Intellectual functioning	• Difficulty with problem-solving • Poor short-term memory • Slow information processing speed • Limited attention span • Difficulty with abstract thinking • Difficulty with generalization and categorization • Difficulty with language and communication skills • Limited ability to learn new skills or information • Difficulty with judgment and decision-making • Impaired reasoning and planning skills • Difficulty understanding cause and effect • Difficulty with math concepts and calculations

Area of functioning	Deficits
Adaptive functioning	• Difficulty with activities of daily living (e.g., bathing, dressing, grooming) • Limited ability to manage personal finances • Difficulty with time management and planning • Limited social skills and difficulty with social cues • Difficulty with problem-solving and decision-making in daily life • Poor judgment and decision-making in social situations • Limited ability to cope with stress or change • Difficulty with using community resources and navigating the environment • Difficulty with following rules and routines • Limited self-awareness and insight into one's own abilities and limitations • Difficulty with communication in social situations (e.g., initiating and maintaining conversations, understanding social norms)

11. Fragile X syndrome is caused by a mutation to the FMR-1 gene. It affects males more than females.
12. Prader-Willi syndrome is caused by several mutations on chromosome 15. Typical signs include learning difficulties, myotonia, small stature, and chronic feeling of hunger. Metabolic disorders can be severe in these children without caretaker education.
13. Cri-du-chat syndrome is a monosomic 5p− mutation causing high-pitched cries, intellectual disabilities, microcephaly, and a flat nose bridge.
14. Noted causes of intellectual disabilities include genetic and chromosomal abnormalities, prenatal and perinatal factors (e.g., prematurity, infections, exposure to toxins), and environmental factors (e.g., malnutrition, lack of stimulation or education, neglect, abuse). Genetics, in utero trauma or deficiencies (oxygen, nutrition), toxins (alcohol, lead), infections, and medical conditions.
15. Fetal alcohol spectrum disorder (FASD) accounts for approximately 80% of intellectual disability cases.
16. Down syndrome is caused by a trisomy (an extra copy) of chromosome 21.
17. The average IQ is 100.
18. Mild intellectual disability describes individuals with an IQ range of 71–84. They require academic accommodations and assistance with the development of social skills.

    Borderline intellectual functioning
19. Fragile X syndrome
20. Tay-Sachs disease is a hereditary metabolic disorder. These individuals have intellectual disabilities.

21.

Level	IQ	Independence	School level	Work
Mild	50–70	Yes, with support	<6th grade	Yes
Moderate	35–50	No	<3rd grade	Yes, with some supervision
Severe	20–35	No, group home, frequent support	Very basic communication, numeracy, literacy (not functional level)	Yes, with intense supervision
Profound	<20	No, constant supervision	Self-care skills, basic communication	Not usually

22. Growth retardation, central nervous system involvement, and facial dysmorphology, such as thin upper lip, micrognathia (small jaw), smooth philtrum, microcephaly, small but wide-set eyes, epicanthal skin folds, short upturned nose, and low/flat nasal bridge. Behavioral and emotional problems, such as difficulty with social interactions, irritability, aggression, anxiety, and depression, are common as well (Fig. 13.1).

23. Mental status exam findings that may be noted for a child with an intellectual disability include:

- Difficulty with abstract thinking and problem-solving
- Limited ability to learn new information
- Impaired reasoning and planning skills
- Difficulty with attention and concentration
- Poor communication skills
- Passive toward and dependent on guardian

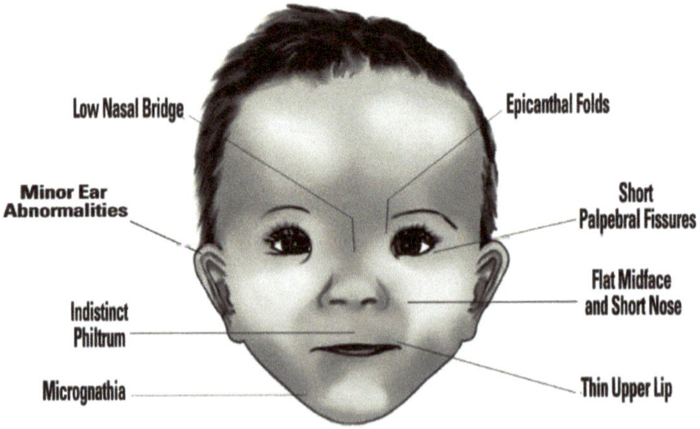

Fig. 13.1 Facial features of fetal alcohol syndrome. (From: Fetal alcohol spectrum disorders: Research challenges and opportunities, Alcohol Research & Health, Vol 34(1):4–14, 2011. https://europepmc.org/article/PMC/3756137. Free full text in Europe PMC)

- Self-injury and/or aggression
- Repetitive movements

24. To receive a diagnosis of global developmental delay, a patient must be no older than 5 years old.
25. Risk factors for the development of a specific learning disorder may include genetics, prenatal exposure to alcohol or drugs, low birth weight, prematurity, perinatal trauma, chronic health conditions, and environmental factors such as poverty, neglect, and lack of stimulation.
26. If restrictive and repetitive behaviors, activities, or interests are also present, the child may receive a diagnosis of autism spectrum disorder.
27. Age, context, gender, family system, growth and developmental stage, and cultural factors, as well as the impact of environmental stressors such as family conflict, poverty, and exposure to violence or trauma.
28. FALSE. The provider should interview the child or adolescent separately from their adult guardians to ensure confidentiality and allow the child to speak openly.
29. FALSE. The mental status examination may need to be modified when working with children to account for their developmental level, attention span, and ability to communicate, as well as the use of play-based assessment techniques and collaboration with parents or caregivers.
30. Ways in which the mental status examination may need to be modified when working with children include:

    - Using age-appropriate language and concepts
    - Incorporating play-based assessment techniques
    - Allowing for breaks and frequent changes in activities
    - Assessing for developmental milestones and age-appropriate behavior
    - Collaborating with parents or caregivers to obtain information about the child's behavior and functioning in different settings

31. 1/D, 2/A, 3/E, 4/B, 5/H, 6/C, 7/G, 8/F, 9/J, 10/I, 11/L, 12/K.
32. Oppositional defiant disorder is less common in females.
33. A child diagnosed with oppositional defiant disorder should be monitored for future development of conduct disorder or antisocial personality disorder.
34. Conduct disorder, ADHD, substance use disorders, antisocial personality disorder, and bipolar I/II disorders.
35. Extreme emotional expressions and harsh or inconsistent parenting is most linked to children's development of ODD.
36. Lead.
37. Parents of children with ODD should seek therapy and education, particularly related to parenting and communication skills.
38. Schizophrenia, mood disorders, substance use disorders especially alcohol use disorder, and antisocial personality disorder.
39. FALSE. Conduct disorder does occur in both boys and girls and in boys more often. Boys also have earlier onset (10–12 years old in boys vs. 16 years old in girls).

40. Antipsychotics, mood stabilizers, SSRIs, and α-agonists.
41. FALSE. Individuals 18 years old or older can have conduct disorder if antisocial personality disorder DSM-5 criteria are not met sufficiently for diagnosis.
42. Disruptive mood dysregulation disorder (DMDD) occurs more often boys <13 years old.
43. To be diagnosed with DMDD, a child must have temper outbursts disproportionate to the provoking circumstance at least three times a week for 12 months.
44. Comorbid disorders to be assessed before a diagnosis of DMDD include ADHD, anxiety disorders, autism spectrum disorder, unipolar and bipolar depressive disorders, and oppositional defiant disorder.
45. One environmental issue that the PMHNP must consider when evaluating a child's negative behavior or developmental delay is exposure to trauma or adverse childhood experiences (ACEs).
46. PMHNP can report suspected child abuse to child protective services or law enforcement agencies.
47. Secondary enuresis is when a child loses bladder control after at least one year of bladder control.
48. Nocturnal enuresis usually occurs during the first half of the night, stages 3 and 4/REM.
49. Parasomnia.
50. Diurnal enuresis is the loss of bladder control during the daytime. It may be a symptom of an underlying medical condition (i.e., anatomical or physiological issue), whereas nocturnal enuresis is usually a developmental issue.
51.

C	Central nervous system, tumors, neural tube defect
A	Anatomical abnormalities in bladder or urethra
P	Psychological
I	Infections, UTI
M	Metabolic, DM, sickle cell trait, anemia

52. Encopresis.
53. FALSE. Enuresis affects boys and girls equally.
54. Treatment options for enuresis may include bedwetting alarms, behavioral interventions such as bladder training, and medication such as desmopressin (DDAVP).
55. Synthetic desmopressin (DDAVP) maintains body fluid balance such as vasopressin. It irritates renal collecting duct V2 receptors, increasing water reabsorption. Urinating is reduced due to less urine production.
56. Separation anxiety disorder is characterized by excessive worry and fear about separation from attachment figures, such as parents or caregivers.
57. FALSE. In some circumstances, such as emergencies, treatment can be provided without guardian consent, and if the minor is emancipated legally or through a life event such as pregnancy.

58. FALSE. In many states, adolescents can consent to these treatments without guardian involvement. Guardians must be notified and consent provided only for substance abuse treatment, although these laws differ by localities and court decisions.
59. Fluoxetine (Prozac) and Escitalopram (Lexapro) are FDA-approved antidepressants for treating major depressive disorder in adolescents.
60. Venlafaxine (Effexor) has strong evidence for treating pediatric anxiety.
61. TRUE. Children often need lower doses of psychotropic medications due to their lower body weights.
62.

TRUE or FALSE	Explanation
FALSE	Medications with adverse effects may be used if the benefits outweigh the risks and careful monitoring is in place
TRUE	Assessment of therapeutic response should include behavior and academic achievement
FALSE	Reassessment should occur more frequently, such as weekly or biweekly, depending on the patient's response to medication
FALSE	A drug holiday should be considered if the patient experiences growth suppression or other adverse effects, not solely based on crossing two percentiles
TRUE	Drug holidays may be considered during low-stress periods, such as school breaks or vacations
FALSE	Medication should be tapered slowly and carefully, and the decision to stop medication should be based on the patient's response to treatment and risk of relapse
FALSE	Non-response to medication may prompt a switch, but other factors such as adverse effects and patient preference should also be considered
TRUE	Behavioral therapy and psychoeducational interventions should be used in conjunction with medication management

63. Reactive attachment disorder is characterized by a child who gravitates away from their caregiver, perhaps due to abuse or neglect at an early age. They have inhibited emotional range and may not seek comfort during negative or threatening interactions.
64. Disinhibited social engagement disorder is characterized by a child who lacks boundaries, is overly friendly with strangers, and may accompany a stranger without informing their caregiver.
65. To receive a diagnosis of Tourette's disorder, a patient must have multiple motor tics and at least one vocal tic lasting for at least one year before the age of 18.
66. FALSE. Tic disorders may cause distress and impairment in social, academic, or occupational functioning, but distress is not required for diagnosis.
67. Rett syndrome disproportionately affects girls more.
68. Rett syndrome is linked to a mutation in the MECP2 gene.

69. 1/B, 2/C, 3/D, 4/A

    - Stage 1 (6–18 months): This stage is characterized by slowed head growth and developmental regression, such as a reduction in eye contact, loss of purposeful hand movements, and a delay in meeting developmental milestones.
    - Stage 2 (1–4 years): During this stage, the child experiences increased irritability, breathing abnormalities, hand stereotypies, and movement disorders. They may also have sleep disturbances and experience seizures.
    - Stage 3 (2–10 years): During this stage, the child may experience a reduction in seizures, but gross motor skills may be lost. They may also have increased hand stereotypies, as well as parasomnias and absence seizures.
    - Stage 4 (>10 years): During this stage, the child may experience a decline in mobility, as well as increased involuntary movements, such as teeth grinding, dystonia, and chorea. They may also experience epilepsy, breathing abnormalities, and cachexia.

70. ADHD can be either inattentive type or hyperactive-impulsive type, or combined type.
71. It is expected by most providers that a diagnosis of ADHD is predicated on symptoms being present before the age of 12.
72. Abnormalities in the neurotransmitters dopamine and norepinephrine are most often associated with ADHD.
73. The reticular activating system (RAS) is involved in maintaining alertness, attention, and arousal. Abnormalities in this system may contribute to ADHD symptoms.
74. The prefrontal cortex and basal ganglia are additional neuroanatomical structures associated with ADHD symptoms.
75. Boys are twice as likely to be diagnosed with ADHD.
76. Inattention symptoms most often persist into adulthood.
77. Symptoms of ADHD must be observed in at least two different settings to qualify for a diagnosis.
78. Symptoms of ADHD include inattention, hyperactivity, impulsivity, forgetfulness, distractibility, and difficulty organizing tasks. Poor attention, increased activity, impulsivity, disruptive behaviors, lack of focus, procrastination, lack of concentration and motivation.
79. Medical conditions that mimic ADHD symptoms include:

    - Seizure disorder
    - Thyroid abnormalities
    - Learning or cognitive disabilities
    - Depression or anxiety
    - Substance abuse
    - Bipolar disorder
    - Autism
    - Low blood sugar levels

- Sensory processing disorder
- Sleep disorders
- Hearing problems

80. Attention-deficit/hyperactivity disorder has a typical onset prior to 12 years old. Symptoms must be present for at least 6 months and in at least two different settings.
81.

Inattentive	Hyperactivity/impulsivity
Lack of attention to details	Fidgets or restlessness
Makes careless mistakes	Constantly moving or changing positions
Difficulty maintaining focus	Difficulty remaining quiet while participating in activities
Appears not to listen	Seems like energized by a motor or battery, which may be an internal sensation
Tends not to follow instructions	Excessive talking
Organization difficulties	Blurts out answers or interrupts
Avoids cognitively demanding tasks	Intrusive
Misplaces or loses items	Impatient
Easily distracted	
Forgetful	

82. Children with ADHD tend to have more injuries caused by accidents.
83. Side effects of stimulants that the PMHNP should share with parents and patients include decreased appetite, insomnia, headaches, stomachaches, and irritability.

    Reduced appetite, weight loss, sleep interruption depending on timing of medication, GI upset, anxiety, irritability, tachycardia, HTN, headache, worsen existing tics, hallucinations, and high doses can lead to seizures, coma, and death.
84.

Generic	Brand	Controlled	Duration (hours)	Key info
Methylphenidate	Ritalin* Metadate* Concerta Methylin* Daytrana	Yes (Schedule II)	3–4, 4–8, 8–10 6–8, 8–10 10–12 3–4, 6–8 10–12	>6 years First-line stimulant Short duration associated with rebound irritability and hyperactivity Long duration may affect sleep Avoid if cardiac issues
(Dextro-) amphetamine	Dexedrine Adderall*	Yes (Schedule II)	4–6, 6–8 4–6, 8–12	>3 years Typical stimulant SE concerns

Generic	Brand	Controlled	Duration (hours)	Key info
Dexmethylphenidate	Focalin*	Yes (Schedule II)	4–6 6–10	Option if SE on methylphenidate
Lisdexamfetamine	Vyvanse	Yes (Schedule II)	10–12	Typical stimulant SE concerns
Atomoxetine	Strattera	No	24	>6 years SE: increased SI, liver damage rare
Guanfacine	Intuniv	No	24	6–17 years Taper on/off SE: hypotension, arrhythmias rare
Clonidine	Catapres	No	4–6, 24 patch	Can be used as adjunct, modulates mood, addresses tics and sleep issues from stimulants SE: hypotension, do not stop suddenly or HTN crisis
Bupropion	Wellbutrin*	No	4–5, 12, 24	Lowers seizure threshold
Imipramine	Tofranil	No	8–24	Get baseline EKG Stop of PR >0.18–0.2 or QRS >0.12 SE: Tachycardia, arrhythmias
Nortriptyline	Pamelor	No	8–24	Same as imipramine

85. Atomoxetine, Bupropion; best for patients with only attention-deficit issues
86. FALSE. Candy, sodas with high fructose corn syrup, and sweetened breakfast cereals have not been shown to be leading causes of ADHD.
87. Two standardized rating instruments for ADHD are the Vanderbilt Assessment Scale and the Conners Rating Scale. Others include the Wender Utah Rating Scale and the Barkley Home Situations Questionnaire.
88. The DSM-5 lists two impairments that constitute autism spectrum disorder (ASD): chronic problems in social communication and interaction across many contexts. Others include confined, repetitive behavior, hobbies, or activities. Early developmental abnormalities must induce clinically substantial social, occupational, or other functioning problems.
89. Neurostructural abnormalities implicated in ASD include increased brain volume, particularly in the frontal and temporal lobes, and reduced connectivity between regions of the brain. Abnormalities in the amygdala, hippocampus, and cerebellar Purkinje cells have also been noted.
90. Imbalances in the neurotransmitters dopamine, serotonin, and gamma-aminobutyric acid (GABA) are linked to ASD. Glutamate also is often implicated.

91. Four times
92. Echolalia refers to an individual repeating exactly what they hear.
93. 3 years old.
94. Modified Checklist for Autism in Toddlers (M-CHAT), Autism Diagnostic Observation Schedule—Generic (ADOS-G), Ages and Stages Questionnaires (ASQ).
95. Patients with ASD may be prescribed atypical antipsychotics, such as risperidone or aripiprazole, to address aggression and tantrums.
96. Self-injurious, hyperactive, obsessive behaviors.
97. Cognitive behavioral therapy. Also, applied behavior analysis (ABA) therapy is recommended for patients with ASD who need assistance with impulsive or aggressive behavior.
98. Neurotransmitters often decreased in patients with eating disorders include dopamine and serotonin. Norepinephrine may also be low.
99. 14–18 years old.
100. Providers should consider admitting patients with anorexia nervosa for acute care when their BMI is 15 or less.
101. The two types of anorexia nervosa are the restrictive type and the binge-eating/purging type.
102. Purging includes self-induced vomiting, laxative use, enemas, and diuretics. Non-purging may include excessive exercise, fasting, and stimulants.
103. Russell's sign refers to abrasions, small lacerations, and calluses on dorsum of the hand overlying the knuckles due to self-inducing vomiting.
104. Undernourished people lack potassium, the main intracellular cation. Refeeding increases cell volume and number, as well as insulin release, which causes an influx of potassium into the cell. This causes hypophosphatemia, hypokalemia, hypomagnesemia, salt retention, and hyperglycemia. The hypophosphatemia, hypokalemia, and hypomagnesemia can cause respiratory and cardiac failure.
105. Hypokalemia (low K^+), lowered level of electrical signals to muscles including cardiomyocytes.
106. Dancers especially ballet, gymnastics, modeling and beauty pageant contestants, wrestlers, and weight lifting.
107. Bupropion (Wellbutrin).
108. Discoloration of tongue/mucosa due to bile from vomit, dental enamel erosion, and hypertrophy of salivary glands.
109. Correct answers are in the right column. Anorexia nervosa is most associated with low BMI, less frequent menstrual cycles, bradycardia, hypotension, inverted T-waves, prolonged QT interval, hypothermia, dry skin, and depressed ST segment on ECG.
110. Lanugo.
111. Anemia, leukopenia, hypokalemia, hypomagnesemia, hypoglycemia, hyponatremia, decreased LH and FSH, and elevated serum amylase in bulimia nervosa.
112. Fluoxetine (Prozac).

113. TRUE. Both anorexia nervosa and bulimia nervosa involve distorted body image and maladaptive behaviors related to food.
114. Patients with anorexia nervosa see themselves as overweight but tend to be underweight.
115. Restrictive eating and food avoidance, excessive exercise, vomiting, laxative or diuretic use, fasting, food rituals and obsessions, calorie counting/dieting, social isolation, body checking, and eating nonnutritional substances (e.g., tissues, cotton balls) to fill the stomach.
116. FALSE. Even after reaching their goal weight, individuals with anorexia nervosa may continue their maladaptive behaviors and have difficulty maintaining their weight.
117. Anorexia nervosa is considered ego-syntonic because individuals with the disorder perceive their behaviors and attitudes as normal and desirable. Individuals do not see their behaviors as excessive or dysfunctional.
118. Obsessive compulsive personality disorder.
119. FALSE. Individuals with anorexia nervosa typically engage in conscious and deliberate efforts to restrict and control their food and eating behaviors. These behaviors are driven by a profound fear of gaining weight or a distorted body image, and individuals with anorexia often plan and execute these actions intentionally as part of their efforts to achieve and maintain extreme thinness.
120. Anorexia nervosa can lead to a range of life-threatening medical issues, including cardiac problems, electrolyte imbalances, organ failure, and suicide.
121. Malnutrition, amenorrhea, osteoporosis, cardiac arrhythmias, electrolyte disturbances, infertility, and gastrointestinal problems.
122. FALSE. While it is more commonly diagnosed in women, anorexia nervosa can affect individuals of any gender. The misconception that anorexia nervosa only occurs in women has contributed to underdiagnosis and delayed treatment for men with the condition.
123. Treatment for anorexia nervosa may include hospitalization, nutritional counseling, and cognitive behavioral therapy. Medications such as fluoxetine (Prozac) and olanzapine (Zyprexa) have shown efficacy in treating the disorder.
124. Patients with anorexia nervosa with a BMI <15 are recommended for hospitalization. However, the specific threshold for hospitalization may vary based on individual factors, including the severity of medical and psychological symptoms and the overall health and stability of the patient. In some cases, individuals with higher BMIs may also require hospitalization if they are experiencing severe medical complications or are at immediate risk to their health.
125. CRAVE—cardiac, renal, arrhythmias, vitals, electrolytes. Suicidal ideation should also be assessed.
126. Binge eating.
127. Purging.
128. Individuals with bulimia nervosa exhibit various binge-eating behaviors, including consuming excessive amounts of food rapidly, feeling a lack of

satiety, hoarding food, and eating in secrecy. Binges are often triggered by emotional distress and are characterized by a loss of control over eating. The episodes continue until the individual feels uncomfortably full, and they may involve a variety of high-calorie foods. Following a binge, individuals typically engage in compensatory behaviors, such as self-induced vomiting, laxative use, excessive exercise, or fasting, to eliminate excess calories and cope with the guilt associated with the binge.

129. Borderline personality disorder.
130. Bulimia nervosa is more common than anorexia nervosa.
131. These may encompass signs of self-induced vomiting, such as dental erosion and enamel damage due to stomach acid exposure, as well as swollen salivary glands (parotid glands) caused by recurrent vomiting. Additionally, examination findings might reveal calluses or scars on the back of the hand or knuckles (Russell's sign) from using the fingers to induce vomiting. Other possible physical exam findings may involve electrolyte imbalances, such as low potassium levels (hypokalemia), which can result from the loss of potassium through vomiting or laxative use, hoarse voice, and damage to the esophagus or throat.
132. Boerhaave syndrome.
133. SSRIs.
134. The reason for avoiding the prescription of the antidepressant bupropion for patients with bulimia nervosa is its potential to lower the seizure threshold, which can increase the risk of seizures, particularly in individuals with a history of eating disorders. In such cases, alternative antidepressant medications that do not carry this seizure risk are usually recommended for individuals with bulimia nervosa who also have co-occurring mood disorders. These alternatives may include selective serotonin reuptake inhibitors (SSRIs), mood stabilizers, or antipsychotics.
135. Binge-eating disorder is similar to bulimia nervosa except there is no compensatory behavior by binge eaters (e.g., purging).
136. ____AN_____Distorted body image

____AN_____Food avoidance

____AN_____Severe medical complications

____AN_____Amenorrhea

____BN_____Purges through vomiting, excessive exercise, laxatives, or strict diets

____BE_____Excessive caloric intake in a short period of time

____AN_____Underweight

____BN_____Normal weight

____BE_____Overweight

____BE_____Strong association with cluster B personality disorders

____BN_____Extremely sensitive to interpersonal rejection

____AN_____Most deadly mental illness

137. Binge-eating disorder.

138. These include the patient's history of dieting, exercise patterns, weight fluctuations, body dissatisfaction, and any purging behaviors they may engage in. Additionally, it is important to explore their eating habits, weight changes over time, the contrast between their self-image and how they believe others perceive them, the role of food in their life, and the extent of control they feel they have over their eating behaviors.

References and Resources

American Psychiatric Association, editor. Diagnostic and statistical manual of mental disorders: DSM-5-TR. 5th ed., text revision. American Psychiatric Association Publishing; 2022.

Barkley RA, DuPaul GJ, McMurray MB. Attention deficit hyperactivity disorder: a handbook for diagnosis and treatment. 4th ed. Guilford Press; 2015.

Evans SW, Owens JS, Bunford N. Evidence-based psychosocial treatments for children and adolescents with attention-deficit/hyperactivity disorder. J Clin Child Adolesc Psychol. 2014;43(4):527–51. https://doi.org/10.1080/15374416.2013.850700.

Goodman R, Ford T, Richards H, Gatward R, Meltzer H. The development and well-being assessment: description and initial validation of an integrated assessment of child and adolescent psychopathology. J Child Psychol Psychiatry. 2000;48(5):429–36.

Hudson JI, Hiripi E, Pope HG, Kessler RC. The prevalence and correlates of eating disorders in the National Comorbidity Survey Replication. Biol Psychiatry. 2007;61(3):348–58. https://doi.org/10.1016/j.biopsych.2006.03.040.

Johnson K, Vanderhoef D, Magrath N. Psychiatric-mental health nurse practitioner review and resource manual. American Nurses Credentialing Center, American Nurses Association; 2020.

Kessler RC, Berglund P, Demler O, Jin R, Merikangas KR, Walters EE. Lifetime prevalence and age-of-onset distributions of DSM-IV disorders in the National Comorbidity Survey Replication. Arch Gen Psychiatry. 2005;62(6):593–602. https://doi.org/10.1001/archpsyc.62.6.593.

Kovacs M. The children's depression, inventory (CDI). Psychopharmacol Bull. 1985;21(4):995–8.

Lock J, Le Grange D, Agras WS, Moye A, Bryson SW, Jo B. Randomized clinical trial comparing family-based treatment with adolescent-focused individual therapy for adolescents with anorexia nervosa. Arch Gen Psychiatry. 2010;67(10):1025–32. https://doi.org/10.1001/archgenpsychiatry.2010.128.

Pelham WE, Fabiano GA. Evidence-based psychosocial treatments for attention-deficit/hyperactivity disorder. J Clin Child Adolesc Psychol. 2008;47(1):3–25. https://doi.org/10.1080/15374410701818681.

Polanczyk G, de Lima MS, Horta BL, Biederman J, Rohde LA. The worldwide prevalence of ADHD: a systematic review and metaregression analysis. Am J Psychiatry. 2007;171(2):130–49. https://doi.org/10.1176/ajp.2007.164.6.942.

Steinhausen HC. The outcome of anorexia nervosa in the 20th century. Am J Psychiatry. 2002;159(8):1284–93. https://doi.org/10.1176/appi.ajp.159.8.1284.

World Health Organization. Improving the mental and brain health of children and adolescents. 2021. https://www.who.int/activities/improving-the-mental-and-brain-health-of-children-and-adolescents

Zakhari R. The psychiatric-mental health nurse practitioner certification review manual. Springer Publishing Company; 2021.

Notes:

Notes:

14 Sleep-Wake Disorders

Test your learning and check your understanding of this book's contents: use the "Springer Nature Flashcards" app to access questions using ▶ https://sn.pub/62J0Ar.

To use the app, please follow the instructions in Chap. 1.

Excellent mental health requires sound sleep. Unfortunately, many of us struggle with getting quality sleep at some point. The Centers for Disease Control and Prevention (CDC 2022) estimate that 70 million Americans experience persistent sleep issues. Sleep disorders can be linked to genetic, social, environmental, neurological, medical, and psychiatric factors. Sleep issues can either be a separate diagnosis or a sign of a mental disorder (e.g., depression, anxiety, or neurocognitive abnormalities).

The DSM lists ten sleep-wake disorders that are divided into dyssomnias and parasomnias. The most prevalent sleep condition is insomnia, which is defined as having trouble falling or staying asleep. About 10–30% of adults have chronic insomnia (Ohayon 2002). A person's mental and physical health can be significantly impacted by insomnia, including an increased risk of depression and anxiety as well as cardiovascular disease, diabetes, and obesity.

Sleep apnea, which is defined by frequent breathing pauses during sleep, has been associated with a higher risk of cardiovascular disease, diabetes, and hypertension (Young et al. 2002). Continuous positive airway pressure (CPAP) therapy is frequently used to treat sleep apnea, although other approaches, such as weight loss and lifestyle changes, may also be successful.

The ability to function on a daily basis and one's quality of life can both be greatly affected by narcolepsy, a condition marked by extreme daytime sleepiness and abrupt, involuntary sleep bouts. In addition to non-pharmacological therapies such lifestyle changes to enhance sleep hygiene, it is frequently treated with stimulant drugs to manage tiredness (Thorpy and Krieger 2014).

T. Stewart, *Psychiatric-Mental Health Nurse Practitioner Program Companion and Board Certification Exam Review Workbook*,
https://doi.org/10.1007/978-3-031-60894-0_14

PMHNPs can provide education, therapeutic interventions, and medications to assist clients who need more restful sleep. Sleep hygiene best practices include establishing a consistent sleep schedule, creating a comfortable sleep environment, and avoiding substances or activities that may interfere with sleep, such as caffeine and electronics before bedtime. Cognitive behavioral therapy for insomnia (CBT-I) (Sateia et al. 2017), clinical interviews, sleep diaries, and objective assessments such as polysomnography (PSG) are examples of therapeutic approaches and diagnostic techniques. Benzodiazepines and Z-drugs are frequently used hypnotic medications, while common wakefulness-promoting medications include amphetamines and modafinil.

A holistic and tailored approach to treating sleep-wake disorders is necessary, taking into account the unique needs and circumstances of each patient. This chapter discusses normal physiology, neuroanatomy, and circadian sleep patterns. Then, variations to these rhythms or dyssomnias and parasomnias are discussed. Sleep hygiene is addressed. Diagnostic criteria, pertinent medications, including wakefulness-promoting medications, and therapies are presented.

14.1 Foundations of Normal Physiology and Anatomy

1. What is sleep?

2. A normal sleep cycle progresses through ____________________ NREM stages and ____________________ REM stage.

3. Complete the following chart on NREM and REM stages of sleep.

Stage	NREM or REM	Description	% of sleep cycle

4. Describe each brain waveform, and include in which stage(s) of sleep the waveform is typically seen. Then, draw an example of the waveform as might be depicted on a polysomnography.

Name	Description	Waveform on EEG
Beta		
Alpha		
Theta		
Delta		

5. A _________________________________ is a burst of activity when the brain is trying to maintain a sleeper's tranquil state. They are found during stage 2 NREM sleep and tend to decrease in frequency and intensity as we age.

6. As noted on an EEG, ______________________________ are characterized by a sharp, high-amplitude wave followed by a slower, lower-amplitude wave. They typically occur during stage 2 of non-rapid eye movement (NREM) sleep and are believed to play a role in protecting sleep by suppressing cortical arousal in response to external stimuli.

7. Sleep stages _____ to _____ occur most often during the first half of sleep.

8. REM cycles occur approximately every ___________ minutes of sleep.

9. The neurotransmitter ___________________________ is most associated with REM sleep.

10. Individuals who wake from ____________________ sleep often have vivid recall of their dreams.

11. Circle when REM is most active.

    Sleep initiation   Middle of night   Toward morning

12. EEGs during sleep studies often show that REM sleep occurs during ______________________________ in individuals with sleep disorders.

13. As we age, light sleep (increases/decreases), and deep sleep (increases/decreases). REM sleep (increases/decreases).

14. When in REM sleep, which of the following vital signs are increased? Mark correct answers with an X.
    _____ Blood pressure
    _____ Heart rate
    _____ Respiratory rate
    _____ Body temperature

15. In which stage of sleep do pediatric populations spend a lot of sleep time? Circle all that apply.
    Stage 1   Stage 2   Stage 3

16. What is the recommended number of hours of sleep for each developmental/age group?

Group	# of hours
Newborns	
Children	
Adolescents	
Adults	

17. How do sleep patterns change as we age?

18. What is orexin? What is its connection to sleep and wakefulness?

19. What neurological structure is known as the body's "master clock"?

14.2 Pathophysiology of Disorders/Mental Illness

20. ____________________ include sleep disorders that make it difficult to fall asleep or result in excessive daytime sleepiness.

21. ____________________ are most common in the pediatric population. They include abnormal behaviors, usually during deep sleep. Somnambulism (sleepwalking), sleep terrors, nightmares, and restless legs syndrome are examples.

22. Identify if each of the following DSM sleep disorders is considered a dyssomnia (D) or a parasomnia (P).
    _____ Insomnia disorder
    _____ Hypersomnolence disorder
    _____ Central sleep apnea
    _____ Sleep-related hypoventilation
    _____ Narcolepsy
    _____ Circadian rhythm sleep-wake disorders
    _____ Non-REM sleep arousal disorders (e.g., sleepwalking, sleep terrors)
    _____ Nightmare disorder
    _____ REM sleep behavior disorder
    _____ Restless leg syndrome

23. An individual with hypersomnolence disorder may report impaired performance and reduced alertness after awakening. This symptom is referred to as sleep ____________________.

24. What is bruxism? During which stage of sleep is it most common?

25. How is bruxism treated?

26. What is insomnia?

27. How is insomnia disorder characterized in terms of signs and symptoms by the DSM?

28. To be diagnosed with persistent insomnia disorder, an individual must have had sleep difficulties for at least ________ months.

29. Is episodic or persistent insomnia most related to stress? Why?

30. Name five key risk factors for insomnia.
    1.
    2.
    3.
    4.
    5.

31. D.E.E.P. is a helpful acronym for remembering causes of insomnia. Complete the table below with each letter's keyword and a brief example/description.

	Keyword	Description and examples
D		
E		
E		
P		

32. What chemical deficiency is associated with narcolepsy, most commonly due to a loss of hypothalamic neurons?

33. Narcolepsy is characterized by at least _______ episodes of sleep latency lasting no more than ______ minutes.

34. ___________________________ is sudden loss of motor tone accompanying a strong emotional response.

35. Hypnagogic hallucinations are experienced between wakefulness and REM.

TRUE FALSE

36. What are five sleep hygiene best practices?
    1.
    2.
    3.
    4.
    5.

37. What types of relaxation and therapy may benefit those with sleep disorders?

38. An individual who reports being groggy, or excessively sleepy, even though they get adequate sleep may have ______________________________________ disorder. This disorder must occur at least _______ times a week over several months. Individuals should be assessed for a _______________________ within the last 12–18 months and comorbidities like MDD, SAD, and BP depressed state.

39. Obstructive sleep apnea (OSA) is characterized by which signs and symptoms?

40. ____________________________ sleep is poor sleep quality that leaves an individual feeling unrested. This problem is often reported by those with breathing-related sleep disorder.

41. What are some risk factors for OSA? Which are more common in children? adults?

42. Compare/contrast "sleep terrors" and "nightmares."

Sleep terrors	
Nightmares	

43. An individual who presents with increased REM sleep, numerous nighttime awakenings, and reduced slow-wave sleep should be assessed for __________ ____________________________.

44. Occurring mostly in males >50 years old, what are common features of REM sleep behavior disorder? What are risk factors?

14.3 Diagnoses and Tools

45. Using the ABCDEFGH mnemonic, list the information points that should be included when taking a client's sleep history.

A	
B	
C	
D	
E	
F	
G	
H	

46. To diagnose a patient with chronic insomnia, they must have had symptoms for at least ____ days a week for ____ months and report a reduced quality of life.

47. ____ is the first-line therapeutic intervention for chronic insomnia.

48. A __________________________ is a visual representation of the cycling of sleep phases over a single night.

49. A ______________________________, also known as a sleep study, is a comprehensive test used to diagnose sleep disorders.

50. An individual with restless legs may have low ________________ levels. However, dopamine agonists and benzodiazepines are first-line treatments.

51. In addition to glucose levels, metabolic causes of sleep disorders can be partially assessed by ________________ and ________________ levels.

52. In addition to a CBC and chemistry panel, a ____________________ hormone function test should be ordered when investigating sleep disorders.

53. A full physical exam should be conducted on an individual who reports sleep disturbances.

    TRUE FALSE

54. What are some psychiatric disorders linked to poor sleep?

55. What signs of insomnia in older adults may be misinterpreted as Alzheimer's disease or another neurodegenerative disorder?

56. What are some nonpsychiatric illnesses linked to poor sleep?

57. Match the three types of breathing-related sleep disorders with their description.

Name	Description
_____ 1. Obstructive sleep apnea hypopnea	A. Variability in respiratory center of brain
_____2. Central sleep apnea	B. Airway obstruction during sleep often due to pharynx closure
_____3. Sleep-related hypoventilation	C. Comorbid with neurological and medication/ substance use

58. ______________________ is a hormone within the brain that helps to regulate the sleep-wake cycle. It increases when it is dark, and it helps us to fall asleep. This hormone is created in the ______________________.

59. "Night owls" may have what type of circadian rhythm sleep-wake disorder?

60. "Early to bed, early to rise" sleepers may have what type of circadian rhythm sleep-wake disorder?

61. Chronic users of opioids may show ________________ breathing in a subtype of central sleep apnea, which presents as a pattern of crescendo-decrescendo variation in tidal volume due to a comorbid medical condition.

14.4 Pharmacological and Therapeutic Interventions

62. Individuals with OSA should avoid sleeping in the ________________ position.

63. What is the most common non-pharmacological approach to addressing sleep apnea?

64. An individual should enjoy their last caffeinated beverage by __________ to avoid sleep disturbances. This is approximately 6 h before bedtime.

65. What is the difference between continuous (CPAP) and bilevel (BiPAP) positive airway pressure devices? How do they help manage OSA?

66. Which medications should be avoided in patients with OSA?

67. Complete the following table on FDA-approved benzodiazepines often used for sleep management, except in OSA. Ideally, these medications would be used for only a few weeks.

Generic	Name brand	Duration	Use
Flurazepam			
Temazepam			
Triazolam			

68. What is the mechanism of action of benzodiazepines with regard to sleep management?

69. Complete the following table on nonbenzodiazepine hypnotics often used for sleep management.

Generic	Name brand	Duration	Use
Zaleplon			
Zolpidem			
Eszopiclone			
Ramelteon			
Suvorexant			

70. Complete the following table on antidepressants often used for sleep management.

Generic	Name brand	Use
Amitriptyline		
Doxepin		
Mirtazapine		
Trazodone		

71. ______________________________ and ______________________________ are antihistamines that cause sedation and are available over-the-counter. Why do these medications have this effect?

72. Why might individuals with low magnesium levels experience insomnia?

73. What are two downsides to using antihistamines for sleep?

74. The non-stimulant wake-promoting drug ________________________________ ___ is used to combat daytime sleepiness, especially related to hypersomnolence disorders.

75. Stimulants are often used to treat which of the following? (select all that apply).
   ______Depression
   ______Enuresis
   ______Narcolepsy
   ______Sleep disorder in depressed patients
   ______Sleep terror disorder

76. What medication is recommended for the treatment of insomnia in children?

77. Which of the following places an infant at increased risk for sudden infant death syndrome? Select all that apply.
   ______Sleeping prone
   ______Sleeping supine
   ______Having numerous blankets and pillows in crib

_____Feeding before being put in crib
_____Sleeping with a light on
_____Smoker in the house
_____Pet in the house

78. ______________________________ therapy can be as effective as medications for some sleep disorders.

79. Depressant medications and substances (e.g., alcohol) reduce quality sleep. Specifically, they reduce which types/stages of sleep?

80. What is desensitization or imagery rehearsal therapy? How is it used to address nightmares?

14.5 Answers and Explanations to Chapter Activities

1. Sleep is a state of rest marked by a decrease in physical activity and an increase in mental relaxation. The individual is unaware of their surroundings, and their bodily functions (e.g., breathing) are slowed. This natural body repair and regeneration process affects mental and physical wellness. Sleep helps memory consolidation, information processing, and well-being by changing our bodies and brains. Good health requires 7–9 h of sleep per night for adults.
2. 3; 1
3.

Stage	Description	% of sleep cycle
1 NREM	Drifting off to sleep (drowsy sleep), lowered brain activity, blood pressure, muscle tone, easy to wake	5
2 NREM	Sleep spindles and K complexes present in EEG, decreased muscle activity, no longer conscious of external environment	50
3 NREM	Slow-wave, deep sleep, parasomnias often present during this stage	20–25
4 REM	Brain activity similar to waking brain, dreaming, later in night, difficult to arouse	Varies (~15)

4.

Name	Description	Waveform on EEG
Beta (β)	Awake, active, alert Fastest waves	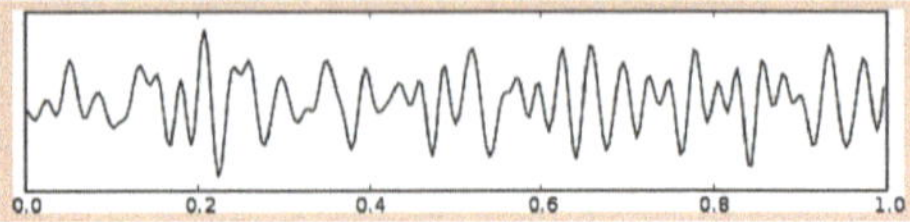
Alpha (α)	Awake, relaxed, closed eyes Neurons firing at different times Stage 1	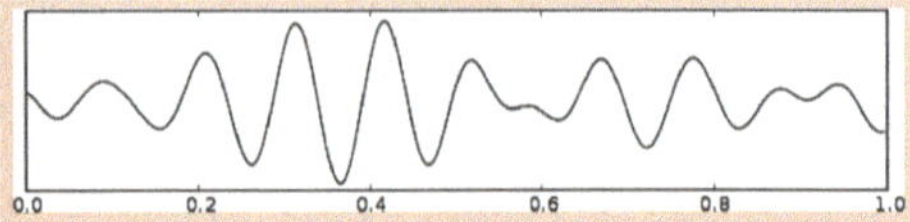
Theta (θ)	Sleepy, already sleeping, or in a sleep transition Hippocampus = memory activity Stage 2 and REM	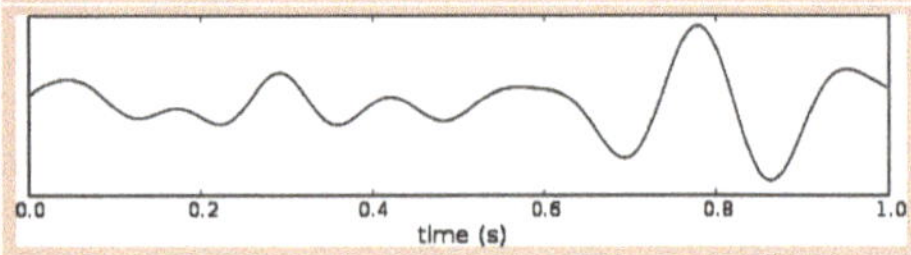
Delta (δ)	Deep sleep Simultaneous firing of neurons, synchronized Waves are large and slow Stage 3	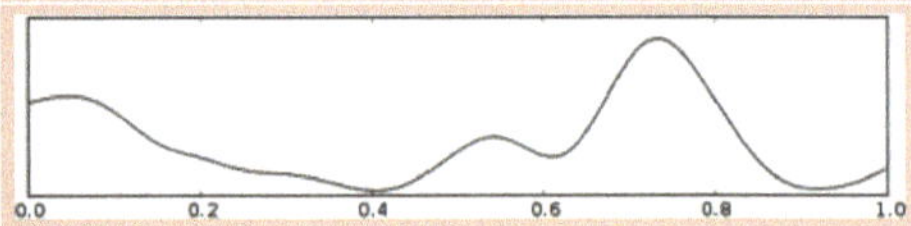

5. NREM stage 2 features sleep spindles, brief brain activity bursts. Fast, repetitive brain oscillations may help limit brain activity and consolidate memories when we sleep. Sleep spindles may help store new memories long-term. They may also protect us from outside stimuli and interruptions, allowing us to sleep regularly. Drugs and sleep disorders can disrupt sleep spindles, impacting memory consolidation and sleep quality.
6. A "K complex" is a type of wave pattern that can be observed on an electroencephalogram (EEG) during sleep. K complexes are characterized by a sharp, high-amplitude wave followed by a slower, lower-amplitude wave (Fig. 14.1).
7. Stages 1–3.
8. 90 minutes.

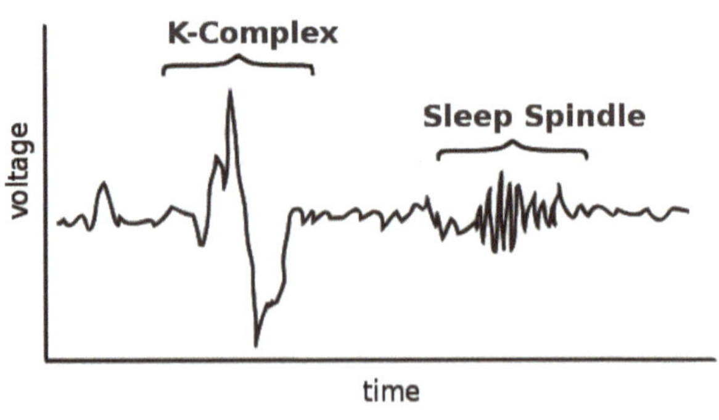

Fig. 14.1 K complex. (With permission from Rakesh Ranjan, et al. A fuzzy neural network approach for automatic K complex detection in sleep EEG signal. https://doi.org/10.1016/j.patrec.2018.01.001, 2018, Elsevier)

9. REM sleep involves acetylcholine. The brainstem manufactures it to control REM sleep. Brain acetylcholine is high, and serotonin and norepinephrine are low in REM sleep. A neurotransmitter change may produce REM sleep's brain activity and muscle paralysis. For learning, memory, and other cognitive activities, acetylcholine may aid memory consolidation during sleeping. Acetylcholine deficit or imbalances can induce REM sleep behavior disorder, which produces vivid, intense dreams and erratic sleep movements. Drugs that regulate brain acetylcholine can treat REM sleep behavior.
10. REM.
11. Toward morning.
12. Sleep initiation. The first few hours of sleep investigations using EEGs commonly indicate REM sleep in those with sleep difficulties. REM sleep may occur earlier and more often in narcolepsy and REM sleep behavior disorder. Daytime fatigue, vivid dreams, and problems falling asleep might result from poor sleep.
13. Increases, decreases, decreases.
14. During REM sleep, all increased, except body temperature. During non-REM sleep, all tend to decrease.
15. Stage 3.
16.

Group	# of hours
Newborns	18 h
Children	10–11 h
Adolescents	8–10 h
Adults	7–9 h

17. As individuals age, they often experience changes in their sleep patterns and quality. These changes can include early wakefulness, drowsiness, reduced REM (rapid eye movement) sleep, and fragmented sleep. One common observation is that older individuals tend to sleep less overall. These alterations in sleep architecture lead to difficulties in both falling asleep and staying asleep. Sleep efficiency, the percentage of nighttime spent asleep, tends to be lower in older adults, resulting in more time spent awake or in lighter sleep stages. Various factors such as medications, underlying medical conditions, and other external influences can contribute to increased awakenings and sleep disturbances in the elderly population.
18. Orexin, also known as hypocretin, is a neuropeptide produced in the hypothalamus of the brain. Orexin is primarily associated with promoting wakefulness and maintaining arousal. It helps to stabilize the sleep-wake cycle by promoting alertness during the day. Reduced orexin production or dysfunction of orexin receptors can lead to conditions such as narcolepsy, which is characterized by excessive daytime sleepiness and disrupted sleep patterns.

19. The suprachiasmatic nucleus controls circadian rhythm, hormone synthesis, and metabolism. The SCN synchronizes the body's clock with the environment via retinal photosensitive ganglion cell light. It then controls daily cycles such as melatonin release by sending signals to other brain and body regions. A SCN or body clock disruption can cause insomnia and circadian rhythm sleep-wake disorders. Daily sunlight and regular sleep schedules control the body's internal clock and increase sleep quality.
20. Dyssomnias.
21. Parasomnias.
22.
    __D___ Insomnia disorder
    __D___ Hypersomnolence disorder
    __D___ Central sleep apnea
    __D___ Sleep-related hypoventilation
    __D___ Narcolepsy
    __D___ Circadian rhythm sleep-wake disorders
    __P___ Non-REM sleep arousal disorders (e.g., sleepwalking, sleep terrors)
    __P___ Nightmare disorder
    __P___ REM sleep behavior disorder
    __P___ Restless leg syndrome
23. Inertia or drunkenness.
24. Nighttime bruxism is tooth grinding. As a common sleep disorder, it affects kids and adults. NREM sleep, especially deep sleep, is bruxism-prone. Wearing down of tooth enamel, jaw pain, and headaches can result from bruxism. Sleep might be disrupted. Tension, worry, and medicines can induce bruxism.
25. Common treatment approaches include the use of nighttime mouth guards or splints to prevent dental damage caused by grinding. Stress management techniques such as meditation and exercise can help reduce bruxism by addressing underlying stressors. In some cases, antidepressants and muscle relaxants may be prescribed to alleviate symptoms. Dental treatment may be necessary if teeth have been damaged due to bruxism, requiring repairs or restorations. Additionally, biofeedback using sensors can assist individuals in recognizing and controlling tooth grinding and clenching behaviors, offering a comprehensive approach to managing bruxism.
26. Insomnia is a common sleep disorder characterized by difficulty falling asleep, staying asleep, or experiencing nonrestorative sleep despite having the opportunity to sleep. It often leads to daytime fatigue, irritability, and impaired cognitive functioning. Insomnia can be a short-term or chronic condition and may be caused by various factors, including stress, medical conditions, medications, or lifestyle habits. Different types of insomnia exist. Acute insomnia can result from stress or environmental changes. Chronic insomnia: three times a week for 3 months. Drugs, medical conditions, and sleep deprivation can cause it. Treatment options for insomnia typically include behavioral interventions, lifestyle changes, and, in some cases, medication.

27. Insomnia, as defined by DSM-5, is characterized by persistent difficulties in falling asleep or staying asleep for more than 30 min on at least three nights a week, leading to significant disruptions in various aspects of life. It is not attributed to underlying medical conditions or the immediate effects of substances such as drugs. Furthermore, the presence of depression alone cannot account for the sleep disturbances. To be diagnosed with insomnia, these symptoms must persist for at least 1 month, and if they last for less than a month, it is considered "short-term insomnia."
28. 3 months.
29. Episodic. Stress disturbs the sleep-wake cycle, making it hard to fall and stay asleep. Traumatic life situations including death, divorce, or job loss can trigger acute insomnia.
30. Female, age, stress, swing-shift work, time zone change, sleep apnea, medications (benzos, stimulants), and substances (caffeine, alcohol) are all risk factors for insomnia.
31.

	Keyword	Description and examples
D	Drugs	Can cause nightmares, excitation, and increased urine output
E	Environment	Noise, stress, snoring partner, irregular work shifts
E	Emotions	Anxiety, depression, mania, agitation, paranoia
P	Physical	Pain, medical conditions

32. Hypocretin (orexin), measured in cerebrospinal fluid. Hypocretin regulates sleep and wakefulness. This impairment may induce narcolepsy's sleepiness and abnormal sleep patterns.
33. 2 episodes; 8 minutes.
34. Cataplexy is sudden muscle tone loss and powerful emotions such as laughter, rage, or astonishment. Cataplexy can cause sudden muscle loss in the face, neck, or limbs, producing weakness, slurred speech, or difficulty standing.
35. TRUE. Wakefulness generates hypnopompic hallucinations. Dreamlike images, sounds, and sensations might be unpleasant or perplexing. REM sleep behavior disorder and narcolepsy produce hypnagogic hallucinations. Medication, alcohol, drugs, and other medical conditions may cause them.
36. A good sleep hygiene routine involves prioritizing only sleep and sex in the bed, avoiding blue light and electronic devices for at least an hour before bedtime. The bedroom should be kept dark and cool, and it is important to maintain a consistent bedtime and wake-up time. Evening consumption of alcohol and caffeine should be limited, and vigorous exercise should be avoided close to bedtime. If unable to sleep, it is advisable not to stay in bed for more than 15 min and to engage in a relaxing activity instead.
37. Meditation, hypnosis, biofeedback, breathing techniques, warm bath, exercise early in day, and CBT.
38. Hypersomnolence (hypersomnia); three times; and head trauma/TBI.

39. Snoring, daytime sleepiness, feeling fatigued despite "slept" well, morning headache, gasping or choking during night, HTN, frequent urination, mood changes, and difficulties concentrating.
40. Nonrestorative.
41. Children: nasopharyngeal anatomical abnormalities (narrow airway), tonsillar and adenoid obstruction; adults: obesity, age, male gender, alcohol use, family history, smoking, and head/neck anatomical issues (thick neck).
42.

Sleep terrors	• Awaken from deep sleep • Loud screaming, frenetic behavior • Benign, self-limiting • Individual usually falls back to sleep and does not realize their terror the following day • Often linked to daytime stress • More common in boys • Potential precursor to temporal lobe epilepsy • Stages 3–4
Nightmares	• Dreams • Late in sleep cycle, REM • Individuals can be wakened easily • Remember nightmare often • Ages 3–7 • Desensitization therapy useful

43. Depression. Depressed people may experience more REM sleep, when most dreams occur. Nighttime awakenings and reduced slow-wave sleep, the deepest stage needed for physical and emotional healing, may occur.
44. Sleep talking, yelling, yanking limbs, punching, self or bed partner injury, and enacting dreams. Narcolepsy, antidepressants, β-blockers, and prodromal neurocognitive deficits are risk factors. Rapid eye movement (REM) sleep behavior disorder generates vivid and violent dreams. Risk factors include: men >50 years old, alcohol consumption, use of antidepressants or antipsychotics, OSA, and Parkinson's disease.
45.

A	Activities that interfere with a restful sleep, usually those completed closest to bedtime
B	Bed partner, including pets
C	Consequences of sleep on daily functioning and quality of life
D	Drug regimen of prescribed medications, not just those for sleep (i.e., hypnotics)
E	Exacerbating or relieving factors
F	Frequency and duration of poor night's sleep
G	Genetic factors, family history
H	Habits with substances (e.g., alcohol, caffeine, nicotine, cannabis, and OTC sleep meds)

46. 3 days; 3 months.
47. Cognitive-behavioral therapy (CBT).
48. A hypnogram illustrates nightly sleep stages. A sleep study (polysomnogram) uses it to examine sleep stages, length, and anomalies. Classic hypnograms involve REM and NREM sleep. NREM sleep contains four stages: 1, 2, 3, and 4. Each level contains separate brain, muscle, and eye activities. REM sleep has quick eye movements, cognitive activity, and muscle tone loss. The hypnogram shows sleep quantity, quality, and interruptions (Fig. 14.2).
49. Polysomnograms are thorough sleep examinations used to diagnose sleep issues. This determines sleep disorder type, severity, and diagnosis. Polysomnograms entail sleeping in a sleep laboratory with sensors and equipment. The sensors monitor brain, eye, muscle, heart, and respiration while sleeping. Polysomnograms diagnose insomnia, restless legs syndrome, and OSA (Fig. 14.3).
50. Ferritin; RLS sufferers may be anemic; thus, iron supplements may assist.
51. B12 and folate levels indicate metabolic sleep problems. Brain and nervous system function require B12. Low vitamin B12 may cause insomnia. Red blood cells and the nervous system require B vitamins like folate. Low folate may induce insomnia. Sleep disturbances can result from abnormal glucose levels.
52. Thyroid hormones regulate metabolism and energy. Sleep disorders such as insomnia and excessive sleepiness may be diagnosed if thyroid hormone levels are abnormal.

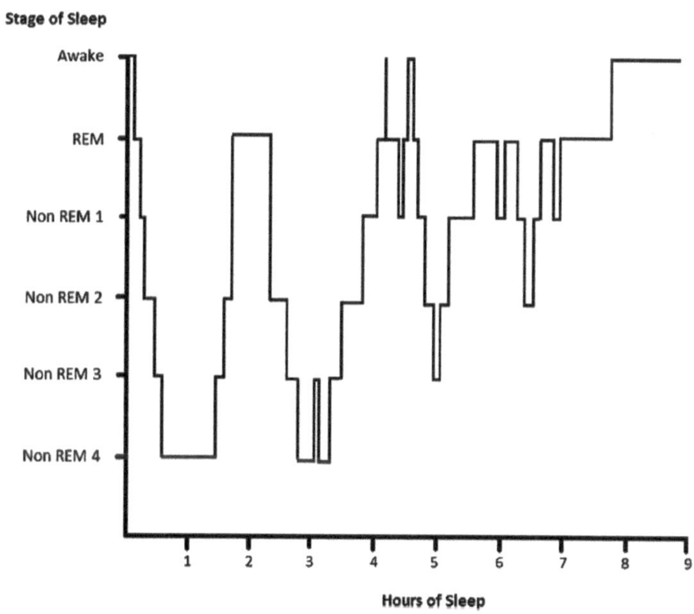

Fig. 14.2 Hypnogram

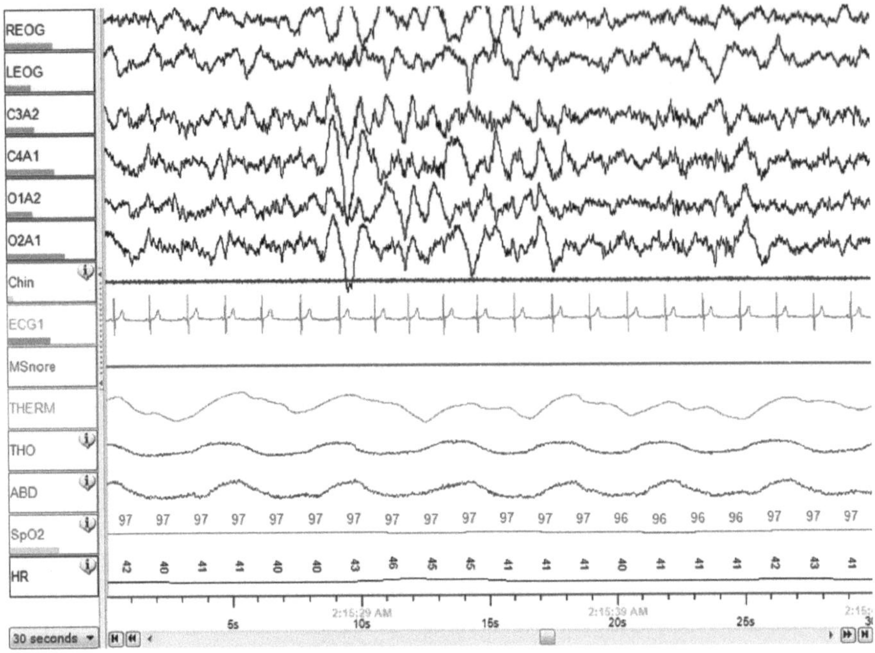

Fig. 14.3 Polysomnography. (With permission from Pandi-Perumal, S.R., Spence, D.W., BaHammam, A.S. (2014). Polysomnography: an overview. In: Pagel, J., Pandi-Perumal, S. (eds) Primary Care Sleep Medicine. Springer, New York, NY. https://doi.org/10.1007/978-1-4939-1185-1_4)

53. TRUE. A thorough physical exam can diagnose sleep apnea, restless leg syndrome, and other sleep disorders. A medical history review, physical exam, and sometimes laboratory tests or other diagnostic procedures comprise the physical exam. Polysomnograms can detect sleep disorders and examine sleep patterns in addition to physical exams.
54. Anxiety and OCD, substance use, depression, mania, ADHD, bipolar disorders, and schizophrenia.
55. Difficulty with memory and concentration, confusion, restlessness, and flipped sleep schedules.
56. Cardiac, GI, pulmonary, GERD, chronic kidney disease, diabetes, and chronic pain (musculoskeletal, nerve).
57. 1/B, 2/A, and 3/C.
58. Melatonin controls sleep-wake cycles and is created in the pineal gland. The pineal gland is in the epithalamus near the third ventricle. After sleeping, melatonin levels drop over the day. People with insomnia may use melatonin supplements.
59. "Night owls," or people who have difficulties sleeping or staying awake, may have delayed sleep phase disorder. DSPD causes trouble falling asleep and staying awake due to its tendency of late rising. DSPD patients may be drowsy in the morning and have problems sleeping until late at night, yet they wake up refreshed

in the afternoon. A mismatch between the body's internal clock and the environment can cause DSPD, which affects sleep and other biological processes. Young adults are more affected and may be hereditary or medical. Chronotherapy (early sleep shifts) and light therapy (strong light at specific times) treat DSPD.

60. Advanced sleep phase disorder. Due to early waking, ASPD makes sleeping and staying awake difficult. ASPD sufferers may struggle to stay awake at night yet wake up refreshed. The body's internal clock and external environment may mismatch, affecting sleep and other biological activities and causing ASPD. It is more common in older people. ASPD can be treated with chronotherapy or light therapy.
61. Cheyne-stokes respiration.
62. Supine. Patients with OSA should not sleep on their backs. Supine sleeping raises sleep apnea risk because gravity pulls tongue and throat soft tissues back and restricts airway. Poor sleep and breathing can ensue. Side sleeping keeps the airway open, reducing sleep apnea risk. A body pillow or other positional device can help OSA patients sleep laterally.
63. Lifestyle change is the most common nondrug sleep apnea treatment. This includes modifying sleep apnea-causing practices such as losing weight, quitting smoking, avoiding alcohol and sedatives, sleeping on your side, and using a humidifier.
64. 3 pm (ideally >6 h before bedtime).
65. These devices overcome breathing restriction by providing air pressure when sleeping. PAP machines blow air through sleeping masks or nasal prongs. Airflow prevents OSA-causing airway blockages. BiPAP inhalation pressure is two-way, higher in inhalation than exhalation pressure. In-and-out air flow pressure is equal in CPAP. OSA is treated with CPAP and BiPAP.
66. Hypnotics. Benzodiazepines and nonbenzodiazepine hypnotics relax airway muscles and increase airway obstruction risk, worsening OSA. Opioids and TCAs should also be avoided in general.
67.

Generic	Name brand	Duration	Use
Flurazepam	Dalmane	Long	Avoid in geriatric populations
Temazepam	Restoril	Intermediate	Sleep maintenance
Triazolam	Halcion	Short	Sleep onset Avoid long-term use

68. GABA/GABA-α agonists increase sleep efficiency and reduce sleep-onset delay and wakefulness to relax (anxiolysis), weariness, and sleep. Benzodiazepines cure insomnia and other sleep disorders, so they are often used temporarily. They can become habit-forming and induce tiredness, dizziness, and impaired cognition, which can be dangerous if the person drives or uses heavy machinery. When benzodiazepines are withdrawn, physical dependence may cause withdrawal (Fig. 14.4).

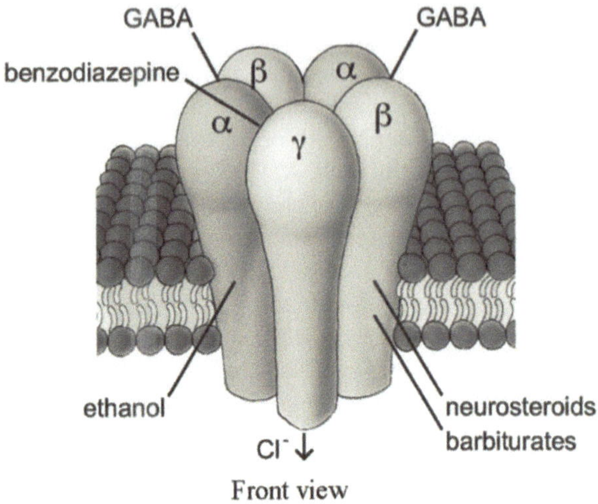

Fig. 14.4 GABA receptor. (With permission from Chen, X., van Gerven, J., Cohen, A. et al. Human pharmacology of positive GABA-A subtype-selective receptor modulators for the treatment of anxiety. Acta Pharmacol Sin 40, 571–582 (2019). https://doi.org/10.1038/s41401-018-0185-5)

69.

Generic	Name brand	Duration	Use
Zaleplon	Sonata	Very short (4 h)	Sleep initiation
Zolpidem	Ambien	Short (6 h)	Take on empty stomach, make sure 8 h of sleep, associated parasomnias well-documented
Eszopiclone	Lunesta	Intermediate (8 h)	Sleep maintenance
Ramelteon	Rozerem	Intermediate	Melatonin receptor agonist, sleep initiation
Suvorexant	Belsomra	Very long	Orexin antagonist

70.

Generic name	Brand name	Use
Amitriptyline	Elavil	For insomniacs or frequent wakers. Amitriptyline should be used for chronic sleep disorders that have failed standard treatment, not acute insomnia. Unsuitable for pregnant, breastfeeding, children, and seniors
Doxepin	Sincquan, Silenor	For insomnia and sleep problems. Lower doses of Silenor treat insomnia. Doxepin works on brain chemicals to improve sleep
Mirtazapine	Remeron	Mirtazapine is sometimes prescribed off-label to assist depressed or nervous persons sleep. It helps start and maintain sleep and is well-tolerated
Trazodone	Desyrel	Due to its sedative qualities, used off-label for insomnia and other sleep disorders. It aids sleep by increasing duration and quality. Trazodone is generally well-tolerated, but dosage should be watched

71. Benadryl, Unisom. Doxylamine (Unisom) and diphenhydramine (Benadryl) bind to brain histamine receptors to sedate. Histamine controls sleep-wake cycles and immune response. Antihistamines inhibit histamine, reducing sneezing, itching, and runny nose. They promote drowsiness and sedation by altering brain chemicals that regulate sleep and wakefulness.
72. Magnesium plays a crucial role in GABA modulation, which is essential for relaxation and sleep. Insomnia and other sleep problems are associated with low magnesium levels, as magnesium is involved in energy metabolism, neuronal transmission, and muscle function, all of which impact sleep-wake cycles. Low magnesium levels can result in disrupted sleep, muscle spasms, cramps, and restlessness, making it challenging to fall and stay asleep.
73. Antihistamines can assist in inducing sleep, but they do not necessarily improve sleep quality. However, it is crucial to use them sparingly because tolerance can develop within as little as three days. One significant drawback of antihistamines is drowsiness, which can impair cognitive function, coordination, and various mental and physical abilities, posing a potential risk for tasks such as driving or operating heavy machinery the following day. Long-term use of antihistamines may lead to physical dependence, and withdrawal from these drugs can result in insomnia and other sleep-related issues. Additionally, antihistamines may have side effects such as dry mouth, constipation, and urinary retention, and they can interact with other medications while potentially exacerbating glaucoma and prostate disorders.
74. (Ar-)modafinil (Nuvigil/Provigil).
75. Narcolepsy.
76. Childhood insomnia is typically related to stress but can sometimes be associated with trauma and hypervigilance. When it comes to treatment, sleep hygiene and behavioral therapy are primary approaches to address pediatric insomnia. Medication is considered a last resort for children with insomnia. If necessary, sleep-inducing medications may be used, with melatonin being the preferred choice for kids. Melatonin helps regulate sleep-wake cycles and is available without a prescription. Benzodiazepines and nonbenzodiazepine hypnotics are generally not recommended for childhood insomnia due to the risk of dependence and other potential side effects.
77. Sleeping prone, having numerous blanket and pillows, and smoker in the house.
78. Cognitive behavior therapy—insomnia (CBT-I).
79. Alcohol and depressants can disturb deep (slow-wave or stage 3) and REM sleep. Depressants diminish deep and REM sleep and cause sleepiness, making it hard to fall or stay asleep. These drugs may cause sleep problems, daytime sleepiness, and poor sleep quality.
80. Pleasant imagery is used to reframe and alleviate repeated nightmares in a therapeutic approach called imagery rehearsal therapy (IRT). This method involves planning and rehearsing the nightmare's storyline and ending during waking hours to reduce its impact. IRT is a form of cognitive behavioral therapy (CBT)

that aims to desensitize individuals to the distressing aspects of their nightmares and help them reinterpret the dreams, ultimately leading to fewer and less intense nightmares. The therapy involves gradual exposure to the frightening elements of the nightmare, relaxation techniques, and creating more positive dream endings. IRT has shown effectiveness in reducing nightmare frequency and intensity, particularly in conditions like posttraumatic stress disorder (PTSD), often complemented by relaxation training or medication.

References and Resources

Akintomide GS, Rickards H. Narcolepsy: a review. Neuropsychiatr Dis Treat. 2011;7:507–18. https://doi.org/10.2147/NDT.S23624.

Alfano CA, Gamble AL. The role of sleep in childhood psychiatric disorders. Child Youth Care Forum. 2009;38(6):327–40. https://doi.org/10.1007/s10566-009-9081-y.

American Academy of Sleep Medicine. International classification of sleep disorders. 3rd ed. American Academy of Sleep Medicine; 2014.

American Psychiatric Association, editor. Diagnostic and statistical manual of mental disorders: DSM-5-TR. 5th ed., text revision. American Psychiatric Association Publishing; 2022.

Broughton RJ. The parasomnias and sleep-related movement disorders—a look back at six decades of scientific studies. Clin Transl Neurosci. 2022;6(1):3. https://doi.org/10.3390/ctn6010003.

Bruni O, Novelli L. Sleep disorders in children. BMJ Clin Evid. 2010;2010:2304.

CDC. Sleep and sleep disorders. Centers for Disease Control and Prevention; 8 Sept 2022. https://www.cdc.gov/sleep/index.html.

Epstein L, Mardon S. The Harvard Medical School guide to a good night's sleep. McGraw-Hill; 2006.

Gauld C, Lopez R, Philip P, Taillard J, Morin CM, Geoffroy PA, Micoulaud-Franchi JA. A systematic review of sleep–wake disorder diagnostic criteria reliability studies. Biomedicines. 2022;10(7):1616. https://doi.org/10.3390/biomedicines10071616.

Jansson-Fröjmark M, Norell-Clarke A. Cognitive behavioural therapy for insomnia in psychiatric disorders. Curr Sleep Med Rep. 2016;2(4):233–40. https://doi.org/10.1007/s40675-016-0055-y.

Johnson K, Vanderhoef D, Magrath N. Psychiatric-mental health nurse practitioner review and resource manual. American Nurses Credentialing Center, American Nurses Association; 2020.

Kalmbach DA, Cheng P, Ong JC, Reffi AN, Fresco DM, Fellman-Couture C, Ruprich MK, Sultan Z, Sagong C, Drake CL. Mindfulness-based therapy for insomnia alleviates insomnia, depression, and cognitive arousal in treatment-resistant insomnia: a single-arm telemedicine trial. Front Sleep Chronobiol. 2023;2:1072752. https://doi.org/10.3389/frsle.2023.1072752.

Kim JH, Elkhadem AR, Duffy JF. Circadian rhythm sleep-wake disorders in older adults. Sleep Med Clin. 2022;17(2):241–52. https://doi.org/10.1016/j.jsmc.2022.02.003.

Ntafouli M, Galbiati A, Gazea M, Bassetti CL, Bargiotas P. Update on nonpharmacological interventions in parasomnias. Postgrad Med. 2020;132(1):72–9. https://doi.org/10.1080/00325481.2019.1697119.

O'Haver Day P, Horton-Deutsch S. Using mindfulness-based therapeutic interventions in psychiatric nursing practice—part II: mindfulness-based approaches for all phases of psychotherapy—clinical case study. Arch Psychiatr Nurs. 2004;18(5):170–7. https://doi.org/10.1016/j.apnu.2004.07.004.

Ohayon MM. Epidemiology of insomnia: what we know and what we still need to learn. Sleep Med Rev. 2002;6(2):97–111. https://doi.org/10.1053/smrv.2002.0186.

Peters AL, Saunders WJ, Jackson ML. Mindfulness-based strategies for improving sleep in people with psychiatric disorders. Curr Psychiatry Rep. 2022;24(11):645–60. https://doi.org/10.1007/s11920-022-01370-z.

Rossman J. Cognitive-behavioral therapy for insomnia: an effective and underutilized treatment for insomnia. Am J Lifestyle Med. 2019;13(6):544–7. https://doi.org/10.1177/1559827619867677.

Sateia MJ, Buysse DJ, Krystal AD, Neubauer DN, Heald JL. Clinical practice guideline for the pharmacologic treatment of chronic insomnia in adults: an American Academy of Sleep Medicine clinical practice guideline. J Clin Sleep Med. 2017;13(2):307–49.

Schutte-Rodin S, Broch L, Buysse D, Dorsey C, Sateia M. Clinical guideline for the evaluation and management of chronic insomnia in adults. J Clin Sleep Med. 2008;4(5):487–504.

Stepnowsky CJ, Ancoli-Israel S. Sleep and its disorders in seniors. Sleep Med Clin. 2008;3(2):281–93. https://doi.org/10.1016/j.jsmc.2008.01.011.

Sun SY, Chen GH. Treatment of circadian rhythm sleep–wake disorders. Curr Neuropharmacol. 2022;20(6):1022–34. https://doi.org/10.2174/1570159X19666210907122933.

Thorpy MJ, Krieger AC. Delayed diagnosis of narcolepsy: characterization and impact. Sleep Med. 2014;15(5):502–7. https://doi.org/10.1016/j.sleep.2014.01.015.

Tobin T, Tobin ML. Staying awake and aware: the importance of sleep in psychiatric nursing practice. Issues Ment Health Nurs. 2017;38(11):924–9. https://doi.org/10.1080/01612840.2017.1341585.

Valerio TD. Much more than a nuisance: health consequences of sleep disorders. Adv Nurse Pract. 2009;17(9):57–60.

Wickwire EM, Geiger-Brown J, Scharf SM, Drake CL. Shift work and shift work sleep disorder: clinical and organizational perspectives. Chest. 2017;151(5):1156–72. https://doi.org/10.1016/j.chest.2016.12.007.

World Health Organization. International statistical classification of diseases and related health problems. 11th ed. WHO; 2022.

Young T, Peppard PE, Gottlieb DJ. Epidemiology of obstructive sleep apnea: a population health perspective. Am J Respir Crit Care Med. 2002;165(9):1217–39. https://doi.org/10.1164/rccm.2109080.

Zakhari R. The psychiatric-mental health nurse practitioner certification review manual. Springer Publishing Company; 2021.

Notes:

Notes:

Sexual Dysfunctions, Gender Dysphoria, and Paraphilic Disorders

15

Test your learning and check your understanding of this book's contents: use the "Springer Nature Flashcards" app to access questions using ▶ https://sn.pub/62J0Ar.

To use the app, please follow the instructions in Chap. 1.

"Let's Talk About Sex," the song goes, yet we hardly ever do so in health care. This is a problem. The brain is the largest sex organ, and sexual behavior, interest, and impact are well within the scope of practice of a PMHNP given their inclusion in the DSM-5. Taboos around sex and patients' own embarrassment about sexual performance dissuade open conversations. More importantly, sexual dysfunctions, gender dysphoria, and paraphilic disorders are important topics for psychiatric-mental health nurse practitioners to understand for several reasons.

First, sexual dysfunctions are common among individuals and can significantly impact an individual's quality of life and relationships. Prevalence rates of sexual dysfunctions in the general population range from approximately 10% to 52% (Laumann et al. 1999). These dysfunctions can include problems with desire, arousal, orgasm, and pain during sexual activity. In some cases, sexual dysfunctions may be related to underlying physical or mental health conditions, such as cardiovascular disease, diabetes, depression, or anxiety (Safarinejad et al. 2009).

Second, gender dysphoria or the distress that an individual experiences as a result of the gender they were assigned at birth not aligning with their gender identity is an increasingly prevalent and important topic in psychiatric-mental health nursing. Gender dysphoria is a recognized psychiatric condition and individuals experiencing gender dysphoria may benefit from gender-affirming care, including hormone therapy and surgery (World Health Organization 2018).

Finally, paraphilic disorders or abnormal sexual interests or behaviors can also impact an individual's mental health and relationships. Paraphilic disorders may include pedophilia, fetishism, and voyeurism (American Psychiatric Association

T. Stewart, *Psychiatric-Mental Health Nurse Practitioner Program Companion and Board Certification Exam Review Workbook*,
https://doi.org/10.1007/978-3-031-60894-0_15

2022). Understanding sexual dysfunctions, gender dysphoria, and paraphilic disorders is crucial for psychiatric-mental health nurse practitioners in order to provide comprehensive and compassionate care to their patients.

This chapter covers sexual dysfunctions, gender dysphoria, and paraphilic disorders. First, we cover some foundations about sexual behavior. Sexual disorders may be categorized as desire disorders, arousal disorders, orgasm disorders, or pain disorders. Sexual dysfunctions such as premature ejaculation and impotence are included. Gender dysphoria including basics of diagnostic assessment and pharmacological treatment and side effects is discussed. Paraphilic disorders, such as fetishistic disorders and pedophilia, are discussed along with their diagnostic criteria, pertinent medications, and therapies.

15.1 Foundations

1. The brain and other sex organs respond to sexual stimuli following the sexual response cycle. Draw and label each phase of the sexual response cycle for men and women. Then, briefly describe each phase in the table that follows.

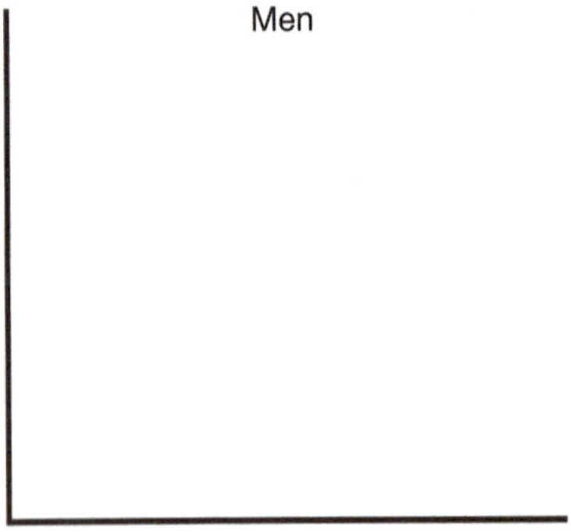

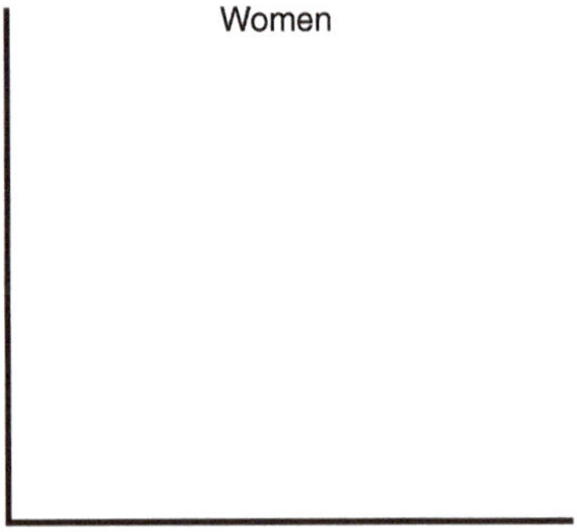

Excitement	

Plateau	
Orgasm	
Resolution	

2. Identify three to five causal factors of sexual dysfunction for each category.

Predisposing factor	Precipitating factors	Maintaining factors

3. As individuals age, sexual desire decreases.
   TRUE FALSE
4. What are age-related physical changes to sexual anatomy and physiological sex drive in men and women?

5. Identify if each of the following substances is associated with enhancing (↑) or inhibiting (↓) libido.

Substance	↑ Libido	↓ Libido
Alcohol—short-term use		
Alcohol—long-term use		
Marijuana		
Cocaine		
Amphetamines		
Narcotics		
Serotonin		
Dopamine		
Testosterone		
Progesterone		

6. What are some medical conditions that are linked to sexual dysfunctions?

7. What are some medications that have sexual side effects?

8. The neurotransmitter ______________________________ enhances libido, while __________________________ inhibits sexual function.

15.2 Sexual Dysfunctions

9. The causes of sexual dysfunctions may be ____________________________ or ________________________.

10. What are some causes of poor sexual desire?

11. Match each DSM sexual dysfunction with its description on the right.

1. _____Delayed ejaculation	A. Persistent deficient or absent sexual thoughts, fantasies, or desires
2. _____Erectile disorder	B. Absent/reduced interest/arousal related to sexual activities, thoughts, encounters, cues, etc.
3. _____Female orgasmic disorder	C. Associated with the use of alcohol, sedatives, hypnotics, anxiolytics, or stimulants
4. _____Female sexual interest/arousal disorder	D. Failure to obtain or maintain erection during partnered sexual activities
5. _____Genito-pelvic pain/penetration disorder	E. Persistent or recurrent pattern of ejaculation during partnered sexual activity within 1 min following penetration or before individual wishes it
6. _____Male hypoactive sexual desire disorder	F. Delay, infrequency, or absence of orgasm or reduced intensity of orgasm sensations lasting more than 6 months

7. _____Premature early ejaculation	G. Difficulties with (a) vaginal penetration during intercourse, (b) pain during intercourse, and (c) fear or anxiety about pain or penetration or contraction of pelvic floor muscles during sex
8. _____Substance/ medication-induced sexual dysfunction	H. A marked difficulty or inability to achieve desired ejaculation lasting more than 6 months during partnered sexual activities

12. Sexual difficulties due to inadequate sexual stimulation would receive a diagnosis of sexual dysfunction.
    TRUE FALSE

13. Complete this table on the onset subtypes of sexual dysfunctions.

Subtypes	Description
Lifelong	
Acquired	
Generalized	
Situational	

14. Which of the following may contribute to an individual's sexual dysfunction? Select all that apply and give an example for that particular category.
    __________Partner (abusive spouse, ostomy bag)
    __________Relationship (poor communication)
    __________Individual vulnerabilities (history of abuse, body image)
    __________Psychiatric comorbidities (depression, bereavement)
    __________Cultural or religious factors (attitudes toward pleasure)
    __________Medical factors (nerve damage)
    __________Developmental factors (advanced age, menopause)

15. Penile erection and vaginal lubrication are examples of sexual ________________.

16. In order to be diagnosed, most sexual disorders require that a client has symptoms for at least _____________.

17. Two medical conditions associated with erectile disorder are _____________ ___________________ and ________________________________.

18. Older men report less distress with erectile disorder than younger men.
    TRUE FALSE

19. During the ______________ stage of sleep men normally experience spontaneous erections.

20. What laboratories should be ordered when diagnosing erectile disorder, particularly secondary erectile disorder?

21. What is the relationship between smoking tobacco and erectile disorder, if any?

22. Orgasm includes contractions of the ____________________ and ____________________ muscles.

23. The ____________________________ period is when men are hesitant to sexual excitement and cannot ejaculate. Women may also experience this period. This period ____________________ with age.

24. Detumescence refers to ____________________________.

25. Label each as being controlled by the parasympathetic (P) or sympathetic (S) nervous system.
    _______Ejaculation
    _______Erection
    _______Vaginal lubrication
    _______Orgasm

26. Label each as being a female (F) or male (M) sexual dysfunction per the DSM-5.
    _______Hypoactive sexual desire disorder
    _______Sexual interest/arousal disorder
    _______Orgasmic disorder
    _______Delayed ejaculation
    _______Erectile disorder
    _______Genito-pelvic pain/penetration disorder
    _______Premature ejaculation

27. For a sexual dysfunction diagnosis, an individual must be symptomatic for at least __________ months, except for sexual dysfunction induced by ___________.

28. What psychiatric medications are commonly associated with substance/medication-induced sexual dysfunction?

29. Premature (early) ejaculation is recurrent ejaculation within _________ minute(s) following penetration.

30. Sexual dysfunction is often a combination of _________________________ and ________________________________ factors. Therefore, any underlying medical conditions should be ruled out first.

31. ______________________________ is avoidance of sexual contact. _________ ______________________________ is deficiency of fantasies/desires, but the individual still has sexual contact.

32. Male patients concerned about erectile dysfunction should avoid which two legal substances?

33. What are some topics that are addressed with those patients who report a lack of sexual desire?

34. ____ is a leading psychological cause of erectile dysfunction.

35. Delayed ejaculation incidence increases around age __________ for men.

36. What age-related physiological changes are linked to delayed ejaculation in older men?

37. Ejaculation is controlled by the ______________________ and ______________________ nerves.

38. Following a transurethral prostatic resection, men are at risk of ______________________ejaculation. This should be differentiated from delayed ejaculation.

39. What are five psychiatric disorders that should be included in the differential for a sexual disorder diagnosis?
    1.
    2.
    3.
    4.
    5.

40. A woman who orgasms through clitoral stimulation, but not during vaginal penetration, meets the criteria for female orgasmic disorder.
    TRUE FALSE

41. Providers treating a patient with hypoactive sexual desire and genito-pelvic pain may consider referring the patient to which medical specialists?

42. Women with ______________________ disorder may report phobia-like avoidance of gynecological examinations and feelings of femininity.

43. What is vaginismus?

44. ________________________ refers to pain before, during, or after intercourse.

45. A diagnosis of genito-pelvic pain/penetration disorder is only given to women.
TRUE FALSE

46. Out of the following, which group most frequently reports genito-pelvic pain with penetration? Circle the correct answer.
Premenopausal Menopausal Postmenopausal

47. While _______________ typically initiate sexual activity, this is not always the case, and may be related to hypoactive sexual desire complaints. It behooves providers to ask about relationship dynamics vis-a-vis sex for this reason.

15.3 Paraphilic Disorders

48. What is a paraphilia?

49. Complete the following table on the eight paraphilic disorders covered in the DSM-5.

Paraphilic disorder	Explanation

Paraphilic disorder	Explanation

50. In which gender are paraphilic disorders most prevalent (based on limited research)?

51. ________________________________ and ____________________________ ________are the two paraphilias most often linked to arrest.

52. Individuals with paraphilic disorders are usually referred for psychiatric help by ________________________________.

53. Individuals usually have only one paraphilia.

    TRUE FALSE

54. Complete the following table by providing good and poor prognostic factors associated with paraphilic disorders.

Good	Poor

15.4 Gender Dysphoria

55. Match each term with its correct definition.

Term	Definition
1. _____Sexual identity	A. Diagnosis of incongruence between experienced and expressed gender and gender assigned at birth
2. _____Gender identity	B. When gender identity does not conform to gender norms
3. _____Gender dysphoria	C. How a person identifies in line with normative constructs of male and female, including biological and social factors
4. _____Sexual orientation	D. Experience and expression of sexuality
5. _____Transgender	E. Individual who identifies as opposite assigned gender and undergoes some hormonal or surgical affirming procedure(s)
6. _____Transsexual	F. Male to female psychological continuum, including sexual attraction
7. _____Sexual behavior	G. Direction of sexual attraction does not always align with gender identity
8. _____Gender nonconforming	H. Somatic features and phenotype do not match societal or historical expectations

56. ____ refers to an individual's feelings of incongruence between experienced and assigned genders.

57. What term is used after an individual has undergone any treatment to support gender reassignment?

58. Name several differential diagnoses for gender dysphoria that should be considered.

59. The ____ __ publishes guidelines to assist clinicians and therapists in working with individuals considering hormone replacement treatment and gender-affirming surgery. They provide sample letters and assessments.

15.5 Treatments

60. Explain sex therapy.

61. Sex therapists use exercises about non-sexual touching and partners recognize and communicate how they like to be touched to address erectile dysfunction. This approach is known as ______________________________.

62. For erectile disorder, a PMHNP might offer a patient a prescription for sildenafil (Viagra). What type of medication is sildenafil? What is its mechanism of action? What other medications are contraindicated to use with sildenafil and other erectile disorder medications?

63. What medications may be offered to help with premature ejaculation?

64. Therapy and pharmacological interventions are the only options to address erectile dysfunction.
    TRUE FALSE

65. Describe approaches to address premature ejaculation.

66. ______________________ is a topical anesthetic that can be applied to the penis to decrease sensation.

67. What are some approaches to addressing painful intercourse and female orgasmic disorder?

68. SSRIs may also delay or inhibit orgasm in women.
    TRUE FALSE

69. ______________________ and ______________________ are not associated with sexual side effects and are often first-line or adjunct medications for patients with depression.

70. First-generation antipsychotics may inhibit sexual desire by raising ______________________________ levels.

71. ______________________________, used for nerve pain, seizures, and depression, has been linked to problems with orgasm.

72. In addition to SSRIs and naltrexone, individuals with paraphilic disorders may be prescribed ______________________________ to lower their sex drive. This use is controversial.

73. What are some treatment options for gender dysphoria?

15.6 Answers and Explanations to Chapter Activities

1. See Fig. 15.1.

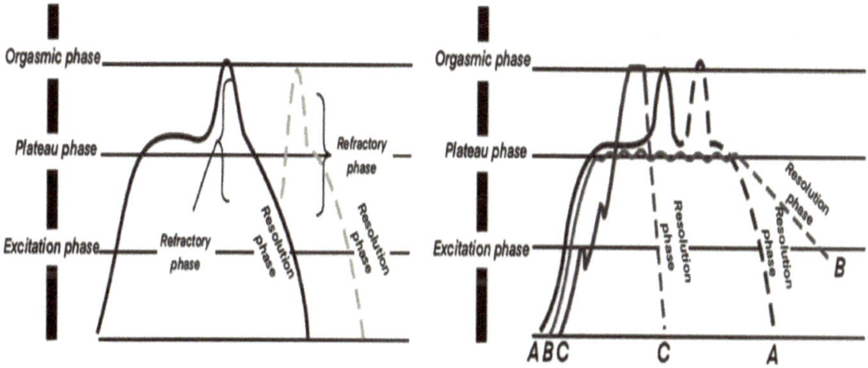

Fig. 15.1 Sexual response cycle (top panel: the male sexual response cycle; lower panel: the female sexual response cycle). (Published in: Zhang, F., Li, Y., Shi, Z. et al. Sexual experience in patients with coronary heart disease: a descriptive phenomenological study. *Sci Rep* 14, 9968 (2024). https://doi.org/10.1038/s41598-024-60496-7. Under Creative Commons Attribution 4.0 International License http://creativecommons.org/licenses/by/4.0/)

Excitement	In the excitement phase, the sympathetic nervous system increases blood flow to the penis, vaginal walls, clitoris, and nipples, elevating heart rate and respiration. Involuntary muscular movements such as grimaces occur during this phase. Body becomes sexually aroused throughout this time. Physical changes include increased heart rate, blood pressure, breathing rate, clitoris and labia enlargement in women, and penile erection in men
Plateau	Breathing, heart rate, and blood flow rise during plateauing. Females feel an orgasmic platform—the outer third of the vaginal walls tightens—and males release healthy sperm cells during "foreplay" (Killick et al. 2011). Birth control with penile withdrawal fails due to early fluid release (Aisch and Marsh 2014). This increases arousal. Vaginal muscle tension and blood engorgement increase
Orgasm	The shortest but most rewarding phase is orgasm. Neuromuscular tension dissipates and oxytocin floods the bloodstream after its peak, fostering emotional attachment. Ejaculation and orgasm muscle contractions are temporally related; however, this link is not necessary because they are physiologically distinct. The sexual response cycle peaks with pleasure and forceful muscle spasms. Men usually ejaculate during orgasm
Resolution	The body returns to a pre-aroused state in the resolution phase. Males enter a refractory period of being unresponsive to sexual stimuli. The length of this period depends on age, frequency of recent sexual relations, level of intimacy with a partner, and novelty. Because females do not have a refractory period, they have a greater potential—physiologically—of having multiple orgasms. Ironically, females are also more likely to "fake" having orgasms (Opperman et al. 2014). After orgasm, the body returns to its pre-arousal state. Men may experience a refractory period, during which they are unable to achieve another orgasm. Women do not have a refractory period and may be able to become aroused and achieve orgasm again more quickly

2.

Predisposing factor	Precipitating factors	Maintaining factors
Predisposing factors enhance sexual dysfunction. Depression, anxiety, neurological illnesses, and hormonal irregularities are examples	Sexual dysfunction at any stage of the sexual response cycle prevents sexual fulfillment. Many causes can cause sexual dysfunction	Sexual dysfunction has causes. These can include major life events such as death or job loss or more specific difficulties such as relationship or communication issues

3. FALSE. A common myth is that sexual desire decreases with age. Hormones, relationships, and life situations affect sexual desire. Sexual desire is personal; therefore, "normal" might differ.
4. Men: increased direct genital stimulation, weaker erections, longer to orgasm, weaker ejaculation, longer refractory time.

   - Lower testosterone: Testosterone drives male sexuality. A decline in testosterone may reduce sexual desire in older men.
   - ED: Older men may have problems getting or holding an erection. Injury to nerves and diminished penile blood supply might cause this.

- The prostate gland near the bladder can enlarge with age, influencing urine and sexual function.

Women: Lower estrogen, vaginal dryness and thinning, sex organ sensitivity, and libido occur.

- Lower estrogen: Estrogen affects female sexual drive. Changing estrogen levels with age might reduce sexual desire and genital tissue changes such vaginal thinning and dryness.
- Menopause, the natural end of a woman's reproductive years, lowers estrogen. Menopause can cause hot flashes, sleep problems, and sexual dysfunction.
- Woman's clitoris and labia may shrink, and labia minora may grow with age.

5.

Substance	↑ Libido	↓ Libido
Alcohol—short-term use	X	
Alcohol—long-term use		X
Marijuana		X
Cocaine	X	
Amphetamines	X	
Narcotics		X
Serotonin		X
Dopamine	X	
Testosterone	X	
Progesterone		X

6. Various medical conditions can contribute to sexual difficulties. Atherosclerosis may lead to arousal and erectile dysfunction due to reduced genital blood flow, while diabetes can result in nerve damage and decreased genital blood flow, affecting sensitivity and erectile function in men. Scar tissue between pelvic organs and tissues can cause sexual pain, affect excitement, and impact orgasm. Hormone imbalances, such as low testosterone levels in men and high prolactin levels in both men and women, can also play a role in sexual problems. Additionally, conditions such as multiple sclerosis, Parkinson's disease, Peyronie's disease, and spinal cord injuries can contribute to sexual difficulties.
7. Certain medications, including antihypertensives used to manage high blood pressure, anticholinergics for conditions such as overactive bladder and Parkinson's disease, antidepressants for mental health issues, and antipsychotics to treat psychotic disorders, can have side effects that impact sexual function. These side effects may include decreased sexual desire, arousal, orgasm, and erectile dysfunction in men.
8. Serotonin and dopamine. Dopamine, a reward and pleasure molecule, boosts libido and sexual desire. Too much serotonin, a mood-regulating neurotransmitter, may reduce sexual activity. Serotonin-boosting medicines such as antidepressants can reduce libido and orgasm.

9. Sexual dysfunction can arise from a combination of mental and physical factors. Physiologically, certain medications, medical conditions such as diabetes and cardiovascular disease, and hormone imbalances can contribute to sexual problems. Psychological and emotional factors, such as depression, anxiety, stress, relationship issues, and past sexual trauma, can also significantly impact sexual function. Given the multifaceted nature of sexual dysfunction, treatment often involves addressing both the physiological and psychological aspects to effectively manage and improve sexual health.
10. Poor sexual desire can have diverse causes that vary from person to person. Some potential factors contributing to low sexual desire include hormonal imbalances, such as low testosterone in men and low estrogen in women, as well as underlying medical conditions such as depression, cardiovascular disease, and diabetes, which can impact sexual desire negatively. Certain medications, such as those for hypertension and depression, can also lead to a decrease in sexual desire. Psychological factors such as stress, anxiety, depression, interpersonal conflicts, and past sexual trauma can play a significant role in diminishing sexual desire. Additionally, the natural aging process can bring hormonal changes that affect sexual desire. For women, variations in sexual drive during menstrual cycles can occur due to lifestyle, dietary factors, and overall health.
11. 1/H, 2/D, 3/F, 4/B, 5/G, 6/A, 7/E, and 8/C.
12. FALSE. Sexual dysfunction is rarely diagnosed by poor sexual stimulation. The sexual response cycle includes desire, arousal, orgasm, and resolution. Insufficient sexual stimulation may affect one or more of these phases, but it is not the main cause of sexual dysfunction.
13.

Subtypes	Description
Lifelong	Present since first sexual experience
Acquired	Disorder(s) develop after period of normal sexual functioning
Generalized	Sexual difficulties not limited to particular situations or partners
Situational	Difficulties occur within particular situations or with certain partners

14. ALL—biological, sociocultural, and psychological factors all may be involved.
15. Sexual arousal.
16. 6 months.
17. Diabetes mellitus and cardiovascular disease.
18. TRUE. Research shows that senior men are less distressed by erectile dysfunction. Older men may accept aging's normal changes or use coping techniques such as talking to their partner or taking erectile dysfunction medicines.
19. REM sleep generally causes spontaneous erections in men. This is a natural sleep cycle component unrelated to sexual desire or dreaming. Brain activity and blood flow changes during REM sleep may trigger erections. Not getting spontaneous erections during REM sleep is not impotence. Not getting or keeping an erection for sexual activity is considered erectile dysfunction.

20. Some key laboratory tests for ED may include hormone assessments such as thyroid, testosterone, and prolactin levels to evaluate hormonal imbalances. Diabetes-related neural and blood vessel damage can contribute to ED, so fasting blood glucose and hemoglobin A1C tests are used to detect high blood sugar. Since ED may be a sign of cardiovascular disease, tests such as stress testing, cholesterol panels, and blood pressure checks assess cardiovascular function. Additionally, basic metabolic and hepatic panels can be conducted to evaluate kidney and liver function, as ED could indicate problems with these organs.
21. Smoking is a significant risk factor for erectile dysfunction (ED). It is closely associated with ED due to the damage it causes to blood vessels and blood flow, which can lead to impaired erectile function. Smoking can also contribute to both psychological and physical ED by promoting anxiety and reducing sexual function. Quitting smoking can have a positive impact on both erectile function and overall health. If you are looking to quit smoking, it is advisable to seek advice and support from a healthcare professional.
22. Perineal and perivaginal muscles.
23. Refractory increases. The refractory period is when men cannot ejaculate and are sexually resistant. The phase can impact women. The time increases with aging. Post-orgasm brain and hormone changes cause it.
24. Loss of erection.
25. S, P, P, S.
26. M, F, F, M, M, F, M.
27. 6, substances/medications.
28. SSRI, SNRI, sedative-hypnotics, and amphetamines.
29. 1 minute.
30. Psychological and physical.
31. Sexual aversion and hypoactive sexual disorder.
32. Alcohol and nicotine.
33. When addressing hypoactive sexual desire disorder (HSDD) with a healthcare professional, discussions can include a thorough medical history, which involves inquiries about current and past medical conditions, medications, surgeries, and lifestyle factors such as alcohol and drug use. A sexual history may be discussed, encompassing past and present sexual experiences, including any history of trauma or abuse. The patient's relationship history, including any concerns related to sexual desire within current and previous relationships, may also be explored. Additionally, the healthcare provider may inquire about the patient's mental health, as conditions such as depression and anxiety can impact sexual desire. Finally, a medical examination may be conducted to rule out any underlying medical causes of sexual aversion or HSDD.
34. Performance anxiety.
35. 50.

36. Several physiological changes in older men can contribute to delayed ejaculation, including lower testosterone levels, decreased genital blood flow, and age-related damage to genital nerves. Lower testosterone levels associated with aging can limit sexual performance by reducing arousal and orgasm. Additionally, aging can lead to a decrease in genital blood flow, further impacting sexual function. The natural aging process may also harm genital nerves, impairing sexual function and potentially delaying ejaculation. In some cases, medical procedures such as prostatectomy or the use of certain medications such as antidepressants and blood pressure drugs can contribute to delayed ejaculation in older men.
37. Hypogastric, pudendal.
38. Post-TURP men risk retrograde ejaculation. Retrograde ejaculation happens when semen enters the bladder instead of the penis. TURP prostate surgery, medicines, and medical conditions may cause it.
39. OCD, PTSD, cognitive delay, traumatic brain injury (frontal lobe), substance abuse, psychoses, cluster B personality disorders, and mania.
40. FALSE. Clitoral orgasms without vaginal penetration do not indicate female orgasmic dysfunction. Female orgasmic dysfunction prevents orgasm following sexual excitement. It must create distress or interpersonal difficulties and not be caused by drugs, sexual arousal absence, or physical conditions. Clitoral stimulation rather than vaginal penetration is common; however, many women do not orgasm every time.
41. Gynecology, urologists, endocrinology, and pain specialists. Others include physical therapists and sexual medicine specialists.
42. Genito-pelvic pain/penetration disorder.
43. Vaginismus is a condition characterized by involuntary vaginal tensing during sexual activity or when attempting to insert a tampon. This muscle tension can lead to pain and discomfort during sexual intercourse. Vaginismus can be triggered by various factors, including sexual anxiety, trauma, or underlying medical conditions. Treatment for vaginismus may involve relaxation techniques, therapy, and the use of vaginal dilators to gradually stretch and relax the vaginal muscles.
44. Dyspareunia can result from infections, injury, worry, or stress.
45. Vaginismus is a condition that can affect individuals of any gender, including men and nonbinary individuals, although it is diagnosed more frequently in women. It is characterized by persistent pelvic discomfort, including pelvic muscle rigidity or spasms during penetration, making sexual activity difficult or impossible. Vaginismus can have both mental and physical components, and it can impact the sexual experience and overall quality of life for those who experience it.
46. Premenopausal.
47. Men.
48. Paraphilia refers to a pattern of distressing, functionally impaired, or nonconsenting sexual attraction to unusual things, activities, or behaviors. It can significantly impact an individual's social, occupational, and overall functioning. Paraphilias encompass various specific attractions, such as pedophilia,

exhibitionism, voyeurism, and fetishism. While some paraphilias may not necessarily involve nonconsensual or illegal behavior, they can still interfere with an individual's daily life and well-being. Treatment options, including therapy and medication, may be considered to address paraphilic tendencies and improve an individual's quality of life.

49.

Paraphilic disorder	Explanation
Exhibitionism	The act of exposing one's genitals to another person, often in a public place, with the intention of achieving sexual arousal or gratification
Fetishism	The use of nonliving objects or a highly specific focus on nongenital body parts in order to achieve sexual arousal or gratification
Frotteurism	The act of touching or rubbing against a nonconsenting individual, often in a public place, with the intention of achieving sexual arousal or gratification
Pedophilia	A sexual focus on children, often leading to abusive or inappropriate behavior
Sexual masochism	The act of undergoing humiliation, bondage, or suffering in order to achieve sexual arousal or gratification
Sexual sadism	The act of inflicting humiliation, bondage, or suffering on another person in order to achieve sexual arousal or gratification
Transvestism	Also known as cross-dressing, involves the act of engaging in sexually arousing cross-dressing
Voyeurism	The act of spying on others in private activities, often with the intention of achieving sexual arousal or gratification

50. Men. Paraphilias may be less stigmatized among men; therefore, they seek therapy more commonly. Cultural or societal norms may make men more paraphilic. Both genders can have paraphilic illnesses, and certain cultures report more of them.
51. Pedophilic, voyeuristic, and exhibitionistic disorders.
52. Courts/legal system.
53. FALSE. Multiple paraphilias are common.
54.

Good	Poor
One paraphilia Self-referral Sense of guilt History of normal sexual activity Willingness to seek treatment Good insight into the problem Effective coping skills No criminal history Good social support Younger age at onset Shorter duration of disorder Lower level of sexual preoccupation	Multiple paraphilias Early age of onset Comorbid substance use High frequency of behavior Referral by law enforcement Nonacceptance of responsibility Lack of insight into the problem Poor coping skills Criminal history Lack of social support Older age at onset Longer duration of disorder Higher level of sexual preoccupation

55. 1/F, 2/C, 3/A, 4/G, 5/B, 6/E, 7/D, 8/H.
56. Gender dysphoria.
57. Gender dysphoria, post-transition.
58. Gender nonconformity, transvestic disorder, body dysmorphic disorder, autism spectrum disorder, dissociative identity disorder, schizophrenia, and delusional disorder.
59. The World Professional Association for Transgender Health (WPATH) publishes guidelines for hormone replacement therapy and gender-affirming surgery applicants. The WPATH standards of treatment (SOC) recommend high-quality, culturally competent treatment for transgender and gender variant people. Clinicians treating transgender and gender-diverse patients can access SOC evaluation guidelines, sample letters, and other materials.
60. Sex therapy is a form of therapy aimed at improving sexual function, behavior, and overall satisfaction in individuals and couples. Typically provided by mental health-trained therapists, counselors, or psychologists, sex therapy addresses a range of sexual concerns, including issues related to sexual desire, arousal, orgasm, sexual orientation or identity, intimacy, and communication. This therapeutic approach employs various techniques to help individuals and couples explore their sexual and intimate thoughts, feelings, and behaviors, considering both past experiences and current situations. Sex therapy may also involve homework assignments to allow clients to practice and apply what they have learned. Ultimately, the primary goals of sex therapy are to enhance sexual functioning, improve communication, and foster greater satisfaction in relationships, with most clients completing therapy within a few months.
61. Sex therapy approaches sexual function and intimacy with sensitivity, allowing both couples and individuals to relax, concentrate, and develop a greater appreciation for their bodies. In the context of therapy, sensate focus exercises may be utilized, encouraging couples to engage in non-sexual touching to emphasize sensory experiences rather than sexual desire or performance. Marriage therapists may also guide couples in discussing their preferences and boundaries regarding touch. These activities can help individuals and couples enhance their connection, sexual satisfaction, communication, and physiological awareness and sensitivity. Sex therapy can address various sexual dysfunctions, including concerns related to erectile dysfunction and low sexual desire, with a focus on improving overall sexual well-being and satisfaction.
62. Viagra is a medication used to address erectile dysfunction (ED) by inhibiting the enzyme PDE-5. By doing so, it relaxes the smooth muscles in the penis, facilitating increased blood flow and promoting erections. Typically, sildenafil tablets are taken orally as needed, about 1 h prior to engaging in sexual activity. It is important to note that this medication should not be taken regularly but rather on an as-needed basis. There can be harmful interactions between sildenafil or other ED treatments and certain pharmaceuticals such as alpha-blockers used for hypertension and prostate conditions, as well as nitrates prescribed for angina.

63. Several medications can be offered to help with premature ejaculation (PE). Common options include selective serotonin reuptake inhibitors (SSRIs), such as sertraline and fluoxetine, which are taken daily to delay ejaculation. Tricyclic antidepressants such as clomipramine can also affect serotonin levels and help with PE. Topical anesthetics containing lidocaine or prilocaine can reduce penile sensitivity when applied before sexual activity. Phosphodiesterase-5 inhibitors such as sildenafil (Viagra) and tadalafil (Cialis) may be prescribed in combination with other treatments. Tramadol, a pain medication, can delay ejaculation and is sometimes used off-label. Some doctors may combine PDE-5 inhibitors with SSRIs to address both premature ejaculation and erectile dysfunction.
64. FALSE. In addition to therapy and medication, there are several other treatment options for erectile dysfunction (ED). Lifestyle changes such as quitting smoking, reducing alcohol consumption, and regular exercise can improve erectile function. Penile injections involve injecting medications directly into the penis to induce erections. Penile pumps create erections by using a vacuum to draw blood into the penis. Surgical penile implants can provide erections for patients with ED. In cases where ED is related to blood flow issues, vascular surgery may be necessary to improve blood flow to the penis.
65. Premature ejaculation, a common sexual issue, can be addressed through various treatments. Behavioral methods aim to enhance ejaculation awareness and delay or prevent it. Medications such as selective serotonin reuptake inhibitors (SSRIs) and topical anesthetics can help in managing premature ejaculation. Therapy, whether individual or couples therapy, may be beneficial for those with mental health issues contributing to premature ejaculation. Techniques such as the "squeeze" technique, involving squeezing the penis to delay ejaculation, and the "stop-start" technique, which involves continuously starting and stopping sexual activity, can also be employed to address premature ejaculation.
66. 1% of dibucaine or benzocaine lowers penile sensation and delays ejaculation. OTC lotions, sprays, and gels can be applied on penile skin. Benzocaine may prolong sexual activity and delay ejaculation by numbing the skin. Benzocaine should not substitute other medical treatments for premature ejaculation.
67. Hegar vaginal dilators, biofeedback, progressive muscle relaxation, CBT to identify underlying beliefs, partner stimulation exploration, anxiety, guilt, trauma, sex education, and couple communication.
68. TRUE. SSRIs may slow or prevent orgasm in some women. Because SSRIs affect brain serotonin levels, they may affect sexual function. This unusual adverse effect may not affect all SSRI users.
69. Bupropion and mirtazapine.
70. First-generation antipsychotic medications, known for their potential to increase prolactin levels, can lead to a decrease in sexual desire. Prolactin is a hormone produced by the pituitary gland and plays a role in regulating menstruation and

breast milk production. Elevated levels of prolactin can have negative effects on sexual function, affecting desire, arousal, and orgasm in both men and women.

71. Gabapentin, commonly known as Neurontin, is a medication used to alleviate symptoms such as depression, seizures, and nerve pain. It works by reducing abnormal brain activity and nerve impulses. However, it is important to note that gabapentin can potentially affect women's orgasms and sexual function. This effect may be related to the medication's impact on brain neurotransmitters, which play a role in various aspects of sexual function.
72. Paraphilic patients may sometimes be prescribed medications such as medroxyprogesterone acetate (MPA), selective serotonin reuptake inhibitors (SSRIs), and naltrexone to help reduce their sex drive. MPA, a synthetic hormone resembling natural progesterone, is used off-label for this purpose, although it is not FDA-approved for treating paraphilic disorders. Its use in this context is somewhat controversial, and research on its safety and efficacy is ongoing. Some studies have suggested that MPA may help lower sexual desire and address paraphilic symptoms, while others have found limited benefit. Therefore, further research is needed to better understand its role and effectiveness in treating paraphilic disorders.
73. Hormone therapy is a common option, involving the use of hormones to induce changes in secondary sexual characteristics. This can include hormone replacement therapy to develop or soften features associated with the identified gender. Gender-affirming surgeries, such as breast augmentation or removal and genital reconstruction, may also be considered. Additionally, counseling, both individually and in group settings, can provide essential support for individuals with gender dysphoria. Social support from friends, family, and the community is crucial in addressing and managing this condition. Ultimately, the choice of treatment depends on the individual's needs and goals in their gender transition journey.

References and Resources

Aisch G, Marsh B. How birth control with withdrawal fails. The New York Times. 2014 July 20. Available from: https://www.nytimes.com/2014/07/21/upshot/how-birth-control-with-withdrawal-fails.html.

American Psychiatric Association, editor. Diagnostic and statistical manual of mental disorders: DSM-5-TR. 5th ed., text revision. American Psychiatric Association Publishing; 2022.

Anderson D, Laforge J, Ross MM, Vanlangendonck R, Hasoon J, Viswanath O, Kaye AD, Urits I. Male sexual dysfunction. Health Psychol Res. 2022;10(3):37533. https://doi.org/10.52965/001c.37533.

Arnone JM, Conti RP, Preckajlo JH. Coprophilia and coprophagia: a literature review. J Am Psychiatr Nurses Assoc. 2024;30(1):8–16. https://doi.org/10.1177/10783903231214265.

Bhatt N, Cannella J, Gentile JP. Gender-affirming care for transgender patients. Innov Clin Neurosci. 2022;19(4–6):23–32.

Bockting WO, Miner MH, Swinburne Romine RE, Hamilton A, Coleman E. Stigma, mental health, and resilience in an online sample of the US transgender population. Am J Public Health. 2013;103(5):943–51. https://doi.org/10.2105/AJPH.2013.301241.

Ettner FM. Primary care for the transgender and gender nonconforming patient. Clin Plast Surg. 2018;45(3):301–6. https://doi.org/10.1016/j.cps.2018.03.001.

Faubion SS, Parish SJ. Sexual dysfunction in women: can we talk about it? Cleve Clin J Med. 2017;84(5):367–76. https://doi.org/10.3949/ccjm.84a.16021.

Hashemi L, Weinreb J, Weimer AK, Weiss RL. Transgender care in the primary care setting: a review of guidelines and literature. Fed Pract. 2018;35(7):30–7.

Johnson K, Vanderhoef D, Magrath N. Psychiatric-mental health nurse practitioner review and resource manual. American Nurses Credentialing Center, American Nurses Association; 2020.

Killick SR, Leary C, Trussell J, Guthrie K. Sperm content of pre-ejaculatory fluid. Hum Fertil (Camb). 2011;14(1):48–52.

Laumann EO, Paik A, Rosen RC. Sexual dysfunction in the United States: prevalence and predictors. JAMA J Am Med Assoc. 1999;281(6):537–44. https://doi.org/10.1001/jama.281.6.537.

Lewis JH. The role of the NP in the diagnosis and management of erectile dysfunction. Nurse Pract. 2000;(Suppl):14–8, 21. https://doi.org/10.1097/00006205-200003001-00006.

Maes CA, Louis M. Nurse practitioners' sexual history-taking practices with adults 50 and older. J Nurse Pract. 2011;7(3):216–22. https://doi.org/10.1016/j.nurpra.2010.06.003.

McCool-Myers M, Theurich M, Zuelke A, et al. Predictors of female sexual dysfunction: a systematic review and qualitative analysis through gender inequality paradigms. BMC Womens Health. 2018;18:108. https://doi.org/10.1186/s12905-018-0602-4.

Opperman E, Braun V, Clarke V, Rogers C. "It feels so good it almost hurts": Young women's experiences of orgasm and sexual pleasure. J Sex Res. 2014;51(5):508–21.

Paradiso C, Lally RM. Nurse practitioner knowledge, attitudes, and beliefs when caring for transgender people. Transgender Health. 2018;3(1):47–56. https://doi.org/10.1089/trgh.2017.0048.

Raveendran AV, Agarwal A. Premature ejaculation—current concepts in the management: a narrative review. Int J Reprod Biomed. 2021;19(1):5–22. https://doi.org/10.18502/ijrm.v19i1.8176.

Safarinejad MR, Kolahi AA, Hosseini SY. Health-related quality of life and sexual functioning in patients with chronic prostatitis/chronic pelvic pain syndrome: A case-control study. J Urol. 2009;181(5):1844–50.

Turner D, Briken P. Treatment of paraphilic disorders in sexual offenders or men with a risk of sexual offending with luteinizing hormone-releasing hormone agonists: an updated systematic review. J Sex Med. 2018;15(1):77–93. https://doi.org/10.1016/j.jsxm.2017.11.013.

World Health Organization. ICD-11—International Classification of Diseases 11th revision. World Health Organization; 2018.

Zakhari R. The psychiatric-mental health nurse practitioner certification review manual. Springer Publishing Company; 2021.

Notes:

Notes:

Trauma, Somatization, Violence, and Forensics

16

Test your learning and check your understanding of this book's contents: use the "Springer Nature Flashcards" app to access questions using ▶ https://sn.pub/62J0Ar.

To use the app, please follow the instructions in Chap. 1.

Trauma refers to a wide range of negative experiences such as physical or sexual abuse, natural disasters, accidents, and other forms of physical or emotional harm. Trauma is a significant contributor to the development of mental health issues, including post-traumatic stress disorder (PTSD), anxiety, and depression (Daniels 2020). PMHNPs must recognize the impact of trauma on an individual's cognitive and emotional functioning, as well as the ways in which trauma can affect relationships and social connections (Kubany et al. 2003).

Somatization manifests psychological distress as physical symptoms (Bremner 2020). Physical pain, fatigue, and other unexplained symptoms may be included. Somatization may be a sign of sadness or anxiety or a defense against trauma. Mental trauma like childhood maltreatment, sexual assault, or battle exposure can induce somatic symptoms. Other factors, such as genetic predisposition, personality traits, and cultural influences, may also contribute to the development of somatization disorders.

Violence may take many forms, including physical assault, sexual assault, domestic violence, and other forms of aggression. PMHNPs may assess and treat individuals who have experienced violence, as well as work with individuals who have a history of perpetrating violence. For this reason, PMHNPs must have a thorough understanding of the impact of violence on mental health, as well as the risk factors and warning signs for violence. Forensics is the application of mental health knowledge and skills in legal and criminal justice settings. PMHNPs may be called upon to provide expert testimony in legal proceedings or to assist in the evaluation

T. Stewart, *Psychiatric-Mental Health Nurse Practitioner Program Companion and Board Certification Exam Review Workbook*,
https://doi.org/10.1007/978-3-031-60894-0_16

of individuals involved in the criminal justice system. So, we must be aware of the legal and ethical considerations involved in addressing violence, such as maintaining patient confidentiality and boundaries while also ensuring the safety of the patient and others (Daniels 2020).

By recognizing the signs and symptoms of trauma, being aware of the impact of psychological distress on physical symptoms, understanding the risk factors and warning signs for violence, and being knowledgeable about the legal and ethical considerations involved in forensic practice, PMHNPs can make a significant impact on the mental health and well-being of our patients.

This chapter presents trauma and trauma-informed care. PTSD is also covered given its manifestation from a traumatic event. Activities will help learners differentiate between somatic symptoms and related disorders, as well as dissociative disorders as related to stress, abuse, and violence. Forensic basics of intimate partner violence, sexual assault, and suicidal and homicidal assessments are included.

16.1 Trauma

1. Define trauma. What qualifies an event as “trauma,” according to the DSM?

2. What are five causes of trauma that one may experience?
    1.
    2.
    3.
    4.
    5.

3. What is vicarious trauma?

4. Most individuals experience at least one trauma in their lifetime.

    TRUE FALSE

5. What mental health disorders may manifest as sequelae to a traumatic event?

6. Use the mnemonic TRAUMA to help remember the signs and symptoms of traumatic disorders, particularly PTSD. Complete the table below with the keywords.

T	
R	
A	
U	
M	
A	

7. What are cued and uncued flashbacks?

8. What are the different ways in which flashbacks may manifest?

9. What mental health disorders almost exclusively stem from trauma?

10. What are key symptoms experienced by someone in a state of hyperarousal?

11. Someone must experience trauma symptoms within the first month after the event to be diagnosed with PTSD.
    TRUE FALSE

12. How is acute stress disorder defined in the DSM?

13. When is adjustment disorder a warranted diagnosis?

14. Men are more commonly affected by traumatic disorders than women.
    TRUE FALSE

15. Who is most at risk of developing PTSD?

16. Why is prazosin effective at reducing nightmares?

17. How are the amygdala and hippocampus linked to trauma disorders like PTSD?

18. What is complex PTSD or complex developmental trauma?

19. What differential diagnoses should be considered for PTSD?

20. ____refer to experiences of abuse, neglect, and household dysfunction that occur during childhood. These can have a lasting impact on mental health and can increase the risk of developing mental health disorders, substance use disorders, and chronic health conditions later in life.

21. ____is an approach to health care that recognizes the impact of trauma on mental health and seeks to create a safe and supportive environment for patients who have experienced trauma. This approach involves building trust with patients, respecting their autonomy and choices, and providing individualized care that is sensitive to their unique needs and experiences.

22. ______________________________refers to a person's ability to adapt and recover from adversity, trauma, and stress. Building this capacity can help individuals cope with traumatic experiences and prevent the development of mental health disorders.

16.2 Somatization

23. Mental distress can be experienced as pain, fatigue, nausea, etc. Disorders that have predominantly bodily symptoms are known as ______________________ _______________ disorders.

24. Why is somatization often a "diagnosis of exclusion"? Why is this problematic?

25. Reported somatic symptoms are most often physically localized in the ______ ___________________________________.

26. What is a key distinction between somatization and factitious disorder or malingering?

27. Why are somatizers, individuals who frequently report physical symptoms without a clear medical cause, at high risk for iatrogenic injuries? How can providers help reduce this concern?

28. Women experience somatoform disorders about __________ times more than men, with most complaints beginning before __________ years old.

29. Individualswithsomatizationappeartohavehyperactive____________________ in their brains, which elevates ones senses or awareness of internal body signals or ______________________________.

30. The misinterpretation of bodily signals in somatoform disorders is linked to the ______________________________ structure in the brain, which recognizes error signals in the brain, and feeling the need to act on the erroneous signals.

31. Another term for functional neurological symptom disorder is _____________ ________________________.

32. Because conversion disorder presents as focused neurologic deficits over which a person has little control, it may be considered _________________________ ____________.

33. When diagnosing conversion disorder, it is important to identify a __________ _______________________, which may be the catalyst to the symptoms.

34. To what does “la belle indifference” refer vis-a-vis conversion disorder?

35. Factitious disorder was previously known as _________________________ _______________________.

36. Why do individuals with factitious disorder intentionally cause illness?

37. Females in their 30's make up most patients with factitious disorder. Overwhelmingly, these individuals work in the ________________________ professional field.

38. What key signs in a patient's history suggest factitious disorder?

39. Are medications or psychotherapy more effective for treating factitious disorder?

40. ______________________ is also intentional production of illness, but for secondary gain like insurance payments, military service discharge, or avoidance of criminal sentencing.

41. Malingering is not a mental disorder.
    TRUE FALSE

42. Depression, personality disorders, obsessive beliefs, and ______________ disorders have strong correlations to somatization.

43. An individual fearing that they have an illness, or fearful of developing an illness, even though there is ample evidence to the contrary may be diagnosed with ______________________________.

44. Women are more likely to be diagnosed with somatic symptom disorders.
    TRUE FALSE

45. An individual who consciously feigns symptoms to avoid responsibility or law enforcement, receive food and shelter, or to earn some form of compensation is ______________________. Therefore, they often refuse to accept a "good prognosis."

46. Psychiatric professionals who treat patients with somatic symptom disorders should maintain working relationships with the patient's ____________ ______________________.

47. According to the DSM, an individual must have experienced somatic complaints for at least __________________ for a diagnosis of somatic symptom disorder.

48. Compare and contrast somatic symptom disorder with conversion disorder by completing the following table.

Characteristic	Somatic symptom disorder (SSD)	Conversion disorder (CD)
Nature of symptoms		
Psychological factors		
Duration of symptoms		
Presence of control		
Medical explanation		

49. Another name for conversion disorder is ______________________.

50. Give two to three common examples of symptoms seen in conversion disorder for each.

Motor	
Sensory	
Speech and swallowing	
Vision and hearing	
Other	

51. In which groups of individuals is conversion disorder most common?

52. Conversion disorder symptoms are often one-time events and do not repeat.
TRUE FALSE

53. An individual who is anxious about either having or developing a serious illness for at least 6 months may be diagnosed with ______________________________ ___________.

54. Individuals with illness anxiety disorder always have somatic symptoms.
TRUE FALSE

55. Individuals with illness anxiety disorder used to be called ________________ ____________________.

56. In addition to regularly scheduled visits to their primary care provider and psychotherapy, individuals with illness anxiety disorder may benefit from ______ ____ medications.

57. Which form of psychotherapy is most often recommended for patients with somatic symptom-related disorders?

58. How does malingering differ from factitious disorder?

59. If an individual produces symptoms in their child, elderly parent, or other person under their care, in order to gain attention and sympathy, then they are diagnosed with ____.

60. What are some common symptoms feigned by individuals with factitious disorder?

61. Men and women engage in malingering for different goals and present often with different symptoms/complaints.
    TRUE FALSE

62. When an individual experiences a disruption to their sense of self, this is known as ______________________________________. It often develops during childhood as a means to buffer a traumatic event (e.g., abuse, religious cults, brainwashing), but may develop during any stressful period.

63. Dissociative amnesia is a lapse in ____ ________ memory, which means that are unable to remember important personal information (e.g., name, address, age, marriage). One's ability to engage in functional, procedural tasks remains.

64. Dissociative memory loss often progresses to complete memory loss, unretrievable overtime.
    TRUE FALSE

65. Individuals with dissociative memory loss often experience comorbid _______ ________________________________ which increases their risk for suicide as the amnesia lifts and traumatic memories are remembered.

66. An amnesic event accompanied by an individual's sudden wandering or travel from normal surroundings is referred to as a ___________________________ _______, if its cause cannot be linked to substance use or another disorder.

67. Men experience dissociation more than women.
    TRUE FALSE

68. What is the primary treatment approach for someone who has experienced a dissociative event?

69. What behaviors/experiences may patients with dissociative amnesia have that echo PTSD patients?

70. As memories return and individuals relive a traumatic experience, they may have a strong emotional reaction known as ________________________ __________.

71. If an individual feels disconnected or detached from one's self, this is called ___________________________. If the detachment is from one's surroundings, then the term ___________________________ is used.

72. The feeling of having an "out-of-body experience" is associated with ___________________________, when an individual feels like they are watching themselves from an external location to their body.

73. ________________________________ experiences are often described as being in a dream or movie because the individual does not interact with the world as if it is real. However, an individual's ability to reality test remains.

74. Depersonalization/derealization disorders affect genders equally. They have an average onset around _______ years old.

75. Describe dissociative identity disorder.

76. Women experience dissociative identity disorder more than men.
TRUE FALSE

77. Dissociative identity disorder is associated with several other psychiatric disorders. Name three of these disorders.
1. ______________________________
2. ______________________________
3. ______________________________

78. While psychotherapy is first-line treatment, several medications can assist individuals struggling with dissociative identity disorder. For nightmares, ______________________ may be prescribed. If the patient engages in self-harm, __________________________ could be useful. And, if the individual experiences depression and/or PTSD, ______________________ may be beneficial.

79. Match each of the following disorders with the best example.

Disorder	Example
_____Somatic symptom disorder	A. A 30-year-old lady has identity uncertainty, amnesia, and mood swings. The patient says she sometimes feels like a different person with different memories and identities. After terrible events, the patient has memory gaps.
_____Illness anxiety disorder	B. A 35-year-old woman suffers chronic back discomfort despite various diagnostic tests and examinations finding no medical explanation. Pain affects her daily life and work, and she worries about it.
_____Conversion disorder	C. A 25-year-old man with chest pain and breathing problems resists diagnosis and treatment. The patient seems more interested in receiving medicines than treating his illness.

Disorder	Example
_____Malingering	D. A 20-year-old lady loses vision in both eyes unexpectedly. Multiple tests and exams have shown no medical explanation for blindness. Due to unexpected blindness, the patient is anxious.
_____Factitious disorder	E. A 40-year-old woman with many medical difficulties visits hospitals and clinics. However, medical examinations often discover no physical cause for her symptoms. The patient fabricated symptoms to gain medical help.
_____Dissociative identity disorder	F. A 50-year-old guy visits his primary care physician for many physiological difficulties despite negative tests. The patient fears a serious illness and spends a lot of time investigating medical issues online. These difficulties worry the patient.

16.3 Violence

80. Individuals with mental illness are more likely to be the victims of violence than the perpetrators of violence.
    TRUE FALSE

81. What is the most important factor in assessing an individual's likelihood for violence in the future?

82. For each type of child abuse, list common red flags, signs, and symptoms.

Abuse	Signs/symptoms
Physical	
Sexual	
Psychological/emotional	
Neglect	

83. Define intimate partner violence (IPV).

84. Provide five reasons an abuser may engage in IPV. Consider abuser characteristics, risk factors, mental health disorders, desired outcomes, and stressors.
    1.
    2.
    3.
    4.
    5.

85. Why might the victims of IPV be less willing to report their experiences?

86. What should a provider investigate in a patient's medical history when considering IPV?

87. How might a victim of abuse act during a mental status exam?

88. For which three populations is a PMHNP required to report suspected abuse or neglect?
    1.
    2.
    3.

89. Draw Lenore Walker's cycle of domestic violence. Explain the different phases and their characteristics.

90. What is a safety plan for victims of IPV or other abuse?

91. What may be included in an escape plan for victims of abuse?

92. Experienced by women more than men, ______________ assault is the most common form of abuse. Perpetrators are most often family members or prospective partners.

93. What physical findings might a provider see on an individual who has experienced sexual abuse?

94. Name five signs that a school-aged child may be considered violent and should be assessed for lethality.
    1.
    2.
    3.
    4.
    5.

95. Place an X before the following behaviors if they are signs of potential homicidal intent.
_____A fascination or preoccupation with weapons, particularly weapons or explosives that could be used for mass destruction, such as semi-automatic guns
_____Being a loner with little or no involvement with other employees
_____Engaging in frequent disputes with supervisors or coworkers
_____Extreme stress from personal problems or a life crisis
_____Identifying with incidents of workplace violence reported in the media and either condoning or sympathizing with the actions of the persons commiting violence
_____Obsessive involvement with one's job, particularly where it occurs with no apparent outside interests
_____Paranoia or easily panicked behavior
_____Persistent violation of company policy
_____Prior history of threatening or violent behavior
_____Volatile or violent home or other personal situation that has the potential to bring violence into the workplace

96. Which of the following patient behaviors would you note as evidencing a potential threat of violence? Place an X in front of your selection(s).
_____Alcohol use increases the risk for violence
_____Attempting to intimidate or harass other persons
_____Behavior indicating that the person is significantly out of touch with reality and that
_____Displaying an intense or obsessive romantic interest that exceeds the normal
_____Making a verbal threat to harm another person or destroy property
_____Making menacing gestures or physical posturing without actually touching the
_____Throwing objects
_____Volatile or violent personal situations such as found in some custody battles bounds of interpersonal interest

16.4 Forensics

97. Explain the term "forensic."

98. Complete the Venn diagram comparing and contrasting forensic vs. correctional nursing. Consider the role of the nurse, the nurse-client relationship, and locations of practice.

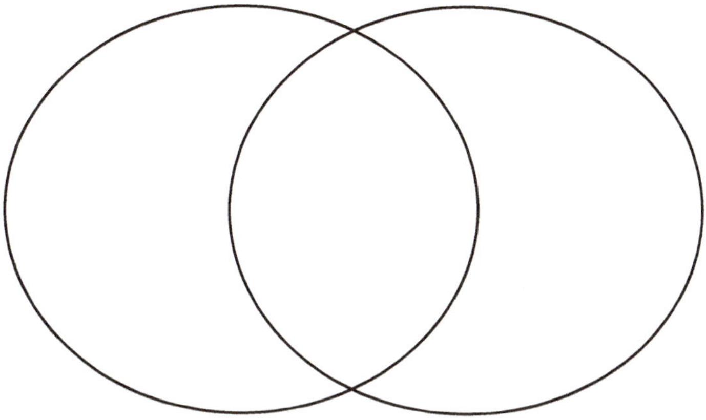

99. Name three to five areas in which forensic PMHNPs can work; each of these areas have an overlap of the mental health and legal systems.
    1. ___
    2. ___
    3. ___
    4. ___
    5. ___

100. Forensic psychiatric-mental health nurse practitioners (PMHNPs) are specialized healthcare professionals who work at the intersection of mental health and legal systems. Name three to five settings in which forensic PMHNPs may work.
    1. ___
    2. ___
    3. ___
    4. ___
    5. ___

16.5 Answers and Explanations to Chapter Activities

1. Trauma can result from various physical, emotional, or psychological events, including exposure to real or threatened death, major injury, or sexual violence. This definition encompasses direct personal experiences of trauma, witnessing traumatic events, or hearing about loved ones being affected by violence or accidents. Those who work as first responders, police, or forensic examiners may be particularly vulnerable to repeated exposure to distressing incident details.

2. Trauma examples:
   - Sexual or physical abuse
   - Domestic violence
   - Sexual assault/rape
   - Natural disasters such as earthquakes, floods, wildfires
   - Being at a horrific accident
   - Battle or military exposure
   - A sudden death of a loved one
   - Psychological abuse or neglect
3. Witnessing another's suffering causes vicarious trauma. Healthcare, social work, and counseling professionals who hear trauma survivors' tales can experience it. Intrusive thoughts, avoidance, and emotional numbing may occur in these occupations. Friends and family of trauma survivors may also experience vicarious trauma.
4. TRUE. Injury, natural disaster, sexual assault, combat, witnessing violence, and other unsettling occurrences can be traumatic.
5. Experiencing a traumatic event can lead to a variety of mental health disorders, such as:
   - Post-traumatic stress disorder (PTSD)
   - Acute stress disorder (ASD)
   - Adjustment disorders
   - Anxiety disorders
   - Mood disorders (such as depression)
   - Substance use disorders
   - Dissociative disorders
   - Personality disorders
6.

T	Trauma
R	Re-experiencing
A	Arousal
U	Unable to function
M	Month
A	Avoidance

7. Individuals with PTSD often experience involuntary or uncued flashbacks, triggered by sensory stimuli like smells, sounds, or images that are related to their traumatic experiences. For example, fireworks on July fourth might evoke memories of combat for military veterans with PTSD. These flashbacks can happen suddenly and unpredictably, transporting the person back to the traumatic event, making it feel as though they are reliving it. Additionally, cued flashbacks can be deliberately induced during therapy sessions, such as those using eye movement desensitization and reprocessing (EMDR), to help process and cope with traumatic memories.

8. Trauma-related flashbacks can manifest in various ways, including vivid visualizations, auditory experiences, sensory sensations, and intense emotional responses. For instance, individuals may vividly imagine and relive the traumatic event, hear sounds related to it, or feel physical sensations reminiscent of the trauma.
9. Trauma can lead to post-traumatic stress disorder (PTSD), characterized by symptoms like flashbacks, nightmares, avoidance, and heightened arousal. Acute stress disorder (ASD) may also follow traumatic events, leading to emotional disconnection and numbness. Adjustment disorder can arise from major life stressors, resulting in symptoms like anxiety, depression, and impaired functioning. Dissociative disorders, such as dissociative identity disorder (DID), can be triggered by trauma and affect memory, identity, and awareness. Complex post-traumatic stress disorder (C-PTSD) often results from chronic trauma, impacting areas like emotional regulation, self-esteem, and relationships. Additionally, trauma can contribute to somatic symptom disorders, which involve physical symptoms without a clear medical cause, influenced by psychosocial and biological factors.
10.
    - Overreaction to shock
    - Anger and irritation
    - Concentration issues
    - Continuously scanning the environment for dangers
    - Trouble falling or staying asleep
    - A beating heart
    - Rapid breathing or ventilation
    - Sweating
    - Shaking
    - Anxious
    - Tense muscles, sleep problems, low energy, restlessness, inattention
11. FALSE. The DSM-5 requires symptoms for 1 month following a traumatic incident to diagnose PTSD. PTSD typically delays symptoms.
12. The DSM-5 defines acute stress disorder (ASD) as a mental illness that starts 1 month after a severe incident and lasts 3–24 days. The person must have observed or suffered a tragic death, catastrophic injury, or sexual violation and felt fear, helplessness, or horror. ASD symptoms include dissociative feelings like numbness, detachedness, or unreality, intrusive memories or dreams, and arousal symptoms including hypervigilance, aberrant startle reaction, irritability, and insomnia.
13. Adjustment disorder may be diagnosed if a stressor causes a substantial emotional or behavioral response within 3 months. Anguish develops when the response surpasses stressor expectations and significantly impacts functioning. It must not be due to another mental illness nor extend beyond 6 months of stress.
14. FALSE. Trauma is reported in women at twice the rate as in men.

15. PTSD can affect anyone who has experienced trauma, but certain factors increase the risk of developing this condition. Those who have been exposed to frequent or prolonged trauma, have a history of mental health disorders or substance addiction, lack social support, or face additional stressors are at a higher risk of developing PTSD. Research also suggests that women are more likely than men to experience PTSD following a traumatic event. Additionally, younger individuals, those who go through traumatic experiences alone, have limited time to process the trauma, and lack social support are among the most vulnerable to developing PTSD.
16. Prazosin decreases nightmares by inhibiting norepinephrine, a "fight or flight" neurotransmitter. Brains exaggerate stress responses in PTSD sufferers, boosting norepinephrine. Under stress, the HPA axis releases cortisol and other stress hormones and the sympathetic nervous system releases adrenaline. Prazosin for nightmares and cortisol-regulating medications may help.
17. Traumatic memories are processed and stored by the amygdala and hippocampus. While the hippocampus stores emotional memories, the amygdala encodes and analyzes them. PTSD sufferers may have amygdala overactivation, creating emotional sensitivity and regulation issues. The hippocampus may be affected, making traumatic memories hard to process. Continuous stress and cortisol exposure may decrease the hippocampus in PTSD sufferers, producing memory and cognitive issues.
18. Complex developmental trauma (C-PTSD) is caused by repeated traumatic events, especially childhood traumas including physical, sexual, or emotional abuse, neglect, or other unpleasant experiences. There may be deeper, long-term effects on emotional, cognitive, social, and self-identity.
19. Some differential diagnoses for PTSD include:

    - Acute stress disorder
    - Adjustment disorder
    - Major depressive disorder
    - Generalized anxiety disorder
    - Panic disorder
    - Substance use disorder
    - Borderline personality disorder
    - Psychotic disorders
    - Dissociative disorders
    - Somatization disorder

20. Adverse childhood experiences (ACEs).
21. Trauma-informed care.
22. Resilience.
23. Somatoform or somatic symptom disorders are mental health issues that cause physical symptoms that cannot be explained by a medical condition. These symptoms may cause serious distress and daily functioning problems.

24. Somatization is considered a "diagnosis of exclusion" when all medical tests have ruled out other bodily diseases, and symptoms without clear biological or physiological explanations are present. However, this diagnosis has its drawbacks. It can lead to diagnostic delays, as it may miss underlying medical issues that share somatization symptoms. Additionally, labeling individuals with somatization can be stigmatizing and dismissive of their distressing physical symptoms that require treatment.
25. Abdomen/gastrointestinal.
26. Somatization refers to the manifestation of physical symptoms without a clear biological or physiological explanation, often stemming from underlying psychological distress, trauma, or mental illness. It is essential to distinguish somatization from factitious disorder and malingering based on the motivations and intents behind the symptoms, as the latter involve intentionally producing or exaggerating symptoms for various purposes, such as seeking sympathy or personal gain.
27. Iatrogenic incidents, which are unintended harm or injuries caused by medical interventions, may be more likely in individuals who present with somatization, exhibiting physical symptoms without a clear medical explanation. Several factors contribute to this increased risk among somatizers. These individuals may undergo excessive medical testing, procedures, and treatments in their quest for a diagnosis, potentially exposing themselves to unnecessary surgical procedures, radiation exposure, and adverse drug effects. Additionally, the challenge of distinguishing between medically unexplained symptoms and underlying medical conditions can lead to delayed or incorrect diagnoses, potentially resulting in inadequate or inappropriate medical care for underlying health issues.
28. Women report somatoform disorders two to three times more than men. Most somatoform disorder symptoms appear before 30 years old.
29. Somatization patients have heightened awareness of internal body signals and sensations due to overactive "interoceptive" brain processes. Interoception plays a crucial role in detecting and interpreting bodily signals such as heartbeat, breathing, and temperature, affecting both the body and emotions.
30. For the "anterior insula/cingulate cortex," which drives action, somatoform illnesses misread physical signals. The anterior insula transmits interoception, emotion, and self-awareness from the insular cortex.
31. Neurological symptoms or impairments without a medical or neurological basis are called functional neurological symptom conditions or "conversion disorder."
32. Functional brain problems beyond control may make conversion disease "dissociative." The DSM-5 includes conversion disorder as a somatic symptom illness, yet its symptoms and causation suggest dissociation.
33. A "psychological stressor" or "triggering event" caused conversion disorder symptoms. Fear or conflict can create physical symptoms or limitations in conversion disorder. Stressors include trauma, emotional problems, life challenges, and psychological triggers. Understanding the psychological stressor before conversion disorder symptoms can assist. It can help create a treatment plan that addresses psychological stressors, emotional conflicts, and psychotherapy or other therapies to relieve symptoms.

34. "La belle indifference" illustrates conversion disorder and other somatoform disorder patients' strange lack of concern about their new physical conditions.
35. The DSM-5 no longer uses "Munchausen syndrome." Factitious disorder, sometimes known as "factitious disorder imposed on self" or "factitious disorder imposed on another" (via proxy), involves intentionally causing symptoms in a dependent or vulnerable person. More objective and descriptive, the phrase now emphasizes planned symptom generation over character or history.
36. Factitious disorder patients feign illness for various reasons, often driven by a complex set of motives. These individuals seek attention, emotional satisfaction, and control through the fabrication of illnesses. Some may use feigned illnesses to gain a sense of control over their lives or manipulate others, as seen in cases of factitious disorder imposed on another (formerly known as Munchausen syndrome by proxy). Factors such as trauma, underlying personality issues, and a strong need for validation can contribute to the development of factitious disorder. For some individuals, identifying as sick and undergoing medical treatment may provide them with a sense of purpose or identity.
37. Most work in the healthcare field, such as physicians, nurses, technicians, and other medical personnel. Knowledge of medical terminology, methods, and settings can help patients feign symptoms.
38. Diagnosing factitious disorder requires a thorough medical evaluation, and certain patterns and indicators in a patient's history may suggest the presence of this condition. Some common signs include inconsistencies in a patient's medical history, such as changing symptoms, conditions, or treatment responses, as well as discrepancies in their medical records. Factitious disorder patients often have a history of frequent hospitalizations or interactions with multiple healthcare providers. They may present with unusual or inexplicable symptoms, sometimes exaggerating or contradicting medical complaints. These individuals may possess knowledge of medical terminology, procedures, and treatments, either from their training, experience, or research. Additionally, factitious disorder patients may resist undergoing examinations that would confirm their absence of illness, and their history may reveal instances of feigned symptoms, self-inflicted injuries, or inexplicable medical events.
39. Multidisciplinary treatment for factitious disorder encompasses both psychotherapy and medication, with the choice of therapy and drugs depending on individual patient characteristics, the severity of the disorder, and the presence of co-occurring psychological conditions such as personality disorders, trauma, mood disorders, or anxiety disorders, which can exacerbate factitious disorder. Cognitive-behavioral therapy (CBT) is a commonly used therapeutic approach for addressing factitious disorder. In therapy, patients explore and understand the underlying psychological issues contributing to their condition, learn effective coping strategies, develop healthier ways of seeking help, and address any

trauma or mental health concerns. Factitious disorder can also lead to conditions like depression, anxiety, and personality disorders, which may be managed with medication. For instance, severe depression may be treated with selective serotonin reuptake inhibitors (SSRIs) or other antidepressants.

40. Malingering is exaggerating symptoms or impairment for gain. To detect malingering impairment, medical records, collateral information, and objective tests must be examined.
41. TRUE. Malingering entails lying about symptoms or impairment for gain. The DSM-5 and ICD-10 do not consider it a mental disorder. Habit or response. Malingering might get money, drugs, or avoid work or legal obligations.
42. Anxiety. Somatization impacts personality, anxiety, melancholy, and obsessive beliefs. Anxiety problems can cause physical symptoms. People confuse normal symptoms for sickness due to physiological awareness caused by anxiety.
43. A person who worries they have or will get a sickness may be diagnosed with "illness anxiety disorder."
44. TRUE. Research suggests that women have more somatic symptom disorders than men. Sociocultural and gender norms can affect symptom expression and diagnosis.
45. Falsely feigning symptoms to evade accountability or law enforcement, acquire food and shelter, or earn money is "malingering." Malingerers fear "good prognosis" or improvement will undermine their aspirations.
46. SSD treatment needs coordination with the patient's "primary care providers" or "other medical specialists." Somatic symptom disorders may require neurologists, gastroenterologists, and pain management experts depending on symptoms and comorbidities. Partnering with these professionals allows for coordinated patient treatment.
47. The DSM-5 requires 6 months of somatic issues for SSD.
48.

Characteristic	Somatic symptom disorder (SSD)	Conversion disorder (CD)
Nature of symptoms	Somatic symptoms causing distress and impairment	Neurological symptoms or deficits without medical explanation
Psychological factors	Excessive preoccupation with health concerns and psychological factors	Symptoms associated with psychological factors or conflicts
Duration of symptoms	At least 6 months	Variable duration, often weeks to months
Presence of control	Perceived as involuntary and beyond control	Not intentionally produced, but influenced by psychological factors
Medical explanation	Symptoms may or may not have a clear medical explanation	Symptoms cannot be explained by a medical condition alone

49. Another name for conversion disorder is functional neurological symptom disorder (FNSD).

50.

Motor	• Paralysis or limb weakness • Shaking, jerking, tremors • Gait or coordination difficulties
Sensory	• Anesthetic or hypoesthesia-induced sensory loss • Glove or stocking distribution sensory loss • Episodic consciousness or movement changes like epilepsy
Speech and swallowing	• Voiceless or dysphonic • Disordered speech • Swallowing disorder without anatomical cause
Vision and hearing	• Vision impairment or functional blindness • Hearing loss
Other	• Convulsions without epilepsy • Psychogenic movement disorders (unrelated, abnormal motions) • Non-physiological psychogenic pain

51. Conversion disorder, a condition characterized by the presence of neurological symptoms with no apparent medical cause, can affect various individuals, with certain groups being more susceptible. Women are more commonly affected, and it often emerges during childhood or early adulthood, possibly due to emotional and psychological changes during these stages. Trauma survivors, including those who have experienced abuse or neglect, have an increased risk of developing conversion disorder, though the precise relationship between trauma and the condition is not fully understood. Mental health factors like depression, anxiety, and personality disorders may also heighten susceptibility. Additionally, there is some suspicion of a genetic component, as it may run in families with a history of conversion disorder or related neurological issues, suggesting a potential genetic predisposition. These factors collectively contribute to a complex understanding of conversion disorder and its varied risk factors.
52. FALSE. Some persons may have recurring conversion disorder symptoms. Conversion disorder symptoms might be brief or permanent. Symptoms may intensify or disappear.
53. Illness anxiety disorder is diagnosed when a person worries about a serious illness for 6 months.
54. FALSE. The symptoms of illness anxiety disorder may not necessarily be physical. Illness anxiety disorder is excessive concern about a serious medical condition, not physical symptoms.
55. Hypochondriacs.
56. Illness anxiety disorder sufferers may benefit from medicines in addition to psychotherapy and doctor visits. SSRIs and SNRIs are typically prescribed. These medications reduce anxiety and obsessive thoughts about a critical illness.
57. Cognitive-behavioral therapy (CBT) is a recommended treatment approach for somatic symptom disorder (SSD) and illness anxiety disorder, formerly known as hypochondriasis. CBT helps individuals identify and address the

psychological roots of their physical symptoms. Treatment for somatic symptoms through CBT typically involves psychoeducation, where therapists educate patients about the connection between mental health and physical symptoms. Cognitive restructuring is used to address biases related to health and illness, promoting a more balanced and realistic perception of symptoms. Behavioral techniques are employed to help patients examine and change illness-related habits, such as excessive checking and seeking reassurance, and develop healthier coping strategies. Techniques like deep breathing, progressive muscle relaxation, and mindfulness are used to reduce symptom-related worry and tension. CBT aims to improve patients' thinking patterns, anxiety regulation, and reduce excessive worry about their symptoms, and it can be delivered through individual or group sessions as needed.

58. The key distinction between malingering and factitious disorder lies in the deceptive motivation; while malingering aims for external benefits, factitious disorder seeks the attention and status of being a patient.
59. A person who produces symptoms in a child or elderly parent to garner sympathy may have factitious disorder imposed on another, formerly Munchausen syndrome by proxy.
60. Individuals with factitious disorder often exhibit a range of feigned symptoms, and pain is a common presentation. These symptoms can encompass gastrointestinal issues such as abdominal pain, nausea, vomiting, diarrhea, and even the presence of blood in the stool. Feigning respiratory problems, including shortness of breath, coughing, and wheezing, is also observed, and they may manipulate or simulate discomfort related to breathing. Neurological symptoms may be fabricated, such as weakness, numbness, paralysis, convulsions, tremors, or alterations in mental status. Additionally, factitious disorder patients may simulate cardiac-related symptoms like chest pain, palpitations, or irregular heartbeats, often describing heart problems or mimicking cardiac episodes. They may even fake allergic reactions, presenting with symptoms such as rashes, hives, swelling, or breathing difficulties, despite a lack of supporting medical evidence.
61. TRUE. Males may malinger to perpetrate crimes, whereas females may pretend physical or psychological distress.
62. Dissociation is psychologically separating from thoughts, feelings, memories, and identity. People feel like they are watching themselves from outside their bodies or have memory gaps.
63. Dissociative amnesia is characterized by a gap in autobiographical memory, resulting in the individual's inability to recall significant personal information, such as their name, address, age, or marital status.
64. FALSE. Dissociative amnesia may not cause permanent memory loss. Personal and meaningful life events are selectively forgotten in dissociative amnesia.
65. Dissociative memory loss, especially in amnesia or DID, may cause PTSD. Traumatic memory recovery after dissociative amnesia or therapy can be upsetting. It can cause strong emotions, flashbacks, and trauma. Pre-existing vulnerabilities and emotional regulation or coping skills issues might enhance psychological suffering and suicide risk.

66. A "dissociative fugue" is an amnesic experience involving unexpected wandering or travel from typical settings that is not related to substance use or another disorder. A subtype of dissociative amnesia, dissociative fugue comprises an abrupt departure from one's typical environment and inability to recollect an identity or past. People may forget their identity, personal history, and events leading up to dissociative fugue episodes.
67. FALSE. Dissociation may affect women more than males.
68. Psychotherapy is the primary treatment for dissociative disorders like amnesia and fugue, focusing on addressing the origins, symptoms, and psychological aspects of the condition to help patients integrate their experiences and regain self-awareness. Trauma-focused psychotherapy is particularly effective, with two main approaches being trauma-focused cognitive-behavioral therapy (TF-CBT) and eye movement desensitization and reprocessing (EMDR). TF-CBT combines cognitive-behavioral techniques with trauma-focused methods to process trauma, challenge dysfunctional thoughts, develop coping strategies, and regulate emotions. EMDR uses bilateral stimulation to help individuals recall and reprocess traumatic memories, reducing distress. These trauma-focused therapies can be supplemented with other supportive and complementary approaches, such as dialectical behavior therapy (DBT) for emotion regulation, mindfulness, body-oriented, and creative arts therapies tailored to specific symptoms and needs.
69. Dissociative amnesia and PTSD share several behavioral and emotional characteristics due to their common association with traumatic experiences. These include experiencing intrusive memories of the trauma, which may manifest as flashbacks, vivid recollections, or distressing mental images. Both disorders can lead to avoidance behaviors, where individuals try to steer clear of triggers or reminders related to the traumatic event and may avoid discussing it. Emotional numbing, characterized by a limited range of emotions, emotional detachment, or a sense of emptiness, can occur in both conditions. Additionally, hyperarousal symptoms such as irritability, heightened startle response, insomnia, and hypervigilance can be present in dissociative amnesia and PTSD.
70. After recalling a traumatic event, people may feel "emotional reactivation" or "emotional flooding." Another name is "abreaction."
71. Isolation from oneself is called "depersonalization." If the separation is from one's surroundings, it is called "derealization." Things may seem twisted, surreal, or meaningless.
72. "Depersonalization," a dissociative symptom, is a sense of unreality or detachment from one's thoughts, feelings, body, or identity. It can feel like being watched, that one's body or actions belong to someone else, or like one is in a dream or fog. PTSD, anxiety, sadness, and depersonalization/derealization disorder can cause depersonalization.
73. Derealization involves a sense of unreality or disconnection from one's surroundings. As if in a dream or movie, derealization can make objects, people, and the environment appear twisted, unnatural, or meaningless.

74. Depersonalization/derealization affects both genders. They usually start around 16 years old.
75. Dissociative identity disorder (DID), formerly known as multiple personality disorder, is a complex and rare dissociative disorder characterized by the presence of two or more distinct personality states or identities within an individual. These different identities, often referred to as "alters," exhibit unique thoughts, feelings, behaviors, and memories. People with DID may experience amnesia when a different identity takes control. DID is often associated with childhood trauma, such as physical, sexual, or emotional abuse, neglect, or other traumatic events, and dissociation may serve as a defense mechanism against overwhelming trauma. Long-term psychotherapy, including trauma-focused therapy and identity integration, aims to improve communication and collaboration among alters while addressing the underlying trauma.
76. TRUE. Research suggests that women are diagnosed with DID more often than men.
77. Dissociative identity disorder (DID) is often associated with several co-occurring psychiatric conditions. Among these, post-traumatic stress disorder (PTSD) is prevalent due to the history of severe childhood trauma in many DID patients, leading to shared symptoms like intrusive thoughts and hyperarousal. Borderline personality disorder (BPD) is another common comorbidity, with both disorders featuring identity fragmentation and emotional dysregulation. Additionally, major depressive disorder (MDD) frequently accompanies DID, stemming from the ongoing trauma, chronic stress, and dissociative symptoms experienced by individuals with the disorder. DID's complexity also puts patients at risk for other psychiatric conditions, including eating disorders and substance use disorders, making comprehensive and tailored treatment crucial for addressing the multifaceted nature of this disorder and its comorbidities.
78. Some medications that may be considered include selective serotonin reuptake inhibitors (SSRIs) like sertraline, fluoxetine, and prazosin, which can help reduce nightmares and improve sleep quality. Mood stabilizers or atypical antipsychotics such as lamotrigine (Lamictal), aripiprazole (Abilify), or olanzapine (Zyprexa) may be beneficial in addressing impulsivity, emotional dysregulation, and self-harming behaviors. Naltrexone can also be an option for certain symptoms. Additionally, SSRIs may be used to manage depressive and PTSD symptoms in individuals with DID.
79.

__B___Somatic symptom disorder
__F___Illness anxiety disorder
__D___Conversion disorder
__C___Malingering
__E___Factitious disorder
__A___Dissociative identity disorder

80. TRUE. Discrimination and stigma may increase mental health patients' risk of violence and victimization. There is no evidence that those with mental health issues are more violent. Actually, they are at risk of self-harm more.
81. While certain factors like a history of violence, youth, maleness, substance use, and lower socioeconomic status are recognized as potential risk factors, predicting future violence is challenging. Research consistently indicates that past violent behavior is the most reliable predictor of future violence. Violence risk assessments also consider present threats, intent to harm, access to weapons, history of aggression, substance misuse, mental health conditions (including psychotic disorders or personality disorders), impulsivity, and the presence or absence of social support.
82.

Abuse	Signs/symptoms
Physical	Nonaccidental injury, severe corporal punishment, breaks, bruises, injuries at various stages of healing, burns, multiple head injuries in different locations or over multiple times
Sexual	Sexual act on minor to provide sexual gratification to abuser Girls > boys as victims, but boys less likely to report STIs, UTIs, bleeding, pregnancy, bruising around genitals, inappropriate sexual knowledge or behavior by minor
Psychological/ emotional	Verbal or symbolic acts to harm recipient, not accidental, withholding affection, or direct verbal abuse
Neglect	Lack of adequate resources, like food, shelter, medical care, education Poor hygiene, malnutrition, developmental delays, death

83. Domestic violence, also referred to as intimate partner violence (IPV), is a pattern of abusive behavior within an intimate relationship where one partner exerts power and control over the other, leading to physical, sexual, emotional, or financial harm. IPV can manifest in various forms, including physical abuse, such as hitting or choking, sexual abuse, which encompasses rape and non-consensual sexual acts, as well as psychological abuse involving intimidation, humiliation, threats, or isolation. Financial abuse is another component, which involves controlling the victim's financial resources and limiting their economic independence. Importantly, IPV can occur in both heterosexual and same-sex relationships, transcending racial, ethnic, socioeconomic, and age boundaries. This pervasive social and public health issue has profound physical and psychological consequences for its victims.
84. Cluster B personality disorders, substance use disorders, childhood violence, cognitive impairment, self-image issues, power, manipulation, intimidation, control, and financial, relationship, and employment stressors may be replied.
85. Victims of intimate partner violence (IPV) often delay reporting their abuse for various complex reasons influenced by personal, cultural, societal, and individual factors. These reasons include the fear of retaliation, as victims worry that reporting the abuse might escalate the violence or endanger themselves and their families. Financial or emotional dependence on the abuser can also be a

significant barrier, with concerns about housing, finances, or child custody hindering reporting. Feelings of shame, guilt, and self-blame may prevent victims from seeking help, as they fear disapproval from family, friends, or their community. A sense of isolation and the belief that no one will believe or assist them can also deter reporting. Additionally, cultural or religious factors, such as preserving family reputation or community disapproval, can discourage victims from coming forward. Immigrant victims may face specific fears related to immigration status or deportation, including concerns about legal and language barriers that could impede their ability to seek assistance.

86. To diagnose intimate partner violence (IPV), healthcare providers must consider physical injuries, unexplained bruises, scars, and trauma using open-ended questions. Providers should delve into the patient's psychosocial history, exploring relationships, living conditions, and behavioral changes. Screening for IPV-related mental health issues like anxiety, depression, and PTSD is crucial, along with assessing previous injuries or hospitalizations related to IPV. Additionally, evaluating substance use, reproductive health issues, and safety concerns, such as threats and access to weapons, is essential for a comprehensive assessment.
87. During mental status assessments, individuals who have experienced abuse may exhibit various emotional, cognitive, and behavioral reactions. These responses can vary among victims and may include signs of stress, avoidance of discussing abuse-related topics, feelings of guilt or shame, low self-esteem, disassociation, and avoidant or defensive behavior. They may avoid eye contact, look only at their abuser, or defer to their abuser when answering questions. Additionally, physical indicators such as unexpected injuries or scars can also provide clues to potential abuse. Recognizing these signs and approaching assessments with sensitivity is essential for healthcare providers to identify and support victims of abuse appropriately.
88. In their role as mandated reporters, PMHNPs have a legal and ethical obligation to report suspected cases of abuse or neglect, especially involving children, vulnerable individuals, and the elderly. PMHNPs must notify the appropriate authorities, such as child protective services for minors, in cases of suspected child abuse or neglect. Additionally, they are also mandated to report instances of abuse or neglect affecting vulnerable individuals, who may include those who are disabled or otherwise defenseless. Elder abuse, which involves mistreatment or neglect of adults aged 60 or older, must also be reported by PMHNPs to ensure the safety and well-being of these populations.
89. In the tension-building phase, conflict and tension gradually increase, leading victims to tread carefully to avoid angering the abuser. The incident or abusive phase involves the actual occurrence of abuse, which can be physical, sexual, emotional, or verbal in nature. Following the abuse, the honeymoon or reconciliation phase occurs, during which the abuser becomes remorseful, apologizes, and attempts to mend the relationship. Finally, the calm or tranquil phase may offer a brief period of normalcy and security, but it is often short-lived as tension begins to build again (Fig. 16.1).

Fig. 16.1 Cycle of abuse

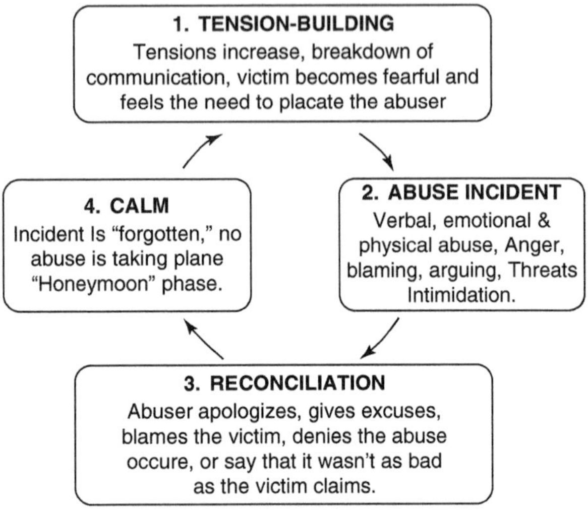

90. To assist a client experiencing intimate partner violence (IPV), creating a safety plan is crucial. This plan involves developing a code word for discreetly seeking help, confiding in a trusted support person, preparing an emergency bag for a quick departure, storing essential phone numbers, monitoring their health, and emphasizing the importance of psychotherapy for coping and healing. Hospitalization may be considered if the client's safety requires it.
91. Emphasize the importance of community support, as abusers often isolate victims and undermine their belief in being believed or helped. Share hotline numbers, police contacts, and emergency medical services for immediate assistance. Encourage the patient to carefully document the development of their abuse and any hospitalizations to ensure safety during health encounters. Assess for suicidal and homicidal thoughts and consider cognitive-behavioral therapy (CBT) as a therapeutic approach. Support groups can be beneficial, and stress the importance of maintaining secrecy during the planning process.
92. Experienced by women more than men, sexual assault is the most common form of abuse.
93. In sexual assault victims, physical signs that an examiner may notice include genital, surrounding skin, STI, or recurrent UTI trauma. These signs can manifest as injuries, bruises, damaged clothes, wounds, swelling, and redness. Even without visible physical injury, sexual assault should be considered. Additionally, sexual assault may lead to the acquisition of sexually transmitted infections (STIs), which can be tested and treated by healthcare providers. Furthermore, a medical examination may reveal the possibility of pregnancy resulting from the sexual assault.
94. If a child engages in serious property damage, petty rage, detailed threats of harm, or displays access to firearms or weapons, immediate action should be taken with the assistance of the school and police. Additionally, children who

threaten suicide or self-harm, engage in bullying, consistently demonstrate extreme anger or rage reactions, repeatedly threaten others, exhibit an obsession with violence or dangerous activities, or display social isolation or withdrawal should all be considered candidates for professional treatment to address their emotional or behavioral concerns.

95.

__X__A fascination or preoccupation with weapons, particularly weapons or explosives that could be used for mass destruction, such as semi-automatic guns
__X__Being a loner with little or no involvement with other employees
__X__Engaging in frequent disputes with supervisors or coworkers
__X__Extreme stress from personal problems or a life crisis
__X__Identifying with incidents of workplace violence reported in the media and either condoning or sympathizing with the actions of the persons committing violence
__X__Obsessive involvement with one's job, particularly where it occurs with no apparent outside interests
__X__Paranoia or easily panicked behavior
__X__Persistent violation of company policy
__X__Prior history of threatening or violent behavior
__X__Volatile or violent home or other personal situation that has the potential to bring violence into the workplace

96.

__X__Alcohol use increases the risk for violence
__X__Attempting to intimidate or harass other persons
__X__Behavior indicating that the person is significantly out of touch with reality and that
__X__Displaying an intense or obsessive romantic interest that exceeds the normal
__X__Making a verbal threat to harm another person or destroy property
__X__Making menacing gestures or physical posturing without actually touching the
__X__Throwing objects
__X__Volatile or violent personal situations such as found in some custody battles bounds of interpersonal interest

97. "Forensic" means using scientific methods to gather, analyze, and interpret evidence for criminal investigations and court trials.
98. Forensic nursing:

- Focuses on direct client care, consulting with healthcare and legal institutions, and providing expert evidence for crime investigations.
- Works in locations such as hospitals, emergency rooms, forensic clinics, and sexual assault examination facilities.
- Often involved in assessing, treating, and supporting crime victims during emergencies.

- May assist police and lawyers as needed.
- Primarily treats legal cases and crime victims.
- Provides care to patients.

Correctional nursing:

- Involves providing care for prisoners in penitentiaries and correctional facilities.
- Works in jails and prisons.
- Provides therapeutic care for inmates, advocates for their health, and offers supervised treatment.
- Focuses on the health and well-being of inmates.
- Primarily treats incarcerated individuals.

Overlapping areas:

- Both forensic nursing and correctional nursing involve working with patients or clients, albeit in different settings.
- They jointly address mental health and crime-related issues, with forensic nurses assisting crime victims and correctional nurses providing therapeutic care to inmates.

99. Correctional psychiatry, competence/decision capability, child custody/visitation, risk assessment, mental disability, malpractice, involuntary treatment.
100. Forensic psychiatric-mental health nurse practitioners (PMHNPs) play a diverse and critical role at the intersection of mental health and the justice system. They work in correctional facilities, where they provide mental health care and assessments for inmates, potentially serving as expert witnesses in legal proceedings. Forensic PMHNPs also offer mental health services in forensic psychiatric facilities, assessing and treating defendants deemed mentally incompetent or facing competency evaluations. Additionally, they collaborate with law enforcement to address the mental health needs of individuals involved in criminal activities. These specialized nurses can work in various settings, including hospitals, mental health clinics, and research institutions, contributing to the evaluation and treatment of mentally ill offenders and the enhancement of mental health services within the justice system.

References and Resources

American Nurses Association. Forensic nursing: scope and standards of practice. 2nd ed. American Nurses Association; 2017.

American Psychiatric Association, editor. Diagnostic and statistical manual of mental disorders: DSM-5-TR. 5th ed., text revision. American Psychiatric Association Publishing; 2022.

Boyer SM, Caplan JE, Edwards LK. Trauma-related dissociation and the dissociative disorders: neglected symptoms with severe public health consequences. Delaware J Public Health. 2022;8(2):78–84. https://doi.org/10.32481/djph.2022.05.010.

Bremner JD. Somatization manifests psychological distress as physical symptoms. Psychosom Med. 2020;82(7):744–51.

Briere J, Scott C. Complex trauma in adolescents and adults: effects and treatment. Psychiatr Clin N Am. 2015;38:515–27. https://doi.org/10.1016/j.psc.2015.05.004.

Campbell MC, Smakowski A, Rojas-Aguiluz M, Goldstein LH, Cardeña E, Nicholson TR, et al. Dissociation and its biological and clinical associations in functional neurological disorder: systematic review and meta-analysis. BJPsych Open. 2022;9(1):e2. https://doi.org/10.1192/bjo.2022.597.

Center for Substance Abuse Treatment (US). Chapter 3: Understanding the impact of trauma. In: Trauma-informed care in behavioral health services (Treatment Improvement Protocol (TIP) series, no. 57). Rockville, MD: Substance Abuse and Mental Health Services Administration; 2014. https://www.ncbi.nlm.nih.gov/books/NBK207191/.

Daniels J. Trauma is a significant contributor to the development of mental health issues, including post-traumatic stress disorder (PTSD), anxiety, and depression. J Trauma Stress Disord. 2020;32(3):213–26.

De Bellis MD, Zisk A. The biological effects of childhood trauma. Child Adolesc Psychiatr Clin N Am. 2014;23(2):185–222, vii. https://doi.org/10.1016/j.chc.2014.01.002.

Dickinson T, Mullan A, Lippiatt K, Owen JA. Nursing people in prisons, forensics and correctional facilities. In: Santos J, Cutcliffe J, editors. European psychiatric/mental health nursing in the 21st century. Principles of specialty nursing. Cham: Springer; 2018. https://doi.org/10.1007/978-3-319-31772-4_16.

Farina B, Liotti M, Imperatori C. The role of attachment trauma and disintegrative pathogenic processes in the traumatic-dissociative dimension. Front Psychol. 2019;10:933. https://doi.org/10.3389/fpsyg.2019.00933.

Fleishman J, Kamsky H, Sundborg S. Trauma-informed nursing practice. Online J Issues Nurs. 2019;24(2) https://doi.org/10.3912/OJIN.Vol24No02Man03.

Gibson LE, Alloy LB, Ellman LM. Trauma and the psychosis spectrum: a review of symptom specificity and explanatory mechanisms. Clin Psychol Rev. 2016;49:92–105. https://doi.org/10.1016/j.cpr.2016.08.003.

Gillig PM. Dissociative identity disorder: a controversial diagnosis. Psychiatry. 2009;6(3):24–9.

Grossman S, Cooper Z, Buxton H, Hendrickson S, Lewis-O'Connor A, Stevens J, et al. Trauma-informed care: recognizing and resisting re-traumatization in health care. Trauma Surg Acute Care Open. 2021;6(1):e000815. https://doi.org/10.1136/tsaco-2021-000815.

Han HR, Miller HN, Nkimbeng M, Budhathoki C, Mikhael T, Rivers E, et al. Trauma informed interventions: a systematic review. PLoS One. 2021;16(6):e0252747. https://doi.org/10.1371/journal.pone.0252747.

Javidi H, Yadollahie M. Post-traumatic stress disorder. Int J Occup Environ Med. 2012;3(1):2–9.

Johnson K, Vanderhoef D, Magrath N. Psychiatric-mental health nurse practitioner review and resource manual. American Nurses Credentialing Center, American Nurses Association; 2020.

Kameg BN, Constantino R. Intimate partner violence in adolescents: preventive strategies for psychiatric-mental health nurse practitioners. J Child Adolesc Psychiatr Nurs. 2020;33(3):163–8. https://doi.org/10.1111/jcap.12286.

Kar N. Cognitive behavioral therapy for the treatment of post-traumatic stress disorder: a review. Neuropsychiatr Dis Treat. 2011;7:167–81. https://doi.org/10.2147/NDT.S10389.

Kloek C, Bossen D, de Bakker DH, Veenhof C, Dekker J. Blended interventions to change behavior in patients with chronic somatic disorders: systematic review. J Med Internet Res. 2017;19(12):e418. https://doi.org/10.2196/jmir.8108.

Kubany ES, Watson SB, Owens JA. Cognitive therapy for trauma-related guilt: Conceptual bases and treatment outlines. Cogn Behav Pract. 2003;10(1):50–61.

Lancaster CL, Teeters JB, Gros DF, Back SE. Posttraumatic stress disorder: overview of evidence-based assessment and treatment. J Clin Med. 2016;5(11):105. https://doi.org/10.3390/jcm5110105.

McLaughlin KA, Conron KJ, Koenen KC, Gilman SE. Childhood adversity, adult stressful life events, and risk of past-year psychiatric disorder: a test of the stress sensitization hypothesis in a population-based sample of adults. Psychol Med. 2010;40(10):1647–58. https://doi.org/10.1017/S0033291709992121.

Morrison AP, Frame L, Larkin W. Relationships between trauma and psychosis: a review and integration. Br J Clin Psychol. 2003;42(Pt 4):331–53. https://doi.org/10.1348/014466503322528892.

Nesset MB, Lara-Cabrera ML, Dalsbø TK, Pedersen SA, Bjørngaard JH, Palmstierna T. Cognitive behavioural group therapy for male perpetrators of intimate partner violence: a systematic review. BMC Psychiatry. 2019;19(1):11. https://doi.org/10.1186/s12888-019-2010-1.

Prior KN, Bond MJ. Somatic symptom disorders and illness behavior: current perspectives. Int Rev Psychiatry. 2013;25(1):5–18. https://doi.org/10.3109/09540261.2012.732043.

Speck PM, Peters S. Forensics in NP practice. Adv Nurse Pract. 1999;7(11):18.

van der Kolk BA, McFarlane AC, Weisaeth L, editors. Traumatic stress: the effects of overwhelming experience on mind, body, and society. Guilford Press; 1996.

Wang SK, Feng M, Fang Y, Lv L, Sun GL, Yang SL, Guo P, Cheng SF, Qian MC, Chen HX. Psychological trauma, posttraumatic stress disorder, and trauma-related depression: a mini-review. World J Psychiatry. 2023;13(6):331–9. https://doi.org/10.5498/wjp.v13.i6.331.

Wheeler K. What do psychiatric nurse practitioners need to know about trauma? Perspect Psychiatr Care. 2022;58(4):2562–9. https://doi.org/10.1111/ppc.13094.

Zakhari R. The psychiatric-mental health nurse practitioner certification review manual. Springer Publishing Company; 2021.

Zeanah CH, Berlin LJ, Boris NW. Practitioner review: clinical applications of attachment theory and research for infants and young children. J Child Psychol Psychiatry. 2011;52(8):819–33. https://doi.org/10.1111/j.1469-7610.2011.02399.x.

Notes:

Notes:

Individual, Group, and Family Therapies 17

Test your learning and check your understanding of this book's contents: use the "Springer Nature Flashcards" app to access questions using ▶ https://sn.pub/62J0Ar.

To use the app, please follow the instructions in Chap. 1.

Individual, group, and family therapies improve mental health, according to emerging data. These therapies are useful for depression, anxiety, substance misuse, and relationship troubles.

PMHNPs often use one-on-one therapy. This therapy comprises regular meetings with a patient to examine their thoughts, feelings, and actions. Individual therapy can benefit patients with low self-esteem, sorrow, or trauma. It can also help patients manage their mental health or make positive life choices A research review indicated that individual treatment reduced depression and anxiety (Cuijpers et al. 2013).

Another essential treatment is group therapy. Individuals with comparable difficulties or challenges meet for group therapy can help patients feel supported and learn from others going through similar problems (May et al. 2016). Group therapy is useful for patients seeking social support and those who benefit from others' perspectives. Group therapy reduces depression and anxiety, improves social skills, and boosts self-esteem.

Family therapy helps family members manage disputes and enhance relationships. Communication, parenting, and other relationship concerns can be addressed in family therapy. Family therapy can help families with loved ones with mental health issues like addiction or depression. Family therapy improves communication, problem-solving, conflict resolution, and family functioning.

PMHNPs and their patients benefit from individual, group, and family therapy in addition to their efficacy. PMHNPs can work closely with patients to teach them mental health coping skills and techniques. They also help PMHNPs develop patient

T. Stewart, *Psychiatric-Mental Health Nurse Practitioner Program Companion and Board Certification Exam Review Workbook*,
https://doi.org/10.1007/978-3-031-60894-0_17

relationships and provide ongoing support. To give patients the greatest care, PMHNPs must be trained in and proficient in these therapies. Individual, group, and family therapy offer patients a secure space to express their thoughts, feelings, and behaviors. They can also help patients improve communication, problem-solving, and mental health management.

PMHNPs should address cost and availability barriers to these approaches to ensure that all patients can receive therapy. Lack of insurance may prevent access to solo, group, and family therapy. Many insurance policies do not cover these therapies or only cover a few sessions, making them pricey for some patients. PMHNPs can push for more insurance coverage for these therapies and help patients locate grants or sliding scale prices (Bohart and Tallman 1999).

The availability of skilled therapists may also limit access to solo, group, and family therapy (Beutler et al. 2016). Many places lack mental health specialists, especially PMHNPs, making it hard for patients to access these therapies. PMHNPs can advocate for mental health professional education and training regulations and work with other providers to make these therapies more accessible in their areas.

PMHNPs treating mental health patients should use individual, group, and family therapy. These interventions have been shown to improve mental health and help PMHNPs and their patients. To give patients the greatest care, PMHNPs must be trained in and proficient in these therapies. PMHNPs should also be aware of cost and availability barriers to these medicines and endeavor to resolve them to ensure that all patients receive therapy. This chapter will focus on individual, group, family, and complementary and alternative therapies.

17.1 Foundations

1. What is a therapeutic relationship between a PMHNP and a client?

2. What are five to seven elements necessary for a successful therapeutic relationship?
    1.
    2.
    3.
    4.
    5.
    6.
    7.

3. Provide a summary for each phase of the therapeutic relationship. Then, provide some behaviors and practices that one might expect from the therapist and the client during each phase.

Phase	Summary	Therapist behaviors/ practices	Client behaviors/ practices
1. Preinteraction phase			
2. Introductory/ orientation phase			
3. Working phase			
4. Termination phase			

4. Distinguish transference from countertransference. Provide an example of each.

Transference	Countertransference

Transference	Countertransference
Example:	Example:

5. What are some key signs that a PMHNP should watch for to detect transference and countertransference?

6. When is a PMHNP obligated to break confidentiality?

7. What are the benefits of nonpharmacological treatments in mental health?

8. While psychiatric-mental health nurse practitioners may combine psychotherapy with medications, one popular model is where one provider prescribes medication and another provides therapy. This is known as ____________________ treatment.

17.2 Individual Therapy

9. What does individual therapy entail?

10. ________________________________ therapy posits that the past shapes present behaviors, often unconscious motivations and instincts. Individuals grow in their personal development by increasing their awareness of __________________ defenses. This therapeutic approach is associated with the theorist and analyst ____________________.

11. Psychoanalysis may be used with clients who are actively psychotic or manic.
    TRUE FALSE

12. In which developmental order are the ID, ego, and superego present?

13. Match each of the following concepts from Freud's theories of the mind to the best explanation on the right.

Concept	Explanation
________1. Unconscious	A. Conscious recall of forgotten childhood memories.
________2. Preconscious	B. The personality aspect that mediates internal and external stimuli, especially in interpersonal relationships. Denial and repression are further ego defenses against anxiety and distress.
________3. Conscious	C. The component of the personality that internalizes social and cultural values, morals, and ideals, and seeks perfection.
________4. Id	D. The most primitive part of the personality, operating on the pleasure principle and seeking immediate gratification of instinctual needs and drives.
________5. Superego	E. Repressed thoughts out of an individual's awareness, including sexual urges and other primitive drives.
________6. Ego	F. Current thoughts and perceptions that are within an individual's awareness.

14. What is the goal of psychoanalysis? Why is it considered insight-oriented?

15. ________________________________ are unconscious psychological strategies that individuals use to protect themselves from unpleasant emotions, thoughts, or situations. These operate at an unconscious level and can distort or deny reality, often resulting in maladaptive or harmful behavior.

16. Identify each of the following defense mechanisms as mature (M), neurotic (N), immature (I), or other (O).

Defense mechanism	Type
Acting out	
Altruism	
Controlling	
Denial	
Displacement	
Humor	
Intellectualization	
Isolation of affect	
Projection	
Rationalization	
Reaction formation	
Regression	
Repression	

Defense mechanism	Type
Splitting	
Sublimation	
Suppression	
Undoing	

17. Complete the crossword puzzle on defense mechanisms.

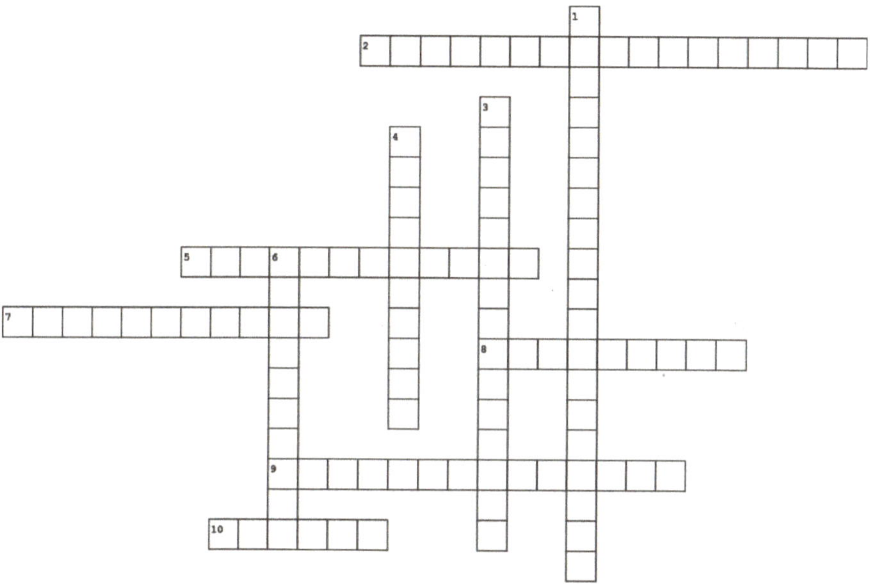

Across		Down	
2.	A patient is angry about the care received but behaves in an ingratiating manner	1.	A parent talks with his child about what love should be like but fails to demonstrate love toward the child
5.	A patient who is angry at his doctor becomes verbally abusive to the nurses	3.	A patient being treated for a drug addiction says he cannot stop taking drugs because he has a "bad marriage"
7.	A mother who lost a son in a drunk-driving accident joins an organization that works to educate the public about the dangers of drunk driving	4.	An accident victim remembers nothing about his accident
8.	A rape victim talks about her rape experience without showing any emotion	6.	A frightened patient lashes out at the nurse, saying the nurse "doesn't know what is going on"
9.	A teenager hospitalized for diabetes wants to become a nurse as a result of his experiences		
10.	A patient who drinks alcohol every day and cannot stop fails to acknowledge that he has a problem		

18. ____________________ therapy argues that an individual's maladaptation is caused by that person's cognitive distortions of their expectations of their reality and events therein. Therapy in this model aims to examine these beliefs objectively and help them to address their misconceptions. _______________ is the theorist associated with this therapy.

19. Arnold Lazarus developed ____________________________ therapy. In this approach, therapists use role-play, exposure, and problem-solving, or very participatory techniques to address various dimensions of an individual's functioning, including behavior, affect, sensation, imagery, cognition, and interpersonal relationships.

20. What is the goal of behavioral therapy?

21. Knowing that behavioral therapy is based on learning theory, define each of the following terms and provide an example.

Type of conditioning	Description	Example
Classical conditioning		
Operant conditioning		

22. What is the difference between negative reinforcement and punishment?

23. Name at least three deconditioning behavioral therapy techniques.

24. What is the goal of cognitive therapy?

25. Explain cognitive-behavioral therapy.

26. Individuals with borderline personality disorder are often engaged in ________ ______________________________ therapy. Marsha Linehan developed this therapeutic approach to assist clients with regulating their behaviors, developing tolerance for distress, engaging with others, and self-introspection techniques.

27. What is dialectical behavioral therapy?

28. Viktor Frankl created ______________________________ therapy, which focuses on a client's responsibility for their current lived experience. Clients ask reflective questions, which may be difficult and indeed to confront long-held beliefs about their sense of self.

29. Humanistic therapy, developed by Carl Rogers, is also known as ___________ ____________________________ therapy. It aims to support an individual's own growth through self-direction. Gratitude journals, positive thinking, and socialization are key techniques in this therapy.

30. Gerald Klerman and Myrna Weissman are associated with _______________ therapy. This therapy approaches that a client's issues within relationships are the basis of their distress. It can be used with a variety of mental health disorders. The approach was developed for depression.

31. EMDR is an abbreviation for ____ __________. It was developed by Francine Shapiro to help individuals with traumatic experiences.

32. Explain how EMDR is conducted during a therapy session using each of the following phases of EMDR.

Phase	Description
Desensitization	
Installation	
Body scan	

33. ______________________________therapy is based on the belief that all individuals must grapple with concepts of freedom, choice, responsibility, isolation, and mortality. A therapist helps clients develop a sense of personal meaning and purpose in their lives. This may involve helping the client to confront their fears and anxieties, to identify their values and priorities, and to find ways to live authentically and in alignment with their own sense of purpose.

34. Developed by Fritz Perls, Laura Perls, and Paul Goodman in the 1940s and 1950s, ______________________________therapy helps clients become more aware of their thoughts, feelings, and behaviors in the present and accept responsibility for their experiences. It invites clients to find their own answers. It helps clients gain self-awareness, self-acceptance, personal progress, and happier relationships.

35. Explain the "empty chair" exercise used in the above therapy.

36. Match each individual therapy with its succinct description.

Therapy	Description
__________1. Psychoanalytic	A. Therapy that focuses on modifying problematic behaviors through learning principles.
__________2. Cognitive	B. Therapy that focuses on improving relationships and communication patterns.
__________3. Behavioral	C. Therapy that focuses on exploring the meaning and purpose of life and the individual's experience of existence.
__________4. Dialectical behavioral	D. Therapy that focuses on the present moment and the client's immediate experience
__________5. Existential	E. Therapy that focuses on identifying and changing negative thinking patterns and beliefs.
__________6. Humanistic	F. Therapy that emphasizes individual potential, self-awareness, and self-actualization.
__________7. Interpersonal	G. Therapy that focuses on exploring the fundamental questions of human existence and the experience of being alive
__________8. EMDR	H. Therapy that focuses on the unconscious mind and childhood experiences.
__________9. Existential	I. Therapy that uses bilateral stimulation to help process traumatic memories.
__________10. Gestalt	J. Therapy that combines cognitive and behavioral techniques with mindfulness to treat emotional dysregulation and borderline personality disorder.

17.3 Group Therapy

37. It is recommended that at least __________ patients must meet with a therapist to be considered a group therapy session.

38. What are some of the advantages to group therapy?

39. Explain Irvine Yalom's group therapy model.

40. Match Yalom's 10 therapeutic factors with their description.

Therapeutic factor	Description
__________1. Instillation of hope	A. Encouraging clients to model the behaviors and attitudes of others in the group who have successfully addressed similar problems.
__________2. Universality	B. Encouraging clients to help and support others in the group, which can improve self-esteem and a sense of purpose.
__________3. Imparting information	C. Helping clients to see that their problems and struggles are not unique and that others share similar experiences.

Therapeutic factor	Description
________4. Altruism	D. Providing clients with a safe and supportive space to express and process their emotions and experiences, which can promote emotional healing and growth.
________5. Corrective recapitulation of the primary family group	E. Helping clients to develop and practice social skills, communication skills, and problem-solving skills.
________6. Development of socializing techniques	F. Fostering a sense of connection and unity among group members, which can provide a supportive and validating environment for growth and change.
________7. Imitative behavior	G. Helping clients to develop a sense of optimism and belief in the possibility of positive change.
________8. Interpersonal learning	H. Providing clients with information about mental health, coping skills, and strategies for managing their symptoms.
________9. Group cohesiveness	I. Helping clients to identify and address patterns of behavior and communication that may have originated in their family of origin.
________10. Catharsis	J. Helping clients to develop insight into their own interpersonal patterns and relationships, and to practice new, more effective ways of relating to others.

41. Provide a brief explanation for each of the following phases of group formation.

Phase	Brief explanation
Forming	
Storming	
Norming	
Performing	
Adjourning	

42. What is reminiscence therapy?

43. What are support groups? What is their purpose in general? Name three to five examples.

17.4 Family Therapy

44. What is the goal of family therapy?

45. A mother may become anxious when her child acts out, which may cause the child to act out more in response to the mother's anxiety. This cycle can continue and intensify, with the child's behavior and the mother's anxiety feeding off of each other. This is an example of ______________________________ __________.

46. A family may resist addressing conflicts or issues because it would upset the balance of power within the family, even if addressing those issues would ultimately lead to greater harmony and well-being. This family would be considered in ____.

47. A family that is able to adjust to the challenges of a new job or move to a new location by maintaining open communication and being flexible in their routines and expectations. This has demonstrated __________________________ ______________.

48. Complete the following table for each aspect of a functional versus dysfunctional family.

	Functional family	Dysfunctional family
Characteristics		
Communication styles		
Use of boundaries		
Traits		
Resolution of problems		
Coping strategies		
Family dynamics		

	Functional family	Dysfunctional family
Family values		
Emotional climate		

49. Match each type of family therapy with its developer(s).

Type of family therapy	Developer(s)
________1. Family systems	A. Murray Bowen
________2. Structural family therapy	B. Jay Haley
________3. Experiential therapy	C. Steve deShazer, Insoo Kim Berg, and others
________4. Strategic therapy	D. Salvador Minuchin
________5. Solution-focused therapy	E. Virginia Satir

50. Explain family systems therapy. How does this model see the family unit? What is the basis of problems within the family? What is the general approach to addressing these problems? What are the goals?

51. ________________________________ refers to the ability of family members to maintain their own identity and emotional stability while still remaining connected to the family system.

52. ____ refers to a dynamic where two family members are in conflict and involve a third person (such as a child) in order to manage the conflict. This practice can perpetuate negative family patterns and make it difficult to address underlying issues.

53. Explain structural family therapy. How does this model see the family unit? What is the basis of problems within the family? What is the general approach to addressing these problems? What are the goals?

54. According to structural family therapy, a pattern of overly close relationships and unclear boundaries within a family system is known as ________________ ____________________________. This dynamic can lead to feelings of suffocation, anxiety, and a lack of individual autonomy.

55. ____refers to a pattern of distant relationships and rigid boundaries within a family system. It can lead to feelings of isolation, detachment, and emotional neglect.

56. In the table below, provide a brief explanation and example for each type of boundary.

Type of boundary	Explanation	Example
Rigid		
Diffuse		
Clearly defined		

57. Name five techniques used in structural family therapy.
    1.
    2.
    3.
    4.
    5.

58. Explain experiential therapy. How does this model see the family unit? What is the basis of problems within the family? What is the general approach to addressing these problems? What are the goals?

59. In experiential therapy, the ____ ___________ concept refers to the notion that people often present a façade to the outside world, while their true feelings and emotions are hidden beneath the surface. By exploring and addressing these hidden emotions, individuals and families could improve their self-esteem and develop more authentic and fulfilling relationships.

60. Explain strategic therapy. How does this model see the family unit? What is the basis of problems within the family? What is the general approach to addressing these problems? What are the goals?

61. ________________________________ involves redefining or reinterpreting a problem or behavior in order to change the family's perception of the problem, so that there is a shift away from blame or negative emotions, and toward more positive and productive solutions (e.g., jealousy relabeled as caring).

62. Explain solution-focused therapy. How does this model see the family unit? What is the basis of problems within the family? What is the general approach to addressing these problems? What are the goals?

63. What is the "miracle question" as used in solution-focused therapy?

64. Write a draft of the "miracle question" as you might use it in your own practice.

65. A therapist guided by solution-focused therapy asks a client, "Was there a time when the problem did not occur?" This is an example of an ______________ ____ question and aims to help the client move toward solutions by assisting them in searching for breaks in the pattern.

66. In solution-focused therapy, a PMHNP might ask a client to rate their progress toward a goal from 1 to 10. This is known as ______________________ __________.

67. Match each of the following types of couples therapy with its definition on the right.

__________1. Conjoint therapy	A. Each member of the couple meets with the therapist separately.
__________2. Concurrent therapy	B. Used in the treatment of sexual problems, two therapists meet with the couple together
__________3. Collaborative therapy	C. Each member of the couple meets with the therapist together
__________4. Four-way therapy	D. Each member of the couple has a separate therapist that they see individually

17.5 Complementary and Alternative Therapies

68. Compare and contrast complementary and alternative therapeutic interventions. Consider definition, examples, purpose, and evidence base.

	Complementary	Alternative
Definition		

	Complementary	Alternative
Examples		
Purpose		
Evidence base		

69. For each of the complementary and alternative therapies, identify if it is mind-body (MB), manipulative physical (MP), or biological (B). Use the column on the right to note two to three pieces of information about each intervention. Blank rows may be used for additional complementary or alternative therapies that you come across during your studies.

Intervention	Category	Description
Acupressure		
Acupuncture		
Aromatherapy		
Biofeedback		
Fish oil		
Guided imagery		
Herbs		

Intervention	Category	Description
Kava		
L-theanine		
Massage		
Meditation		
Melatonin		
Nutraceuticals		
Reflexology		
Sam-e		
Tryptophan		
Vitamins		
Yoga		

17.6 Answers and Explanations to Chapter Activities

1. A psychiatric-mental health nurse practitioner (PMHNP) and client form a professional collaboration to improve mental health. A trusting, respectful, empathetic, and collaborative therapy partnership helps clients achieve their treatment goals. Therapeutic relationships require active listening, good communication, and nonjudgmental treatment of client issues. The PMHNP provides a secure space for clients to explore their thoughts, feelings, and behaviors and overcome obstacles. Setting limits, honoring client autonomy, and ensuring confidentiality are also part of the therapeutic interaction. The PMHNP tracks the client's development, changes the treatment plan, and assures the optimum care.
2. Answers will vary, but can include: trust, empathy, respect, attentiveness, active and reflective listening, affirmation, authenticity, collaboration, clear communication, cultural competence, confidentiality, boundaries.
3.

Phase	Summary	Therapist behaviors/ practices	Client behaviors/ practices
1. Preinteraction phase	Assessing personal biases, assumptions, and expectations to prevent potential harm to clients.	Self-reflection, identifying personal biases and assumptions, understanding cultural differences, maintaining professional boundaries.	N/A
2. Introductory/ orientation phase	Introductions, building rapport and trust, establishing goals, and setting expectations.	Active listening, establishing boundaries, explaining confidentiality, building rapport, setting goals.	Sharing background, identifying concerns, asking questions, establishing trust.
3. Working phase	Working on treatment goals, exploring issues, building insight and awareness, and making progress.	Applying evidence-based treatments, encouraging expression, providing support and guidance, challenging negative behaviors, and monitoring progress.	Participating actively in therapy, exploring thoughts and feelings, practicing new behaviors, and learning new coping strategies.
4. Termination phase	Consolidating gains, summarizing treatment outcomes, reviewing goals, planning for future maintenance, and termination of therapy.	Reviewing progress, reinforcing gains, preparing for termination, and ensuring a smooth transition.	Consolidating treatment gains, reviewing goals, planning for maintenance, preparing for termination, expressing gratitude.

4.

Transference	Countertransference
A client subconsciously transfers feelings, emotions, and attitudes from past major relationships onto the therapist. These favorable or negative feelings may be based on parental, sibling, or authority figure experiences.	Countertransference is the therapist's unconscious emotional response to the client based on personal history and unsolved difficulties. The therapist's objectivity and treatment effectiveness may be affected by this reaction.
Example: A client had a poor connection with their father and still feels angry toward him, they may unconsciously project their resentment onto the therapist, viewing them as a father figure.	Example: A therapist may feel overly protective of a client, wanting to rescue them from their difficulties or solve their problems for them. This reaction may be rooted in the therapist's own unresolved issues related to control or anxiety, rather than in the client's needs or treatment goals.

5. To avoid harming the therapy relationship or treatment outcomes, PMHNPs must be cognizant of transference and countertransference. Watch for these signs:

   - Intense emotions: A client may show exaggerated wrath, affection, or terror toward the PMHNP.
   - Resistance: A client may react defensively or hostilely to PMHNP interventions or comments.
   - Overdependence: A client may rely on the PMHNP for emotional support and comfort.
   - Overidentification: The PMHNP may identify with the client's feelings, behaviors, or experiences.
   - Avoidance: PMHNPs may avoid sensitive topics or emotions.
   - Overinvolvement: The PMHNP may want to save the client or address their difficulties.
   - Discomfort: The PMHNP may feel uneasy with the client for no reason.

6. Maintaining confidentiality is a vital aspect of a PMHNP's role in preserving the therapeutic relationship and enhancing client well-being. However, there are situations in which a PMHNP may need to breach confidentiality to ensure the safety of the client or others. These instances include when there is a risk of harm to the client or someone else, in which case actions such as calling emergency services or involving the client's family may be necessary. Reporting allegations of abuse or neglect of children or vulnerable adults is another circumstance that requires breaching confidentiality. Additionally, legal proceedings or ethical misconduct by other mental health providers may compel the PMHNP to disclose certain information. Finally, in cases of reportable communicable diseases, confidentiality may be breached to protect public health.
7. Nonpharmacological treatments offer a holistic approach to addressing mental health concerns, taking into account environmental stressors, interpersonal relationships, coping strategies, and other psychological factors. They can be more

accessible and affordable for individuals without health insurance or limited financial resources. Some people prefer nonpharmacological therapies due to concerns about medication side effects or personal preferences. Combining nonpharmacological treatments with medication can lead to more comprehensive and effective therapy. These therapies are particularly beneficial in addressing mental health issues such as grief, interpersonal conflicts, phobias, underlying causes, and existential crises that may not be fully addressed by medication alone. Additionally, nonpharmacological therapies may be preferred or mandated in specific situations, such as for children, pregnant individuals, geriatric populations, or in legal and forensic matters, as they may be more suitable for addressing personality disorders and other complex psychological conditions.

8. Split treatment involves psychiatric-mental health nurse practitioner managing medicine and a certified therapist or counselor providing psychotherapy.
9. Individual therapy, also known as psychotherapy, talk therapy, or counseling, involves a mental health professional working one-on-one with a client to address emotional, relationship, behavioral, or mental health issues. Improve the client's health and quality of life.
10. Psychoanalysis therapy posits that the past shapes present behaviors, often unconscious motivations and instincts. Individuals grow in their personal development by increasing their awareness of psychological defenses, particularly maladaptive defenses. This therapeutic approach is associated with the theorist and analyst Sigmund Freud.
11. FALSE. Psychoanalysis is a long-term, insight-oriented therapy that demands stability and insight into one's own emotions and experiences. Actively psychotic or manic clients may struggle with reality checking, impulse control, and self-stability, making psychoanalysis less successful or even dangerous. For acute psychotic or manic symptoms, cognitive-behavioral therapy may be better.
12. Freud's psychoanalytic theory states that the id, ego, and superego evolve in a definite order. Id, the innate and unconscious aspect of personality, is present at birth. The ego—the conscious, reasoning element of personality—develops between 6 months and 2 years. Three to five years old is when the moral and ethical superego emerges. Thus, the id, ego, and superego grow in order.
13. 1/E, 2/A, 3/F, 4/D, 5/C, 6/B.
14. Psychoanalysis aims to reveal underlying conflicts and motivations and resolve them for emotional healing and personal growth. Psychoanalysis is insight-oriented because it explores the unconscious mind and the intricate id, ego, and superego relationships. Free association, dream analysis, and transference and resistance analysis help clients understand their unconscious thoughts and behaviors. Clients can grasp their emotional suffering and find new solutions by understanding these patterns.
15. Psychoanalytic theory and therapy are based on defense mechanisms.

16. Identify each of the following defense mechanisms as mature (M), neurotic (N), immature (I), or other (O).

Defense mechanism	Type
Acting out	I
Altruism	M
Controlling	N
Denial	I
Displacement	N
Humor	M
Intellectualization	N
Isolation of affect	N
Projection	I
Rationalization	N
Reaction formation	N
Regression	I
Repression	N
Splitting	O
Sublimation	M
Suppression	M
Undoing	O

17. Complete the crossword puzzle on defense mechanisms.

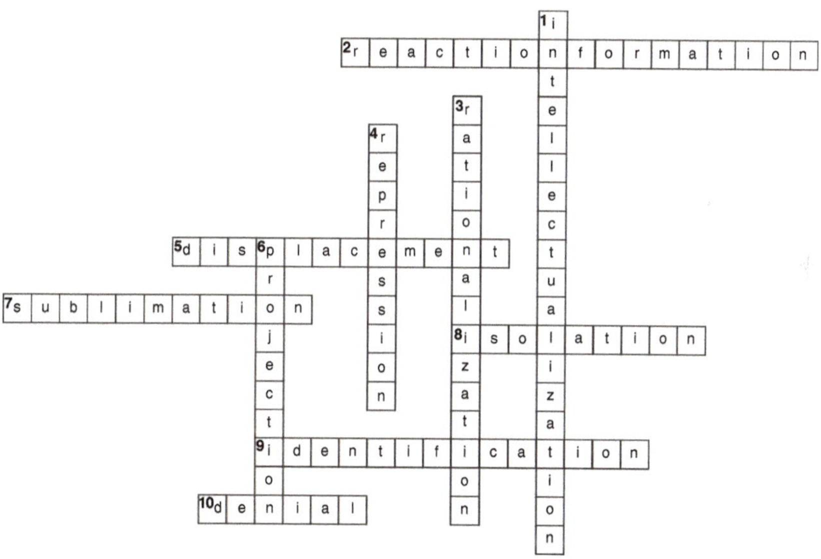
1 intellectualization
2 reaction formation
3 rationalization
4 repression
5 displacement
6 projection
7 sublimation
8 isolation
9 identification
10 denial

18. Cognitive, Aaron Beck.
19. Multimodal therapy.
20. Behavioral therapy aims to help patients change maladaptive behaviors that contribute to their symptoms by replacing them with healthy alternatives.

21.

Type of conditioning	Description	Example
Classical conditioning	A type of learning where a neutral stimulus becomes associated with a specific response after being paired with a stimulus that naturally evokes that response. The neutral stimulus eventually comes to evoke the same response as the natural stimulus.	An adult with anxiety may learn to associate a certain location, such as a hospital waiting room, with feelings of panic and anxiety, even if there is no immediate danger present. Over time, the neutral stimulus of the location becomes a conditioned stimulus that elicits the conditioned response of anxiety.
Operant conditioning	Involves learning through consequences, specifically reinforcement and punishment. Behaviors that are reinforced with positive consequences (such as rewards) are more likely to be repeated in the future, while behaviors that are punished or receive negative consequences are less likely to be repeated.	An adult with depression who engages in enjoyable activities (such as spending time with loved ones or pursuing a hobby) that are positively reinforced with feelings of pleasure and satisfaction is more likely to repeat these activities in the future, as they serve as a source of positive reinforcement. On the other hand, an adult with OCD who engages in compulsive behaviors (such as hand washing) that are negatively reinforced by reducing anxiety is more likely to repeat these behaviors, as they serve as a source of negative reinforcement.

22. A negative reinforcement, a behavior is encouraged by removing an aversive stimulus. Punishment is the application of in aversive response to an undesirable behavior.
23. Systematic desensitization, flooding and implosion, aversion therapy, token economy, biofeedback.
24. Cognitive therapy aims to correct faulty assumptions, or cognitive distortions, and negative feelings that exacerbate psychiatric symptoms by identifying maladaptive thoughts and replacing them with positive ones.
25. Cognitive-behavioral therapy (CBT) is a structured and goal-oriented approach that explores the interaction between thoughts, emotions, and behaviors in the context of mental health. It is based on the premise that negative thought patterns and behaviors can contribute to and perpetuate mental health conditions, and by modifying them, individuals can enhance their mental well-being. Typically consisting of 12–20 weekly sessions, CBT involves a collaborative effort between the therapist and client to identify and challenge harmful thought patterns and behaviors and replace them with more positive and adaptive ones. The therapy includes cognitive restructuring to address negative beliefs,

behavior activation to modify detrimental behavior patterns, and skills training to help clients manage their thoughts, emotions, and behaviors effectively. CBT has been found effective for treating conditions like anxiety, depression, PTSD, and eating disorders, making it particularly suitable for motivated individuals seeking short-term, goal-focused therapy.

26. Dialectical behavioral therapy.
27. DBT is a structured therapy that develops mindfulness, distress tolerance, emotion control, and interpersonal effectiveness. Through individual, group, and homework treatment, clients learn these skills and are encouraged to use them daily. DBT changes harmful behaviors into better ones, making it a behavioral treatment. It also uses Zen Buddhist mindfulness and acceptance techniques to assist clients become more self-aware and accepting of their circumstances. DBT has been demonstrated to treat borderline personality disorder, depression, anxiety, eating disorders, and substance use disorders. DBT is ideal for trauma survivors and those who struggle to control their emotions since it emphasizes acceptance and validation.
28. Existential.
29. Person-centered therapy.
30. Interpersonal.
31. Eye movement desensitization and reprocessing.
32.

Phase	Description
Desensitization	Therapists help clients recognize painful memories that cause distress. After that, the client is asked to focus on the memory while bilaterally stimulating their hands by tapping, following the therapist's fingers, or utilizing headphones with alternating noises.
Installation	The therapist helps the client replace traumatic memory-related negative beliefs with positive ones. The client must focus on the traumatic memory and the good belief they want. In this phase, the therapist may employ bilateral stimulation to reinforce the positive belief.
Body scan	The therapist helps the client discover traumatic memory-related physical and emotional symptoms. As they recall the memory, the client is urged to scan their body for sensations and emotions. The therapist will help the client process remaining feelings and sensations utilizing bilateral stimulation.

33. Existential therapy.
34. Gestalt therapy.
35. Gestalt therapy uses the empty-chair practice often. The client is shown an empty chair and asked to envision someone or something important sitting in it. The client is then asked to share their thoughts and feelings with the imaginary person or item. The empty-chair exercise is used to address the client's unresolved issues, such as anger or sadness. It helps clients communicate their thoughts and feelings in a secure and supportive setting. The empty-chair exercise helps individuals understand their emotions and behaviors and create better coping techniques for stressful situations. Clients can practice assertiveness and

communication skills for their relationships outside of treatment. The empty-chair exercise helps clients process complex emotions and experiences in a meaningful and transforming way.

36. 1/H, 2/E, 3/A, 4/J, 5/C, 6/F, 7/B, 8/I, 9/G, 10/D.
37. Group therapy sessions should have three to four patients. Group therapy uses member interactions to provide support, feedback, and encouragement. The group may lack the diversity of ideas and experiences needed for meaningful therapeutic interactions with less than three to four members. However, interpersonal process groups and psychoeducational groups may have various group size guidelines.
38. Group psychotherapy involves regular meetings of a small group of individuals under the guidance of a qualified therapist to address emotional and psychological issues. This form of therapy offers several advantages, including peer support, as it allows participants to connect with others facing similar challenges, reducing feelings of isolation and enhancing a sense of belonging. Additionally, group therapy is cost-effective compared to individual therapy, making it more accessible to those with financial constraints. Exposure to diverse perspectives within the group fosters learning and the development of coping skills, while also providing an opportunity for skill-building in areas such as social interaction, assertiveness, communication, and problem-solving. Group therapy enables participants to receive constructive feedback from both the therapist and fellow group members, aiding in self-awareness and personal growth.
39. Yalom's group therapy approach places a strong emphasis on the significance of group dynamics and interpersonal relationships as a means for personal growth and healing. Yalom contends that group therapy holds equal importance to individual therapist-client therapy. Within Yalom's framework, there are ten therapeutic components, including instilling hope, developing socializing skills, and promoting group cohesiveness. Authenticity, honesty, and self-disclosure are central to his existential and humanistic approach to group therapy. Yalom's group therapy is open-ended, with regular meetings over an extended period, and it can encompass a wide range of mental health issues. It can be utilized either as a standalone therapy or in conjunction with individual therapy, and has shown effectiveness in addressing conditions such as depression, anxiety, and substance use problems. This approach creates a supportive and validating environment that fosters connections, sharing, and learning among group members.
40. 1/G, 2/C, 3/H, 4/B, 5/I, 6/E, 7/A, 8/J, 9/F, 10/D.
41.

Phase	Brief explanation
Forming	In this initial phase, group members are getting to know each other and establishing the purpose and goals of the group. Members may be polite and tentative in their interactions, and may be hesitant to express their opinions or needs.
Storming	In this phase, conflicts and disagreements may arise as group members begin to assert their opinions and vie for leadership or influence within the group. This can be a challenging and potentially stressful phase for the group, but can also be an opportunity for growth and learning.

Phase	Brief explanation
Norming	In this phase, the group begins to establish norms, values, and expectations for behavior within the group. Members may start to develop a sense of cohesion and camaraderie, and may begin to work together more effectively toward the group's goals.
Performing	In this phase, the group is working effectively toward its goals and members are collaborating well. Members are comfortable with each other, and the group is able to make progress toward its objectives.
Adjourning	In this final phase, the group is coming to an end, and members may be experiencing feelings of sadness or loss. The group may reflect on its accomplishments and take time to celebrate its successes before moving on.

42. Reminiscence therapy is a therapeutic approach that harnesses the power of past memories to enhance mental health and overall quality of life, particularly among older individuals. This form of therapy can be conducted individually or in group settings and typically involves activities such as reviewing old photographs, listening to nostalgic music, or sharing personal memories. Reminiscence therapy has been shown to have several positive effects, including boosting self-esteem, improving mood, reducing feelings of loneliness, and imparting a sense of purpose and meaning to life. By reflecting on past achievements and challenges, individuals can gain insights into their present issues and develop a more positive outlook for the future. This therapeutic approach has proven effective in addressing conditions such as depression, anxiety, and dementia, and it also plays a valuable role in preventing social isolation among the elderly by fostering social connections and participation.
43. Support groups are groups of people who share their thoughts, feelings, and experiences with others facing similar issues. They offer a secure space to share feelings, receive support, and learn from others with similar experiences. Support groups can address mental health, addiction rehabilitation, chronic illness, grieving and loss, parenting, and other topics. They can be peer-driven or led by a qualified facilitator in person or online. Participating in a support group can reduce isolation and loneliness, improve coping skills, boost self-esteem and self-awareness, and offer practical advice from people who have faced similar issues. Support groups can inspire and motivate persons suffering with challenging challenges and provide a sense of community. Examples include Alcoholics Anonymous, Parents without Partners, Grief Support Groups, NAMI Support Groups, Cancer or other chronic illness groups (for caregivers as well), LGBTQI groups at local centers.
44. Family therapy improves family functioning rather than individual members. Family therapy seeks to detect and correct dysfunctional family communication, behavior, and interaction and foster healthy, supportive connections. Family therapy is based on the idea that family dynamics and relationships affect mental health and behavior and that resolving family issues can enhance mental health. Family therapy provides a safe space for family members to discuss their issues and solve them.

45. Circular causality states that familial events reinforce one another. Thus, family members impact and are influenced by each other. This dynamic might create a "feedback loop" of family issues and behaviors.
46. Family homeostasis is the tendency of families to retain stability or equilibrium despite disturbance. Thus, families may reject system change even if it benefits them. Family homeostasis can lead to undesirable behavior to maintain the status quo.
47. Family adaptability means its ability to handle changes and challenges. Flexible families can adapt to new events and challenges while remaining stable and healthy.
48.

	Functional family	Dysfunctional family
Characteristics	Positive, respectful, and supportive interactions among members. Clear roles and expectations, mutual respect, and a sense of shared values and purpose.	Tense, negative, and conflictual interactions among members. Unclear roles and expectations, lack of respect, and a sense of disconnection and mistrust.
Communication styles	Open and honest communication, active listening, and respectful expression of feelings and needs.	Poor communication, including blaming, defensiveness, stonewalling, and invalidation of feelings and needs.
Use of boundaries	Clear and flexible boundaries that respect individual needs while also maintaining a sense of connectedness and belonging.	Rigid or diffuse boundaries that either restrict or lack respect for individual needs, leading to a lack of intimacy and trust.
Traits	Empathy, cooperation, respect, and trust.	Hostility, defensiveness, lack of empathy, and mistrust.
Resolution of problems	Collaborative problem-solving that respects individual needs and seeks to find win-win solutions.	Blame, defensiveness, and avoidance of problems, leading to ongoing conflicts and resentment.
Coping strategies	Healthy and adaptive coping strategies, such as seeking support, problem-solving, and self-care.	Dysfunctional and maladaptive coping strategies, such as substance abuse, avoidance, or aggression.
Family dynamics	A sense of balance and equity in decision-making, with each member contributing their strengths and respecting others' contributions.	Imbalanced dynamics, such as scapegoating, triangulation, or enmeshment, with certain members dominating or manipulating others.
Family values	Clear and shared values that guide decision-making and behavior.	Conflicting or unclear values, with members having different priorities or goals.
Emotional climate	Positive and nurturing emotional climate that supports each member's growth and development.	Negative and critical emotional climate that undermines each member's sense of self-worth and potential.

49. 1/A, 2/D, 3/E, 4/B, 5/C.

50. Murray Bowen's family systems therapy treats the family as a complex system of interconnected pieces. Bowen felt that family dynamics substantially influence individual behavior and that systemic solutions are ideal for family issues. Bowen's family therapy involves recognizing and resolving family emotional and relational patterns. He felt that complex family relationships might affect behavior and mental health. Treatment goals are to raise family awareness of each member's role and self-differentiation (the level to which one's sense of self-worth is not dependent on other connections, situations, or events).
51. Differentiation.
52. Triangulation.
53. Salvador Minuchin established structural family therapy to address family dynamics and relationships systemically and structurally. To promote healthy family functioning, this approach considers the family as a linked system with different roles, rules, and boundaries and stresses understanding and treating these structural features. Minuchin's family therapy is founded on the idea that power imbalances, unclear boundaries, and poor communication generate family issues. Structural family therapy reorganizes family roles and boundaries, improves communication and problem-solving, and balances power relations.
54. Enmeshment.
55. Disengagement.
56. In the table below, provide a brief explanation and example for each type of boundary.

Type of boundary	Explanation	Example
Rigid	Overly restrictive boundaries hinder family communication and connection. A strict family may have established duties and expectations with limited possibility for negotiation or flexibility. A diffuse barrier is too permeable and allows dysfunctional familial codependency. In a diffusely defined family, family members may lack healthy autonomy and independence.	A family with rigid boundaries may have a parent who is very controlling and domineering, and who does not allow children to express their own opinions or make their own decisions.
Diffuse	A diffuse boundary is too permeable and allows dysfunctional familial codependency. In a diffusely defined family, family members may lack healthy autonomy and independence.	A family with diffuse boundaries may have a parent who is overly involved in the lives of their children, and who has difficulty separating their own emotions and needs from those of their children.
Clearly defined	A clear border is flexible and facilitates healthy family communication and engagement while respecting individual individuality and independence. In a family with clear boundaries, duties and expectations may be negotiated and altered, and closeness and distance can be balanced.	A family with clearly defined boundaries may have parents who provide guidance and support to their children, while also allowing them to make their own decisions and express their own opinions.

57.

- Joining: developing a rapport with each family member.
- Boundary Setting: clarifying roles and expectations within the family system.
- Enactments: recreating problematic family interactions in order to identify and address dysfunctional patterns.
- Structural Mapping (genogram): creating a visual representation of the family system.
- Reframing: shifting the family's perspective on a problem or issue.
- Restructuring: changing the way that family members interact and communicate.
- Unbalancing: temporarily disrupting the family's power dynamics.
- Externalizing: separating the individual from the problem or issue to promote a sense of agency and control.

58. Virginia Satir's humanistic and systemic family therapy emphasizes emotional and experiential relationships. Satir thought that people require connection and healthy relationships and that relationship issues might cause mental health issues. Experiential therapy helps family members explore their emotions and build more honest and healthy connections in a safe and supportive atmosphere. The therapist may utilize role-playing, guided imagery, and other experiential exercises to assist family members understand and express their emotions. Being real, liberated, validated, and savoring the moment are priorities.
59. "Self-esteem iceberg".
60. Strategic therapy, established by Jay Haley, is a brief, solution-focused family therapy that uses particular techniques and treatments to solve family issues. The problem is seen as an opportunity to alter the family's interactions and connections through targeted and planned interventions. The therapist exercises control and uses particular methods to break bad habits and promote transformation.
61. Reframing.
62. Solution-focused therapy (SFT) is brief, goal-oriented therapy that focuses on solutions rather than problems. SFT, developed by Steve de Shazer, Insoo Kim Berg, and others, holds that individuals and families can solve their own problems and that the therapist's responsibility is to help them.
63. The PMHNP asks the customer to visualize their problem solved overnight in the "miracle question." This question helps the customer focus on solutions rather than the problem and identify goals and solutions.
64. Example answer: "If a miracle were to happen tonight while you were asleep, and tomorrow morning you awoke to find that the problem no longer existed, what would be different?" "How would you know the miracle took place?" "How would others know?"
65. Exception-finding question.
66. Scaling.
67. 1/C, 2/A, 3/D, 4/B.

68.

	Complementary	Alternative
Definition	Complementary therapies supplement conventional medicine. They are supposed to improve standard treatment, manage adverse effects, and increase patient well-being.	Alternative medicine uses non-conventional methods to treat or cure a health condition. Unlike conventional medicine, these therapies use different theories and principles.
Examples	Acupuncture, massage therapy, yoga, meditation, guided imagery, aromatherapy, herbal supplements, and nutritional counseling.	Homeopathy, naturopathy, traditional Chinese medicine, Ayurveda, energy therapies (e.g., Reiki), and chiropractic.
Purpose	Complementary therapies promote healing, reduce stress, and increase quality of life. They may assist patients manage sickness or treatment symptoms, side effects, and stress.	Alternative therapies try to prevent, treat, or cure certain health disorders by addressing the cause rather than just managing symptoms.
Evidence base	Complementary therapy evidence varies widely. Acupuncture for pain and meditation for stress reduction have strong evidence bases, whereas others have mixed or inadequate data.	Alternative remedies often have less, mixed, or contentious evidence than traditional medicine. Some alternative medicines have conflicting or equivocal scientific evidence of their efficacy.

69.

Intervention	Category	Description
Acupressure	MP	Involves applying pressure to specific points on the body to relieve pain or promote healing; based on traditional Chinese medicine principles.
Acupuncture	MP	Involves inserting thin needles into specific points on the body; can help with pain relief and various health conditions.
Aromatherapy	B	Use of essential oils for their therapeutic properties; can help with stress reduction, mood enhancement, and symptom relief.
Biofeedback	MB	Technique that uses monitoring devices to provide feedback on physiological processes; helps individuals gain control over bodily functions.
Fish oil	B	Rich in omega-3 fatty acids, which have anti-inflammatory properties; can support heart health and cognitive function.
Guided imagery	MB	Uses mental visualization to promote relaxation and healing; can help reduce anxiety, stress, and pain.
Herbs	B	Plant-derived substances used for their medicinal properties; can interact with medications and have varying levels of evidence for effectiveness.
Kava	B	Herbal supplement derived from the kava plant, used for its sedative and anxiolytic effects; can interact with medications and has potential liver toxicity concerns.
L-theanine	B	Amino acid found in tea leaves, known for its relaxing and stress-reducing effects; can be used as a supplement to promote relaxation without drowsiness.

Intervention	Category	Description
Massage	MP	Manipulation of soft body tissues to relieve tension, reduce pain, and promote relaxation; can improve circulation and support the immune system.
Meditation	MB	A variety of practices aimed at focusing the mind and promoting relaxation; associated with reduced stress and improved mental health.
Melatonin	B	Hormone that regulates sleep-wake cycles; used as a supplement to improve sleep quality and treat sleep disorders.
Nutraceuticals	B	Products derived from food sources with potential health benefits; may include probiotics, antioxidants, and other functional food components.
Reflexology	MP	Application of pressure to specific points on the feet, hands, or ears; believed to correspond to organs and systems in the body, promoting healing and balance.
Sam-e	B	Naturally occurring compound involved in various biochemical processes; used as a supplement to support mood, joint health, and liver function.
Tryptophan	B	Amino acid that is a precursor to serotonin, a neurotransmitter involved in mood regulation; can be used as a supplement to improve mood and sleep quality.
Vitamins	B	Essential nutrients that support various bodily functions; can be used to address deficiencies or support overall health.
Yoga	MB	A practice that combines physical postures, breathing exercises, and meditation; can improve flexibility, strength, and mental well-being.

References and Resources

American Psychiatric Association, editor. Diagnostic and statistical manual of mental disorders: DSM-5-TR. 5th ed., text revision. American Psychiatric Association Publishing; 2022.

Beutler LE, Someah K, Kimpara S, Miller K. Selecting the most appropriate treatment for each patient. Int J Clin Health Psychol. 2016;16(1):99–108. https://doi.org/10.1016/j.ijchp.2015.08.001.

Bohart AC, Tallman K. How clients make therapy work: the process of active self-healing. American Psychological Association; 1999.

Cuijpers P, Donker T, van Straten A, Li J, Andersson G. Is guided self-help as effective as face-to-face psychotherapy for depression and anxiety disorders? A systematic review and meta-analysis of comparative outcome studies. Psychol Med. 2013;43(5):423–35. https://doi.org/10.1017/S0033291710000772.

Egan G. The skilled helper: a problem-management and opportunity-development approach to helping. 10th ed. Brooks/Cole; 2014.

Jacobson NS, Martell CR, Dimidjian S. Behavioral activation treatment for depression: Returning to contextual roots. Clin Psychol Sci Pract. 2001;8(4):255–70. https://doi.org/10.1093/clipsy.8.3.255.

Johnson K, Vanderhoef D, Magrath N. Psychiatric-mental health nurse practitioner review and resource manual. American Nurses Credentialing Center, American Nurses Association; 2020.

Linehan MM. Cognitive-behavioral treatment of borderline personality disorder. Guilford Press; 1993.

May JM, Richardi TM, Barth KS. Dialectical behavior therapy as treatment for borderline personality disorder. Mental Health Clin. 2016;6(2):62–7. https://doi.org/10.9740/mhc.2016.03.62.

Segal ZV, Williams JMG, Teasdale JD. Mindfulness-based cognitive therapy for depression: a new approach to preventing relapse. New York: Guilford Press; 2002.

Zakhari R. The psychiatric-mental health nurse practitioner certification review manual. Springer Publishing Company; 2021.

Notes:

Notes:

Culturally Competent Care

18

Test your learning and check your understanding of this book's contents: use the "Springer Nature Flashcards" app to access questions using ▶ https://sn.pub/62J0Ar.

To use the app, please follow the instructions in Chap. 1.

Culturally competent care entails being aware of and sensitive to cultural differences, as well as adapting behaviors and approaches accordingly. Cultural competency is especially important for psychiatric-mental health nurse practitioners (PMHNPs) because cultural beliefs and values can heavily influence how patients perceive and express mental health symptoms. Some cultures, for example, may regard mental illness as a sign of weakness or as deserving of shame, whereas others may regard it as a spiritual issue or attribute it to supernatural causes (Paniagua 2014).

Cultural competency can lead to improved patient outcomes in mental health care (Sue and Sue 2012), including improved patient satisfaction and treatment outcomes, especially for ethnic minority patients. Cultural competency, according to Giger et al. (2008), also can improve patient trust and the therapeutic relationship, resulting in better mental health outcomes. Cultural competency is also essential for reducing health disparities. Minority populations are frequently underserved in mental health care, and cultural competency can improve access to care and reduce treatment barriers (Giger et al. 2008).

Cultural competency is an ongoing process, and PMHNPs should continue their education and training to better understand different cultural beliefs, practices, and values. Learning about different cultural groups and their specific healthcare needs, as well as understanding the impact of racism and discrimination on mental health, is part of this education. PMHNPs should also be willing to learn from their patients and adjust their treatment strategies as needed.

T. Stewart, *Psychiatric-Mental Health Nurse Practitioner Program Companion and Board Certification Exam Review Workbook*,
https://doi.org/10.1007/978-3-031-60894-0_18

This chapter provides an overview of the fundamental concepts of culturally competent care. Special populations and how mental illness manifests differently depending on culture are covered (e.g., evil eye, ataque de nervios).

18.1 Practice Activities

1. Define culture.

2. What are race and ethnicity? How do they compare and contrast?

3. What is the cultural formulation interview (CFI) available in the DSM? Name the four domains of assessment in the CFI.

4. Individuals only belong to one cultural group at a time, so the practitioner can focus on those behaviors and beliefs.

   TRUE FALSE

5. List at least five different examples of cultural groups to which an individual may belong.
   1.
   2.
   3.
   4.
   5.

6. Approximately ______% of adults in the United States have low health literacy.

7. ________ in 10 adults struggle to communicate in English, and nearly __________ of U.S. hospitals often fail to offer interpreters.

8. Mental health providers, like psychiatrists and nurse practitioners, are overwhelmingly White at __________%. This complicates what we know from research that patients prefer and do better when cared for by someone who looks like them, or shares cultural elements.

9. The first step in providing culturally competent care is for the PMHNP to learn everything they can about their client's culture.
   TRUE FALSE

10. Why is being cognizant about a patient's culture central to providing correct care, particularly in mental health?

11. Match each term with the best definition.

_____1. Cultural competence	A. Continuum of attitudes, behaviors, and policies supporting cross-cultural environments and interactions; includes PMHNP's awareness of their biases and those of their patient
_____2. Cultural syndromes	B. Efforts to include a patient's culture in their care, acknowledging the power and positivity that their beliefs and attitudes may have long-term; development of skills to work with diverse clientele
_____3. Cultural proficiency	C. A pattern of mental illness and abnormal behavior that is unique to a specific ethnic or cultural population and does not conform to standard classifications of psychiatric disorders; is not seen as an illness within the native culture
_____4. Cultural explanation or perceived cause	D. Cultural way of talking about suffering within a group that is not necessarily connected to symptoms or disorders; can be everyday language
_____5. Cultural idiom of distress	E. Cultural-based etiology for symptoms or illness

12. For each culture-bound syndrome, or cultural conceptualizations of distress, provide a brief description. While this list is not exhaustive, it is representative of the most often tested culture-bound syndromes listed in the DSM-5 and International Statistical Classification of Diseases and Related Health Problems (ICD).

Name	Description	Geographic/ethnic group
1. Ataque de nervios		
2. Khyâl cap (wind) attacks		
3. Dhat syndrome		
4. Ghost sickness		
5. Shenjing shuairuo		
6. Susto (fright)		
7. Taijin kyofusho		
8. Amok		
9. Koro		
10. Kufungisisa		
11. Maladi moun		

13. ______________________________ is a belief that intense looks/stares by others can cause sickness (e.g., diarrhea) by transferring negative energy to the recipient. To counter the evil eye, a practitioner may tie a red bracelet or ribbon around the child's wrist, dote on how handsome/beautiful the child is, among others.

14. There is usually a one-to-one correspondence between cultural concepts and DSM diagnoses.
    TRUE FALSE

15. ______________________________ patients are more frequently hospitalized involuntarily, placed in seclusion, diagnosed with schizophrenia and substance abuse than White patients.

16. Check which of the following are best practices when working with interpreters.
    _____Gender, age, religion, and other demographics of the interpreter are not important.
    _____Use family members if possible.
    _____Meet with interpreter to review procedures.
    _____The interpreter can take liberty with translation; however, they think the PMHNP will best understand.
    _____Short, simple sentences are best.
    _____The interpreter may ask a question in different ways, translating as literally as possible.
    _____The PMHNP should sit behind the interpreter, directing the questions in their ear.
    _____Direct eye contact with the client is key, unless culturally inappropriate.
    _____It takes the same amount of time to meet with a patient when working with an interpreter.

17. The ______________________________ consists of 17 questions to help the PMHNP to assess and understand a client's mental health issues framed within the client's culture. It covers identity, conceptualizations of distress, stressors, vulnerability, and resilience, and clinical relationship expectations. It is included in the DSM.

18. ______________________________identity is how the individual sees themself, while ______________________________ identity is formed according to what society values and how it perceives the individual's behaviors. The latter can be stressful for individuals adjusting to another culture.

19. If a practitioner over-identifies with a client's culture and loses objectivity, they may be experiencing ______________________________________.

20. Refugees emigrate against their will due to displacement by war, famine, and natural catastrophes. Two psychiatric illnesses to which this group is particularly susceptible are ______________________________________ and ______________________________________.

18.2 Answers and Explanations to Chapter Activities

1. Culture refers to the shared beliefs, values, customs, traditions, behaviors, symbols, and practices that characterize a particular group of people, community, or society. It encompasses the way individuals within a group perceive the world, interact with each other, and interpret their experiences. Culture can include elements such as language, religion, art, cuisine, social norms, and rituals, and it often plays a significant role in shaping people's identities, worldviews, and social interactions. Culture can be passed down through generations and can vary widely between different regions, ethnicities, and communities around the world.
2. Race typically refers to physical characteristics such as skin color, hair type, and facial features, while ethnicity is more related to cultural factors like language, ancestry, nationality, and shared traditions. It is important to note that both race and ethnicity are social constructs, meaning they are categories created by society rather than being based on scientific or biological criteria. These classifications can vary across different societies and time periods and have been used, at times, to justify discrimination or oppressive practices. In modern discussions, ethnicity often focuses on cultural diversity and heritage.
3. The cultural formulation interview (CFI) is an assessment tool found in the DSM-5, designed to assist clinicians in understanding cultural factors relevant to a person's mental health. It comprises four key domains of assessment: (1) Cultural Definition of the Problem, which explores how individuals perceive and define their mental health issues within their cultural context; (2) Cultural Perceptions of Cause, Context, and Support, which delves into beliefs about the origins of their issues, cultural context, and support systems; (3) Cultural Factors Affecting Self-Coping and Past Help Seeking, focusing on cultural coping strategies and past experiences with help-seeking; and (4) Cultural Factors Affecting Current Care, examining how cultural factors may impact an individual's current engagement with mental health services and treatment preferences. The CFI helps clinicians provide culturally sensitive and effective care by considering these domains during psychiatric evaluations.
4. FALSE. Individuals can belong to multiple cultural groups simultaneously, as people often have intersecting identities related to race, ethnicity, nationality, religion, gender, sexual orientation, and more. Recognizing these intersecting identities is essential for a comprehensive understanding of an individual's cultural background and its influence on their beliefs and behaviors. Therefore, a practitioner should consider the various cultural groups to which an individual may belong to provide more nuanced and culturally competent care.
5. SES, age, religion, sexual orientation, race, gender, ethnicity, ability, mental illness/medical diagnosis, country, occupation, ceremonies, customs, death concept.
6. About 35% of U.S. adults lack health literacy, or the ability to understand and use health information and services to make appropriate health decisions. Medical misunderstanding, difficulty following recommendations, and poor health outcomes can result from a lack of health literacy.

7. The U.S. Census Bureau reports 10% of adults speak English "less than very well." Thus, in complex or new circumstances, English may be difficult to communicate. Nearly one-third of U.S. hospitals do not supply non-English translators. Poor English may hamper communication and access. Interpretation services assist patients understand and participate in healthcare decisions, enhancing treatment quality.
8. 65%; lack of diversity in mental health may make patients prefer or feel more comfortable with a culturally similar practitioner. Patients who share cultural qualities with their caregivers may feel understood and have better outcomes, research says. The mental health business needs more diverse doctors to serve diverse patients.
9. FALSE. Assuming a provider can learn everything about a client's culture and making assumptions about their ideas, attitudes, and behaviors can lead to cultural misunderstandings. The provider must first admit their own cultural biases and be open to learning about and embracing their customers' cultures to deliver culturally competent care. Open-ended questions, active listening, and openness to seek help may be needed. Each person is unique and may have different cultural ideas and experiences; thus, the provider must recognize this.
10. Understanding a patient's culture is essential to providing mental health care since it affects beliefs, attitudes, and actions. Culture influences mental health symptoms and therapy. Some cultures treat mental health help differently and disagree on its causes. Cultural differences might also affect symptom expression and treatment preferences. Mental health professionals can provide culturally appropriate care by respecting patients' needs and choices. Quality of care and patient outcomes can improve.
11. 1/A, 2/C, 3/B, 4/E, 5/D.
12.

Name	Description	Geographic/ethnic group
Ataque de nervios	Shaking, screaming, crying Loss of family bond or trauma In front of others	Latin America
Khyâl cap (wind) attacks	Panic attacks and psychosis, somatic complaints like tinnitus and neck myalgias	Cambodia
Dhat syndrome	Belief that passing "vital fluid" semen in urine Sluggishness, low energy, and low temperament, impotence	India, Southeast Asia
Ghost sickness	Malaise, anorexia, loss of breath, nightmares Attributed to ghosts or magic	Native American, Polynesian
Shenjing shuairuo	Nerve weakness, stress related	China
Susto (fright)	Somatic suffering and depression Witness of trauma causes soul to leave the body	Latin America, Latinos in USA
Taijin kyofusho	Social anxiety Fear of displeasing others through interpersonal interactions, body odor	Japan
Amok	Dissociation behavior Sudden assault against people or objects	Southeast Asia, Austronesians

Name	Description	Geographic/ethnic group
Koro	Fear of penis retracting into body Genital retraction syndrome Panic attacks	Asia
Kufungisisa	Over thinking, anxiety, dizziness, headache, brain fatigue/fog	Zimbabwe
Maladi moun	Sickness caused by jealousy, lose recent successes	Haiti

13. The belief described is known as "mal de ojo" or "the evil eye." This belief suggests that intense or envious stares from others can bring harm or sickness to the person being stared at. To counteract the effects of the evil eye, various protective practices may be employed, such as tying a red bracelet or ribbon around the child's wrist or offering compliments about their appearance to ward off negative energy.
14. FALSE. DSM diagnosis and culture do not always have a direct correspondence. US and international mental health experts diagnose with the DSM. Heredity, brain chemistry, and neurotransmitter imbalances are linked to mental disease in this scientific paradigm. However, different cultures may describe mental health concerns differently than DSM. Other cultures may view DSM mental illnesses as normal or useful. Cultural values and attitudes can also affect mental health understanding and expression, which can affect diagnosis.
15. African-American patients are more likely than White patients to be hospitalized, secluded, and diagnosed with schizophrenia and substance abuse. Racial bias in mental health is well-known. Mental health providers' unconscious prejudices, access to care disparities, and healthcare system structural imbalances may cause this bias. Although they have identical symptoms as White patients, African-Americans are more likely to be diagnosed with schizophrenia and given antipsychotics. Even if harmless, individuals are more likely to be hospitalized and sequestered without consent. Disparities can impair patients' mental health.
16.

    __x___Meet with interpreter to review procedures.

    __x___Short, simple sentences are best.

    __x___The interpreter may ask a question in different ways, translating as literally as possible.

    __x___Direct eye contact with the client is key, unless culturally inappropriate.
17. Cultural formulation interview (CFI).
18. A person's personal identity is how they see themselves, while ascribed/assigned identity is based on society's ideals and deeds. Personal experiences, values, beliefs, and objectives impact self-perception and self-concept. Personal identity influences behavior and decision-making. Society assigns identities

based on race, ethnicity, gender, age, and socioeconomic class. People are often coerced into these identities, which affects how others view them. Adapting to a new culture can be hard if their identity is unknown. Marginalization can harm mental health. Personal identities must be expressed independently of identity.

19. Countertransference. Over-identifying with a client's culture compromises objectivity. These emotions affect therapist-patient contact and treatment. If a practitioner becomes too associated with a client's culture and accepts dysfunction or poor behavior as standards, countertransference can be extremely harmful.
20. Major depression, PTSD. War, starvation, and natural disasters drive refugees from their homes. They typically emigrate without wanting to, enduring hardships and stress. Refugees risk PTSD and serious depression. Major depression causes sadness, hopelessness, and dullness. It can impair function and necessitate treatment. PTSD can develop from combat, torture, or natural disasters. Flashbacks, nightmares, and avoiding trauma triggers are symptoms. Mental health can suffer, requiring medication and therapy.

References and Resources

Aggarwal NK, Cedeño K, Guarnaccia P, Kleinman A, Lewis-Fernández R. The meanings of cultural competence in mental health: an exploratory focus group study with patients, clinicians, and administrators. Springerplus. 2016;5:384. https://doi.org/10.1186/s40064-016-2037-4.

American Psychiatric Association, editor. Diagnostic and statistical manual of mental disorders: DSM-5-TR. 5th ed., text revision. American Psychiatric Association Publishing; 2022.

Bhui K, Warfa N, Edonya P, McKenzie K, Bhugra D. Cultural competence in mental health care: a review of model evaluations. BMC Health Serv Res. 2007;7:15. https://doi.org/10.1186/1472-6963-7-15.

Boyer CJ, Rice MJ, Sorrell TR, Spurling AM. Advancing racial/ethnic and cultural sensitivity among PMHNP students through education, practice, and experience. J Am Psychiatr Nurses Assoc. 2019;25(6):487–95. https://doi.org/10.1177/1078390318824651.

Dixon LB, Lewis-Fernández R, Isom J, Bellamy C, Gaba A, Rossom RC, Adams L, Legha RK, Carlo AD, Sokol Y, Norquist GS, Roy M, Jackson D. Reporting on and reviewing for race/racialization, ethnicity, and culture. Psychiatric Serv (Washington, DC). 2022;73(5):482–3. https://doi.org/10.1176/appi.ps.20220099.

Giger JN, Davidhizar R, Purnell LD. Transcultural nursing: assessment and intervention. 6th ed. Mosby Elsevier; 2008.

Hernandez M, Nesman TM, Mowery D, Acevedo-Polakovich I, Callejas LM. Cultural competence: a literature review and conceptual model for mental health services. Psychiatric Serv (Washington, DC). 2009;60(8):1046–50. https://doi.org/10.1176/appi.ps.60.8.1046.

Johnson K, Vanderhoef D, Magrath N. Psychiatric-mental health nurse practitioner review and resource manual. American Nurses Credentialing Center, American Nurses Association; 2020.

Kirmayer LJ. Rethinking cultural competence. Transcult Psychiatry. 2012;49(2):149–64. https://doi.org/10.1177/1363461512444673.

Mollah TN, Antoniades J, Lafeer FI, Brijnath B. How do mental health practitioners operationalise cultural competency in everyday practice? A qualitative analysis. BMC Health Serv Res. 2018;18(1):480. https://doi.org/10.1186/s12913-018-3296-2.
Moran M. Impact of culture, race, social determinants reflected throughout new DSM-5-TR. Psychiatr News. 2022;57(3) https://doi.org/10.1176/appi.pn.2022.03.3.20.
O'Connor K. Culture as treatment: some indigenous people wary of evidence-based treatment. Psychiatr News. 2022;57(8) https://doi.org/10.1176/appi.pn.2022.08.8.17.
Paniagua, FA. Assessing and treating culturally diverse clients: A practical guide (4th ed.). Sage Publications, Inc.; 2014. https://doi.org/10.4135/9781506335728.
Pope-Davis DB, Coleman HLK, Liu W, Toporek RL, (Eds.). Handbook of multicultural competencies in counseling & psychology. SAGE Publications Inc.; 2003. https://doi.org/10.4135/9781452231693.
Rathod S, Gega L, Degnan A, Pikard J, Khan T, Husain N, Munshi T, Naeem F. The current status of culturally adapted mental health interventions: a practice-focused review of meta-analyses. Neuropsychiatr Dis Treat. 2018;14:165–78. https://doi.org/10.2147/NDT.S138430.
Rice AN, Harris SC. Issues of cultural competence in mental health care. J Am Pharm Assoc. 2021;61(1):e65–8. https://doi.org/10.1016/j.japh.2020.10.015.
Sharan P, Hans G. Cultural issues related to ICD-11 mental, behavioural and neurodevelopmental disorders. Consortium Psychiatricum. 2021;2(2):7–15. https://doi.org/10.17816/CP67.
Sue DW, Sue D. Counseling the culturally diverse: Theory and practice (6th ed.). John Wiley & Sons, Inc.; 2012.
Trinh N-H, Jahan AB, Chen JA. Moving from cultural competence to cultural humility in psychiatric education. Psychiatr Clin North Am. 2021;44(2):149–57. https://doi.org/10.1016/j.psc.2020.12.002.
World Health Organization. International Classification of Diseases (ICD-10). 11th ed. World Health Organization; 2022.
Zakhari R. The psychiatric-mental health nurse practitioner certification review manual. Springer Publishing Company; 2021.

Notes:

Notes:

Public Health, Biostatistics, and Research Foundations

19

Test your learning and check your understanding of this book's contents: use the "Springer Nature Flashcards" app to access questions using ▶ https://sn.pub/62J0Ar.

To use the app, please follow the instructions in Chap. 1.

Psychiatric-mental health nurse practitioners (PMHNPs) play a vital role in addressing the mental health needs of their patients and the larger community. In order to effectively do so, PMHNPs must have a strong understanding of public health concepts, such as social determinants of health and health equity (American Nurses Association 2023). Mental health is closely connected to overall health and well-being (World Health Organization 2014). For example, depression has been linked to an increased risk of heart disease (National Institute of Mental Health 2021), and chronic stress has been linked to digestive issues, high blood pressure, and weakened immune system function (Mayo Clinic 2021).

Further, PMHNPs often work with vulnerable or underserved populations, who may be at higher risk for mental health problems (American Nurses Association 2023). Individuals living in poverty may experience mental health problems due to the stress and strain of financial insecurity, lack of access to quality health care, and other social and economic challenges. PMHNPs may use health promotion strategies such as education, advocacy, and community outreach to promote mental health awareness and to identify and address factors that may be impacting the mental health of their patients and the larger community.

T. Stewart, *Psychiatric-Mental Health Nurse Practitioner Program Companion and Board Certification Exam Review Workbook*,
https://doi.org/10.1007/978-3-031-60894-0_19

Finally, PMHNPs need to have a solid understanding of public health concepts in order to effectively advocate for the mental health needs of their patients and the broader community (American Nurses Association 2023). This may involve working with community organizations, policymakers, and other stakeholders to promote mental health awareness and access to care. PMHNPs may work with local schools to provide mental health education and resources, or advocate for policy changes that increase access to mental health care for underserved populations.

Psychiatric-mental health nurse practitioners (PMHNPs) similarly need a working knowledge of biostatistics, the branch of statistics that deals with the collection, analysis, and interpretation of data related to health and biology (Centers for Disease Control and Prevention 2023). PMHNPs rely on research to make evidence-based decisions about the care of their patients, or to identify risk factors for certain mental health conditions. In order to accurately interpret and apply research findings, PMHNPs need to be able to understand and evaluate statistical concepts such as sample size, statistical significance, and confounding variables.

In addition to using research evidence to inform their practice, PMHNPs may also be involved in conducting research or collaborating with researchers on studies. In these cases, a strong understanding of biostatistics is essential for designing and analyzing research studies and interpreting the results. Furthermore, PMHNPs often work with large data sets, such as electronic health records, to track and monitor the health of their patients and the larger population. PMHNPs may use biostatistical methods to analyze electronic health record data to identify trends in the prevalence of certain mental health conditions, or to evaluate the effectiveness of a particular treatment approach.

PMHNPs need to be knowledgeable consumers of research studies in order to evaluate the quality and relevance of research studies and apply the findings to their practice in order to provide the best possible care to their patients. This requires a strong understanding of the various types of research studies, including experimental studies, observational studies, and systematic reviews, as well as the strengths and limitations of each type. PMHNPs may use the results of a randomized controlled trial to inform their decision about which treatment approach is most effective for a particular patient population, or they may use the findings of an observational study to identify risk factors for a certain mental health condition. PMHNPs conducting research need to use research methods such as sampling techniques, data collection and analysis methods, and statistical analyses in order to answer a specific research question.

Lastly, PMHNPs may be called upon to contribute to policy or practice guidelines, or to advocate for evidence-based approaches to mental health care. In these roles, a strong understanding of research studies is essential for identifying and synthesizing the best available evidence and for making informed, evidence-based recommendations. PMHNPs may be asked to review the literature on a particular topic and provide recommendations for best practices based on the evidence.

A strong foundation in public health, biostatistics, and research allows nurse practitioners to make informed decisions about treatment, advocate for the health of their communities, and stay up to date on the latest evidence-based practices in nursing. Additionally, being proficient in these areas can also enhance your credibility and leadership skills within the nursing profession. In this chapter, we will explore the various ways in which public health, biostatistics, and research can impact the work of a nurse practitioner and how to apply these concepts in practice.

19.1 Public Health

1. Match each phase of the FDA clinical trial with its description.

________Phase 1	A. Adverse effects and efficacy data collected in a larger sample across years. Prevalence and incidence rates calculated
________Phase 2	B. Safety and adverse effects of drug tested in healthy volunteers
________Phase 3	C. Efficacy dose and tolerability tested in group of individuals with target disease
________Phase 4	D. Focus on efficacy and continuous monitoring of adverse effects in larger patient sample

2. What are social determinants of health? Provide examples.

3. Label each description as primary, secondary, or tertiary prevention.

Prevention level	Objective
	Decrease the incidence (number of new cases) of mental disorders.
	Decrease the prevalence (number of existing cases) of mental disorders.
	Decrease the disability and severity of a mental disorder.

19.2 Biostatistics

4. ______________________________ is the rate at which new events occur in a population.

5. ______________________________ is the rate at which everyone in a population experiences an event.

6. How do public health practitioners calculate incidence rates?

7. How do public health practitioners calculate the prevalence rate?

8. A diagnostic test's ______________________________ refers to its probability of correctly identifying a case of the disease. A test's ________________ ________________, in contrast, is its probability of correctly identifying individuals who do not have the disease.

9. ______________________________ tells us how much more likely an individual/group is of contracting a disease compared to a comparison group.

10. Match the following biostatistics terms with the most appropriate description.

____Internal validity	A. Tests the relationship between two variables.
____External validity	B. Numerical values that enable one to reach conclusions that extend beyond the immediate data alone; generated by quantitative research designs.
____Descriptive statistics	C. The sample is representative of the population and the results can be generalized.
____Standard deviation	D. Also known as level of significance; describes the probability of a particular result occurring by chance alone (if $P = 0.01$, there is a 1% probability of obtaining a result by chance alone).
____Variance	E. Measure of dispersion of data from its mean.
____Inferential statistics	F. Likelihood of an event occurring; lies between 0 and 1; an impossible event has a probability of 0, and a certain event has a probability of 1.
____*t*-Test	G. The independent variable (the treatment) caused a change in the dependent variable (the outcome).
____Analysis of variance (ANOVA)	H. Tests the differences among three or more groups.
____Pearson's *r* correlation	I. How the values are dispersed around the mean; the larger the variance, the larger the dispersion of scores.
____Probability	J. Used to describe the basic features of the data in the study; numerical values that summarize, organize, and describe observations; can be generated by either quantitative or qualitative studies.
____*P*-value	K. Assesses whether the means of two groups are statistically different from each other.

11. A test that is able to measure a variable consistently has high ______________________________. If this test's measures capture the true value of what it is intending to measure, then it also has high ______________________.

12. On the following bullseye images, label each as valid or not valid, and reliable or unreliable (Figs. 19.1–19.4).

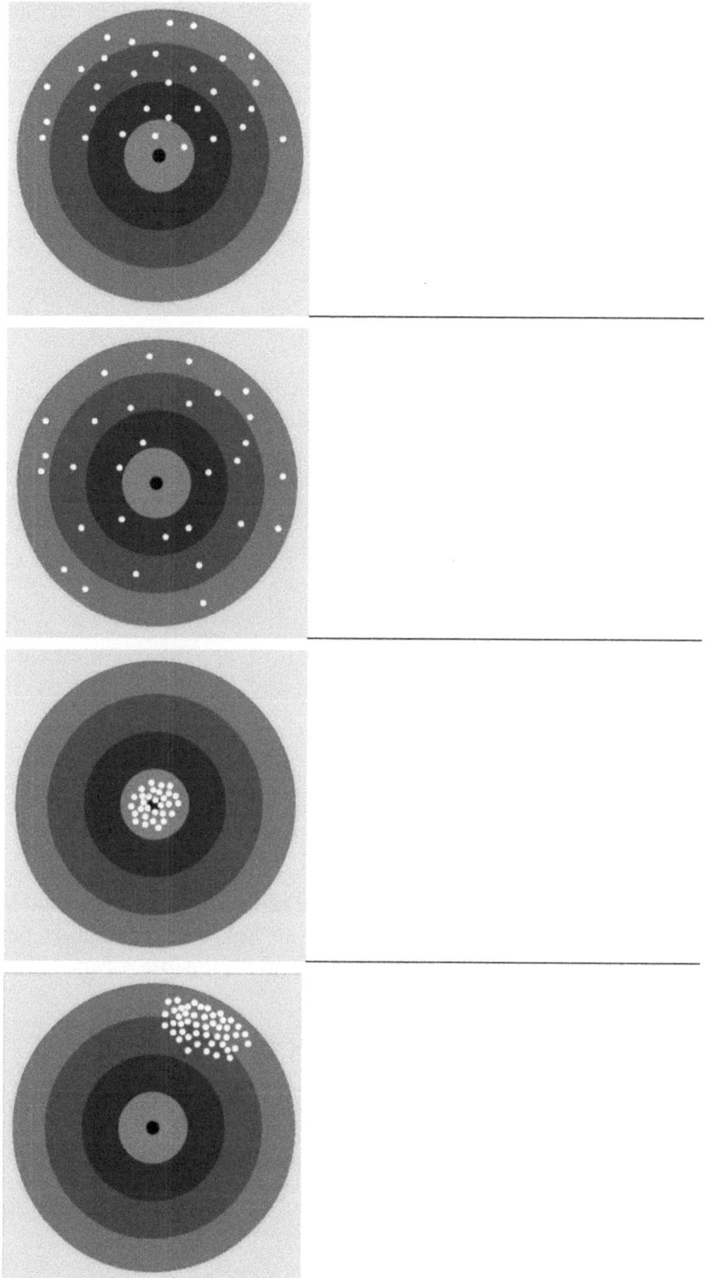

Figs. 19.1–19.4 Validity and reliability. (Published in: Lenka Benova et al. What is meant by validity in maternal and newborn health measurement? A conceptual framework for understanding indicator validation. PLoS One, May 2020, 15(5):e0233969. https://doi.org/10.1371/journal.pone.0233969. © 2020 Benova et al. under the terms of the Creative Commons Attribution License, which permits unrestricted use, distribution, and reproduction in any medium, provided the original author and source are credited)

13. A(n)________________________________measures the intensity and direction of the link between two binary (yes/no) variables in statistics. A high number indicates a high risk of disease if exposed to a risk factor. It is often used in case-control studies and other retrospective research to compare the probabilities of an outcome with and without an exposure.

14. For each example, how would you interpret the odds ratio?

Example	Occurrence	Interpretation
Smoking and lung cancer	OR = 3.0	
Vaccination and disease occurrence	OR = 0.2	
Exercise and heart disease	OR = 0.5	
High-fiber diet and colon cancer	OR = 2.5	
Seatbelt use and car accident fatalities	OR = 0.1	

15. ________________________________ are a range of values produced from statistical analysis of data used to estimate an unknown population parameter. They give us a 95% or 99% confidence interval for the true parameter. Narrower intervals suggest more precise estimations.

16. For each example, how would you interpret the confidence interval?

Example	Finding	Interpretation
Average height	Suppose a study measures the average height of a sample of 100 adult men and finds it to be 175 cm with a 95% CI of 173–177 cm.	

Example	Finding	Interpretation
Medication effectiveness	A clinical trial investigating a new drug reports that the average decrease in blood pressure is 10 mmHg, with a 95% CI of 8–12 mmHg.	
School performance	A study on a new teaching method reports an average score improvement of 5 points, with a 95% CI of 2–8 points.	

17. For the following research and epidemiology terms, match each term with the correct description. Write the correct answer letter in the space provided.

Terms	Descriptions
_____1. FALSE positive	A. The proportion of actual positives correctly identified by a test or screening method.
_____2. FALSE negative	B. The proportion of actual negatives correctly identified by a test or screening method.
_____3. TRUE positive	C. The number of new cases of a disease or condition in a population during a specific period.
_____4. TRUE negative	D. The total number of cases of a disease or condition at a particular time in a given population.
_____5. Sensitivity	E. A test result that incorrectly indicates that a particular condition or attribute is present in the subject being tested.
_____6. Specificity	F. A test result that incorrectly indicates that a particular condition or attribute is absent in the subject being tested.
_____7. Prevalence	G. A test result that correctly identifies the presence of a condition or attribute.
_____8. Incidence	H. A test result that correctly identifies the absence of a condition or attribute.

18. When researchers conclude that there is a statistically significant effect, when there is actually none, this is known as a ____________________ error, or error of commission.

19. ____________________ errors are when researchers conclude that there is no statistically significant effect on the sample, but there actually is. This error is also known as an error of omission.

20. Name three ways in which the statistical power of a study may be increased.
    1. ____________________
    2. ____________________
    3. ____________________

21. For the following data set, provide the mean, median, and mode.

Data	Mean	Median	Mode
20, 10, 40, 10, 70			

22. Confidence intervals provide an estimate of what the data value for the population may be, based on data collected from a representative sample. If the confidence intervals do not overlap, then we assume that the means are ___________________________.

19.3 Research Foundations

23. Name at least five roles of an Institutional Review Board (IRB).
    1. ___________________________
    2. ___________________________
    3. ___________________________
    4. ___________________________
    5. ___________________________

24. Label each type of observational study as either case-control, cohort, or cross-sectional.

	Retrospectively compares cases of COVID delta variant with cases of COVID omicron variant to determine causal relationships.
	Captures the prevalence of PTSD among female Veterans in June 2022.
	Follows two groups of individuals over 3 years. One group has HIV and one does not. The study compares the incidence rate of dementia among the two groups.

25. The ___________________________ group in a study is composed of individuals who do not receive an intervention.

26. Number needed to treat/harm tells us how many individuals have to be treated/harmed in order for ____ patient(s) to benefit.

27. Match each type of research bias with its definition.

Types of research bias	Definitions
_____Selection	A. Unforeseen factors affect results.
_____Measurement	B. Study sample is not representative of the target population.
_____Expectancy	C. Researchers confuse early detection with increased survival.
_____Lead-time	D. Parts of the study do not fit together to provide data on which to draw conclusions.
_____Recall	E. Study participants are not able to remember accurately.
_____Confounding	F. The researcher's beliefs affect the outcomes.
_____Design	G. Data are distorted during collection.

28. To reject the null hypothesis, the calculated P-value would typically need to be ________.

29. Rank the following types of studies from least rigorous (6) to most rigorous (1). Consider the study's structure, the control over variables, and the ability to minimize bias. When completing this ranking, think about the extent to which each type of study is able to provide clear, unbiased, and comprehensive answers to research questions. Consider the methodologies used, the scope of the study, and the degree of analysis and critique applied to the evidence.

	Case-control
	Meta-analysis
	Cohort
	Randomized controlled trial
	Case series
	Systematic review

30. The PICOT clinical question framework is a method used to formulate and direct the search for obtaining evidence in clinical research. Each letter in the acronym PICOT stands for a different aspect of the clinical question you are interested in exploring. Identify what each letter in PICOT stands for and provide an example of the type of information that may be used for each letter.

	Description	Example
P		
I		
C		
O		
T		

31. Label the following quantitative evidence types from least (1) to most rigorous (5).

__________Evidence from RCT without randomization
__________Randomized controlled trials (RCT), meta-analysis, or systematic review
__________Evidence from expert opinion or committee reports
__________Evidence-based guidelines based on systematic review
__________Evidence from systematic review of descriptive and qualitative studies

32. Label the following qualitative evidence types from least (1) to most rigorous (6).

__________Evidence from well-designed controlled trials without randomization
__________Evidence from a single descriptive or qualitative study

__________Evidence from systematic reviews of descriptive and qualitative studies
__________Evidence-based guideline based on systematic review of RCTs
__________Evidence from at least one well-designed RCT
__________Evidence from expert opinion or committee

19.4 Answers and Explanations to Chapter Activities

1.
 ____B_____Phase 1
 ____C_____Phase 2
 ____D_____Phase 3
 ____A_____Phase 4
2. Social determinants of health play a significant role in shaping individuals' well-being throughout their life stages, influencing health outcomes and disparities. These determinants encompass a range of nonmedical factors tied to global, national, and local resource allocation, which impact birth, growth, living, working, and aging. Addressing these socioeconomic factors is crucial for improving overall health and eliminating healthcare disparities. Key elements include a stable economy, access to quality education, healthcare access and quality, neighborhood and built environment, social context, access to healthy food, and reliable transportation.
3.

Prevention level	Objective
Primary prevention	Decrease the incidence (number of new cases) of mental disorders.
Secondary prevention	Decrease the prevalence (number of existing cases) of mental disorders.
Tertiary prevention	Decrease the disability and severity of a mental disorder.

4. Incidence.
5. Prevalence.
6. # of new events in period of time/# at risk of having new event in period of time.
7. # of individuals within a population with a disease at specified time/period/total population at risk at specified time/period.
8. Sensitivity; specificity,
9. Relative risk.
10.
 _G__Internal validity
 _C__External validity
 _J__Descriptive statistics
 _E__Standard deviation
 _I___Variance
 _B__Inferential statistics

_K__*t*-Test
_H__Analysis of variance (ANOVA)
_A__Pearson's *r* correlation
_F__Probability
_D__*P*-value

11. Precision (reliability); accuracy (validity).
12. See Fig. 19.5.

    A measure's reliability is its consistency and stability over time and settings. The graphic shows reliability as three overlapping "consistency" circles. This means a metric is dependable if it yields consistent results across administrations and settings. For instance, an anxiety scale should yield identical scores whether given to the same person at different periods or to others with similar anxiety levels. A measure's validity is its accuracy in judging the notion it is meant to measure. The bullseye in the center of the three circles symbolizes legitimacy. Valid measures accurately measure the concept they measure. For instance, an anxiety scale should appropriately assess anxiety, not depression.

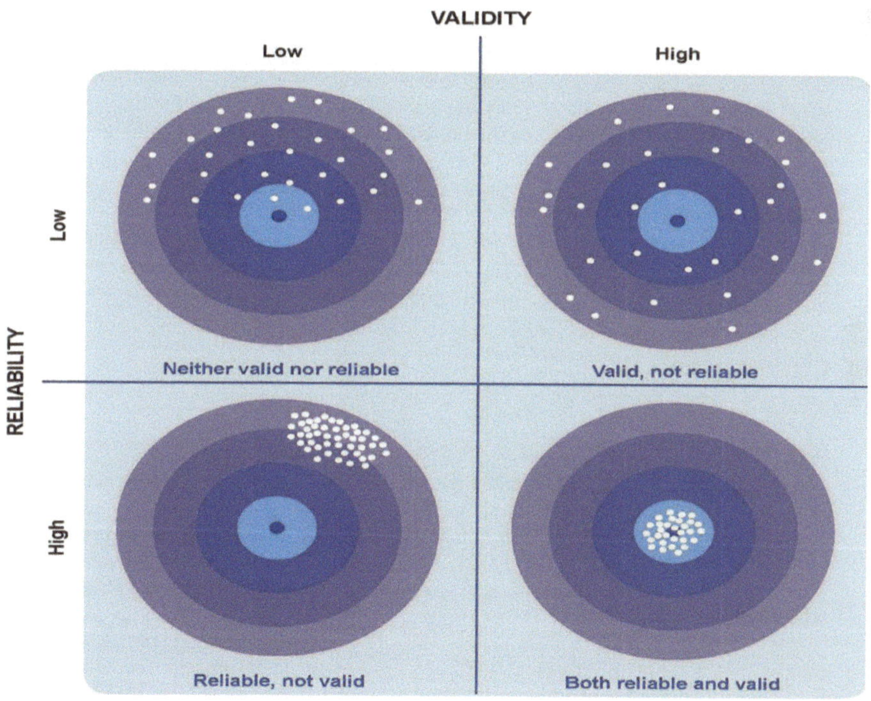

Fig. 19.5 Validity and reliability answers. (Published in: Lenka Benova et al. What is meant by validity in maternal and newborn health measurement? A conceptual framework for understanding indicator validation. PLoS One, May 2020, 15(5):e0233969. https://doi.org/10.1371/journal.pone.0233969. © 2020 Benova et al. under the terms of the Creative Commons Attribution License, which permits unrestricted use, distribution, and reproduction in any medium, provided the original author and source are credited)

13. Odds ratio

- OR = 1: The odds of the outcome occurring are the same for both groups. There is no association between the exposure and the outcome.
- OR > 1: The odds of the outcome are higher in the group with the exposure than in the group without the exposure. This indicates a positive association.
- OR < 1: The odds of the outcome are lower in the group with the exposure than in the group without the exposure. This indicates a negative association or a protective effect.

14.

Example	Occurrence	Interpretation
Smoking and lung cancer	OR = 3.0	Smokers are three times more likely to develop lung cancer compared to non-smokers. This indicates a positive association between smoking and lung cancer.
Vaccination and disease occurrence	OR = 0.2	Individuals who are vaccinated have 0.2 times the odds, or an 80% lower chance, of getting the disease compared to those who are not vaccinated. This suggests a protective effect of the vaccine.
Exercise and heart disease	OR = 0.5	Individuals who exercise regularly have half the odds of developing heart disease compared to those who do not exercise. This indicates a protective effect of exercise against heart disease.
High-fiber diet and colon cancer	OR = 2.5	Individuals with a high-fiber diet have 2.5 times the odds of developing colon cancer compared to those with a low-fiber diet. This suggests a positive association between a high-fiber diet and colon cancer.
Seatbelt use and car accident fatalities	OR = 0.1	Individuals who wear seatbelts have 0.1 times the odds, or a 90% lower chance, of fatality in car accidents compared to those who do not wear seatbelts. This indicates a strong protective effect of wearing seatbelts.

15. Confidence intervals

16.

Example	Finding	Interpretation
Average height	Suppose a study measures the average height of a sample of 100 adult men and finds it to be 175 cm with a 95% CI of 173–177 cm.	This means we are 95% confident that the average height of all adult men in the population is between 173 and 177 cm.
Medication effectiveness	A clinical trial investigating a new drug reports that the average decrease in blood pressure is 10 mmHg, with a 95% CI of 8–12 mmHg.	This suggests that we can be 95% confident that the true average decrease in blood pressure for the population taking the drug is between 8 and 12 mmHg.
School performance	A study on a new teaching method reports an average score improvement of 5 points, with a 95% CI of 2–8 points.	This indicates that the true average improvement in scores due to the teaching method is likely between 2 and 8 points.

17.

__E_1. FALSE positive
__F_2. FALSE negative
__G_3. TRUE positive
__H_4. TRUE negative
__A_5. Sensitivity
__B_6. Specificity
__D_7. Prevalence
__C_8. Incidence

18. Type I (α).
19. Type II (β).
20. Increase sample size, expected effect size, precision of measurement.
21. The mean, often known as average, is a measure of central tendency determined by adding all the values in a collection of numbers and dividing by their count. The median is the middle number in an ascending or descending list. If there are even observations, the median is the middle two numbers averaged. The mode of a data set is its most frequent value. A set of numbers can have one, several, or no mode.

Data	Mean	Median	Mode
20, 10, 40, 10, 70	30	20	10

22. Significantly different.
23. The Institutional Review Board (IRB) plays a crucial role in ensuring the ethical conduct of research involving human participants. It does so by accepting, modifying, or rejecting research studies based on ethical standards and participant welfare considerations. The IRB has several key responsibilities, including minimizing risks to participants by reviewing research designs, ensuring fair participant selection and protection of vulnerable populations, reevaluating adverse events and risk-benefit ratios, overseeing the informed consent process to ensure clarity and comprehensiveness, and implementing data and safety monitoring plans for high-risk research projects. These functions collectively help safeguard the rights, well-being, and ethical treatment of research participants.
24.

Case-control	Retrospectively compares cases of COVID delta variant with cases of COVID omicron variant to determine causal relationships.
Cross-sectional	Captures the prevalence of PTSD among female Veterans in June 2022.
Cohort	Follows two groups of individuals over 3 years. One group has HIV and one does not. The study compares the incidence rate of dementia among the two groups.

25. Control (placebo).
26. One patient to benefit.
27.
    __B__Selection
    __G__Measurement
    __F__Expectancy
    __C__Lead-time
    __E__Recall
    __A__Confounding
    __D__Design
28. Rejecting the null hypothesis means that the findings are unlikely due to chance <0.05.
29.

5	Case-control
1	Meta-analysis
4	Cohort
3	Randomized controlled trial
6	Case series
2	Systematic review

30.

	Description	Example
P	Population/disease	Age, gender, ethnicity, with a certain disorder
I	Intervention or variable of interest	Exposure to a disease, risk behavior, prognostic factor
C	Comparison	Could be usual care; a placebo or no disease, absence of risk factor, prognostic factor B
O	Outcome	Risk of disease, the accuracy of a diagnosis, rate of occurrence of adverse outcome
T	Time	Days, weeks

31.
    __3__Evidence from RCT without randomization
    __5__Randomized controlled trials (RCT), meta-analysis, or systematic review
    __1__Evidence from expert opinion or committee reports
    __4__Evidence-based guidelines based on systematic review
    __2__Evidence from systematic review of descriptive and qualitative studies
32.
    __3_Evidence from well-designed controlled trials without randomization
    __2_Evidence from a single descriptive or qualitative study
    __6_Evidence from systematic reviews of descriptive and qualitative studies
    __5_Evidence-based guideline based on systematic review of RCTs
    __4_Evidence from at least one well-designed RCT
    __1_Evidence from expert opinion or committee

References and Resources

American Nurses Association. Nursing: scope and standards of practice. 4th ed. American Nurses Association; 2023.

American Psychiatric Association, editor. Diagnostic and statistical manual of mental disorders: DSM-5-TR. 5th ed., text revision. American Psychiatric Association Publishing; 2022.

Baghi H, Kornides ML. Current and future health care professionals' attitudes toward and knowledge of statistics: how confidence influences learning. J Nurs Educ Pract. 2013;3(7):24–9. https://doi.org/10.5430/jnep.v3n7p24.

Bebell C, Haines DL. Public health nursing: practicing population-based care. 3rd ed. Jones and Bartlett Publishers; 2017.

Burns N, Grove SK. The practice of nursing research: appraisal, synthesis, and generation of evidence. 8th ed. Elsevier; 2023.

Centers for Disease Control and Prevention. Data and statistics. 2023. Retrieved from https://www.cdc.gov/datastatistics/index.html.

Chernick MR. The essentials of biostatistics for physicians, nurses, and clinicians. John Wiley & Sons; 2013.

Creswell JW. Research design: qualitative, quantitative, and mixed methods approaches. 5th ed. Sage Publications; 2018.

Johnson K, Vanderhoef D, Magrath N. Psychiatric-mental health nurse practitioner review and resource manual. American Nurses Credentialing Center, American Nurses Association; 2020.

Mayo Clinic. Chronic stress puts your health at risk. 2021. Retrieved from https://www.mayoclinic.org/healthy-lifestyle/stress-management/in-depth/stress/art-20046037.

National Institute of Mental Health. Depression and heart disease. 2021. Retrieved from https://www.nimh.nih.gov/health/publications/depression.

Nies MA, McEwen M. Community/public health nursing: promoting the health of populations. 7th ed. Elsevier; 2018.

Polit DF, Beck CT. Nursing research: generating and assessing evidence for nursing practice. 10th ed. Lippincott Williams & Wilkins; 2016.

Stanhope M, Lancaster J. Public health nursing: population-centered health care in the community. 9th ed. Mosby; 2015.

World Health Organization. Mental health: a state of well-being. 2014. Retrieved from https://www.who.int/news-room/fact-sheets/detail/mental-health-strengthening-our-response.

Zakhari R. The psychiatric-mental health nurse practitioner certification review manual. Springer Publishing Company; 2021.

Notes:

Notes:

Leadership, Advocacy, Policy, and Quality Improvement

20

Test your learning and check your understanding of this book's contents: use the "Springer Nature Flashcards" app to access questions using ▶ https://sn.pub/62J0Ar.
To use the app, please follow the instructions in Chap. 1.

In addition to providing clinical care to individuals with mental health conditions, PMHNPs may also engage in leadership, advocacy, and policy work, as well as quality improvement efforts (American Association of Nurse Practitioners 2021).

Leadership is an essential aspect of the role of PMHNPs in providing high-quality health care. Nurse practitioners are often leaders within their organizations and can play a key role in shaping the direction of the healthcare system (Baggs 2018). Their leadership abilities can have a significant impact on patient outcomes and the overall success of their organizations. PMHNPs may hold positions of authority, such as serving as department heads or program directors. They may also serve as mentors or role models for other nurses and healthcare providers.

Advocacy is another important aspect of the PMHNP role. Nurse practitioners are advocates for their patients, working to ensure that their needs and preferences are met (National Association of Clinical Nurse Specialists 2023). They also advocate for the profession, working to increase recognition and respect for nurse practitioners and their contributions to health care. PMHNPs may also advocate for the rights and needs of individuals with mental health conditions.

Policy is another important area for PMHNPs to consider in their practice. Nurse practitioners must be aware of and adhere to relevant policies and regulations in their practice, including those related to scope of practice, prescribing, and patient privacy (American Association of Nurse Practitioners 2023). They must also be aware of policy developments at the local, state, and national levels that may impact their practice and the healthcare system as a whole (Fitzpatrick and Alfes 2022). This may

T. Stewart, *Psychiatric-Mental Health Nurse Practitioner Program Companion and Board Certification Exam Review Workbook*,
https://doi.org/10.1007/978-3-031-60894-0_20

involve working with policymakers to develop and implement policies that support mental health care, or collaborating with community organizations to promote mental health awareness and access to care. By staying informed about policy developments and advocating for policies that support high-quality care, nurse practitioners can play a key role in shaping the direction of the healthcare system.

Quality improvement is another aspect of the PMHNP role. Nurse practitioners have a responsibility to continuously assess and improve the quality of care they provide to patients (Institute for Healthcare Improvement 2023). This may involve implementing evidence-based practices, using quality improvement tools and techniques, and collaborating with other healthcare professionals to identify and address areas for improvement. PMHNPs may collaborate with other healthcare providers to develop and implement evidence-based practices, or use data to track and measure the outcomes of mental health care.

The role of a PMHNP is multifaceted; leadership, advocacy, policy, and quality improvement are all important aspects of this role. Nurse practitioners must be able to lead interprofessional teams, advocate for their patients and the profession, adhere to relevant policies and regulations, and continuously assess and improve the quality of care they provide. These skills are essential for nurse practitioners to provide high-quality health care to their patients and to advance the nursing profession (American Nurses Association 2021).

This chapter examines the concepts of leadership, advocacy, and policy with regard to the role of a nurse practitioner. Quality improvement models and safety extend this information to the clinical setting.

20.1 Leadership and Conflict Resolution

1. Define leadership.

2. What qualities do effective leaders possess?

3. Match the following leadership theories with their description.

Theory	Description
_____Trait theory	A. Emphasizes that the effectiveness of a leader depends upon or depends on various situational factors, rather than a one-size-fits-all approach to leadership. In other words, it emphasizes that there is no single best leadership style, and the most effective leadership style depends on the specific circumstances or situations.

Theory	Description
_____Behavioral theory	B. Posits that effective leadership depends on the readiness or maturity level of followers and that leaders should adapt their leadership style to match the needs of their followers and the specific situation. This theory is often depicted as a two-dimensional model, considering both leadership behavior and follower readiness.
_____Contingency theory	C. Emphasizes the importance of being true to oneself and one's values. Authentic leaders are transparent and open about their beliefs and values, and they encourage their followers to do the same.
_____Transformational leadership	D. Emphasizes the importance of innate characteristics, such as intelligence, confidence, and charisma, in effective leadership.
_____Situational leadership	E. Emphasizes the importance of helping others and putting their needs before one's own. Such leaders focus on creating a culture of empathy and compassion, and they prioritize the needs of their followers above their own personal interests.
_____Servant leadership	F. Emphasizes the importance of inspiring and motivating followers to achieve their full potential. These leaders focus on creating a vision for the organization and empowering their followers to achieve that vision.
_____Authentic leadership	G. Emphasizes the importance of observable behaviors and actions in effective leadership. The theory suggests that effective leaders demonstrate certain behaviors, such as providing clear direction and support to their followers.

4. Match each leadership style with the best description.

Leadership style	Description
_____Autocratic	A. Focuses on the exchanges that occur between the individual and followers. Provides clear instructions and expectations and rewards or punishes team members based on their performance. It is often used where routine and structure are important.
_____Democratic	B. Has a strong vision for the future and the ability to communicate this vision. Focused on moving the organization toward this future and can inspire and motivate the team to work toward this shared vision.
_____Transformational	C. Focuses on developing individuals, showing them how to improve their performance, and helping to connect their goals to the organization's goals. Often provides plenty of feedback and nurtures long-term development.
_____Transactional	D. Encourages, inspires, and motivates others to innovate and create change that will help grow and shape future success. Often achieved through setting challenging goals, demonstrating commitment to the goals, and supporting others in achieving them.
_____Laissez-faire	E. Adjusts the approach according to the situation, considering the ability and willingness of followers. This flexible approach means choosing between being more directive or supportive as needed, making it very adaptive.
_____Servant	F. Characterized by individual control over all decisions with little input from group members. Typically, choices are made based on personal judgments and ideas, rarely accepting advice from others. It often leads to high productivity but can reduce morale.

Leadership style	Description
_____Situational	G. Gives team members a lot of freedom in how they do their work and set their deadlines. Provides tools and resources needed but does not oversee the process; may provide feedback if requested.
_____Charismatic	H. Involves group members in the decision-making process. The final decision-making authority is maintained while gathering information and opinions from team members, fostering a sense of collaboration and respect.
_____Visionary	I. Inspires and motivates others through magnetic personality and charm. Often able to instill both reverence and trust, which helps to influence others and to drive change.
_____Coach-style	J. Emphasizes the role as a doer first, who contributes to the Well-being of team members. Focuses on followers' needs and helps them perform as highly as possible, often leading by example to gain loyalty and trust.

5. What are three to five key ways to keep patients motivated?
   1. ____ __________
   2. ____ __________
   3. ____ __________
   4. ____ __________
   5. ____ __________.

6. What are S.M.A.R.T. goals? Write one example.

	Letter meaning	Example
S		
M		
A		
R		
T		

7. Motivation and team building are important concepts. Match each of the following key theories and principles related to motivation and team building with its description.

_____Maslow's hierarchy of needs	A. This theory states that expectations of results inspire people to behave. The hypothesis states that expectation, instrumentality, and valence influence motivation. In team development, this theory states that members should understand how their actions affect outcomes to be motivated to succeed.
_____Herzberg's two-factor theory	B. People learn by watching and copying others, according to this belief. This theory proposes that team members can learn from other competent team members and model their behavior to help the team succeed.
_____Expectancy theory	C. This idea states that self-actualization requires meeting a hierarchy of wants. The hierarchy covers physiological, safety, belongingness, love, esteem, and self-actualization requirements. This notion indicates that team members' basic needs must be satisfied to succeed in team development.
_____Tuckman's stages of group development	D. This hypothesis states that cleanliness and motivators affect job satisfaction and motivation. Salary, working environment, and job stability can avoid unhappiness but they may not motivate. Success, recognition, and responsibility can boost job happiness. In team building, this notion advocates giving team members motivators rather than hygienic aspects to help them succeed.
_____Social learning theory	E. This model shows how groups form and collaborate. The stages are developing, storming, norming, performing, and adjourning. This concept proposes that teams must go through these stages to achieve good teamwork and collaboration.

8. Match each of the following developmental steps to team formation with its description.

Development	Description
_____ Forming	A. The group reaches its peak effectiveness, with members working together seamlessly to achieve shared goals. Members trust each other and are committed to the success of the group.
_____ Storming	B. The group is just starting to come together, and members are getting to know each other. They may be polite and hesitant to express their opinions or ideas.
_____ Norming	C. The group disbands, either because its goals have been achieved or because its members move on to other projects or organizations. This stage may involve feelings of sadness or loss as well as recognition of the group's accomplishments.
_____ Performing	D. The group starts to establish shared expectations for behavior. Members begin to work together more effectively and may develop a sense of camaraderie or loyalty.
_____ Adjourning	E. The group begins to experience conflict as members start to express their opinions and vie for leadership or power. There may be disagreements about goals, roles, or approaches.

9. Label each level of the pyramid with the appropriate level of Maslow's hierarchy.

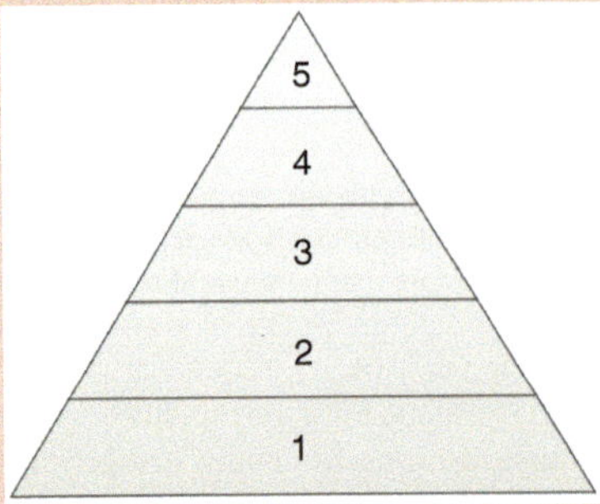

5.
4.
3.
2.
1.

10. Decision-making and problem-solving are important. Here are some key models related to decision-making and problem-solving. Match each model with its description.

_____Rational decision-making model	A. This model proposes systematic problem-solving. According to the approach, problem-solving entails recognizing the problem, acquiring information, generating options, assessing them, choosing the best one, and implementing and monitoring it.
_____Intuitive decision-making model	B. This paradigm helps strategic planners identify problem or decision strengths, weaknesses, opportunities, and threats. The analysis helps people evaluate internal and external aspects that may affect a decision or solution.
_____Problem-solving model	C. The intuition model suggests people make decisions based on their gut feelings. The paradigm says that people make decisions based on past experiences and emotions rather than a systematic consideration of options.
_____SWOT analysis	D. This approach suggests people make judgments by systematically analyzing alternatives and their effects. According to the paradigm, decision-making comprises identifying the problem, acquiring information, developing options, assessing them, and choosing the best one.
_____Bounded rationality model	E. This model suggests people cannot process or make judgments completely. The approach implies that humans reduce complex judgments with heuristics or mental shortcuts and use past experiences or patterns to make decisions.

11. Shared governance and decision-making are models of decision-making that involve collaboration and shared responsibility among members of a group or organization. List at least three pros and cons of shared governance and decision-making.

Pros	Cons

12. Match each of the following key theories and models related to conflict management and resolution with its description.

_____Thomas-Kilmann conflict mode instrument (TKI)	A. This model suggests mediation using a neutral third party to help conflicting parties negotiate. By providing a secure and structured atmosphere for parties to communicate their wants and concerns, mediation may help resolve disagreements.
_____Interest-based relational (IBR) approach	B. This model suggests identifying each party's interests and needs and finding a solution that meets them. Communication, active listening, and negotiation are suggested to achieve this.
_____Negotiation theory	C. This model suggests that conflict parties negotiate by giving and taking to reach a compromise. According to the philosophy, negotiating entails establishing common ground, building rapport, and finding mutually beneficial solutions.
_____Mediation model	D. This model suggests balancing self- and other-concerns to resolve conflict. According to the approach, conflict resolution requires resolving both parties' concerns.
_____Dual concerns model	E. This model suggests fighting, collaborating, compromising, avoiding, and accommodating to resolve conflicts. According to the paradigm, conflict resolution styles depend on goals, situation, and personal preferences.

13. As a nurse practitioner, conflict management and resolution skills are important to maintain positive relationships with patients, colleagues, and other health-care professionals. Place the following steps of conflict management in the correct order from first step (1) to last step (7).

_____Communicate effectively
_____Consider possible solutions
_____Evaluate the outcome
_____Gather information
_____Identify the issue
_____Implement the solution
_____Negotiate and find common ground

14. Match each of the following terms related to conflict resolution with its description.

_____Conflict	A. Occurs when a person believes his or her needs, interests, or values are incompatible with others
_____Conflict resolution	B. Behavior that shows respect toward another person
_____Negotiation	C. Directed by a neutral third party who facilitates a "win-win" situation
_____Mediation	D. Process in which a third party reviews evidence from both sides and makes a decision to settle the case
_____Arbitration	E. Voluntary and confidential process in which a third party facilitates discussion to reach an agreement
_____Professional civility	F. Discussion among two or more people with the goal of reaching an agreement

15. Describe change management and how it pertains to a nurse practitioner.

16. What is reflective practice and its utility to a PMHNP?

20.2 Advocacy

17. What is advocacy? What is the role of nurses and nurse practitioners in advocacy?

18. Name at least five advocacy principles and practices.
    1. ____________________
    2. ____________________
    3. ____________________
    4. ____________________
    5. ____________________
    6. ____________________
    7. ____________________

19. What are five ways in which PMHNPs advocate for patient rights and needs?
    1. ____________________
    2. ____________________
    3. ____________________
    4. ____________________
    5. ____________________

20. What community-based approaches to mental health care support advocacy for patients?
    1. ____________________
    2. ____________________
    3. ____________________
    4. ____________________
    5. ____________________

20.3 Policy

21. What are the main goals of the Affordable Care Act (ACA)? How does it seek to increase access to healthcare services?

22. Who are the beneficiaries of Medicare and Medicaid, and what are the key differences between these two programs?

23. What is the primary purpose of the Health Insurance Portability and Accountability Act (HIPAA), and how does it protect patients' privacy?

24. Explain how the Mental Health Parity and Addiction Equity Act (MHPAEA) affects coverage for mental health and substance use disorder services.

25. Healthcare delivery models and systems refer to the different ways that health care is organized, financed, and delivered to patients. There are many different models and systems in use around the world, each with their own strengths and weaknesses. Match each of the following payment models with its description.

Payment model	Description
_____Fee-for-service (FFS)	A. Providers work together to coordinate care for a group of patients. Aimed at providing high-quality care at lower costs, with incentives for patient involvement.
_____Capitation	B. Care is provided through remote consultations using technology. Useful for patients in remote areas or with travel difficulties.
_____Accountable care organizations (ACOs)	C. Healthcare providers are paid for each service or procedure performed. Incentivizes more services, but may lead to overuse and unnecessary procedures.
_____Patient-centered medical homes (PCMHs)	D. Patients receive coordinated care from a primary provider. Focuses on preventive care, chronic disease management, and patient education.
_____Telemedicine	E. Providers offer comprehensive care across specialties and settings, improving coordination and potentially reducing costs but may reduce competition.
_____Integrated delivery systems	F. Providers are paid a fixed amount per patient, regardless of the services provided. Encourages preventive care and cost-effective treatments but may lead to underuse of necessary procedures.

26. Describe the role of accreditation in health care. Name at least two accrediting bodies in psychiatric-mental health nursing and discuss what aspects of health care they evaluate.

27. Explain why licensure is essential for PMHNP. Discuss how licensure requirements can vary and what they generally include.

28. Define certification and its importance in health care. Provide an example in psychiatry-mental health where certification might be particularly important and explain why.

29. List at least three patient safety regulations or guidelines in psychiatry-mental health and describe how each contributes to patient safety.

30. Explain what quality improvement initiatives are and their significance in psychiatric-mental health care.

31. Discuss the purpose of electronic health record (EHR) regulations and how they contribute to patient safety and care quality in psychiatry-mental health.

32. What types of scientific evidence are typically used to develop evidence-based practice guidelines in psychiatry-mental health? How is the quality and relevance of this evidence evaluated?

33. Who might be included on the teams that develop evidence-based practice guidelines in psychiatry-mental health, and why is a multidisciplinary approach important?

34. What does it mean for the guideline development process to be transparent? How does transparency benefit clinicians and patients in psychiatry-mental health?

35. Describe the consensus-building process involved in developing practice guidelines. Why is it crucial to integrate different expert perspectives in psychiatry-mental health?

36. Explain what it means for practice guidelines to be dynamic in psychiatry-mental health. How often should evidence-based practice guidelines be updated, and why?

20.4 Quality Improvement

37. Quality improvement (QI) theories refer to the principles and methodologies used to improve the quality of healthcare services and outcomes. There are several QI theories that have been developed over time, each with its own unique approach and emphasis. Match each theory and model with its description.

Theories and models	Description
_____Lean management	A. Involves a four-step approach to problem-solving and continuous improvement: Planning a change, implementing the change, studying the results, and acting on the results to further improve the process.
_____Six sigma	B. Focuses on promoting a culture of safety within healthcare organizations, with an emphasis on identifying and reporting errors, learning from mistakes, and continuously improving safety practices.
_____Plan-do-study-act (PDSA)	C. Emphasizes the importance of ongoing monitoring and evaluation of processes and outcomes, with a focus on making incremental improvements over time.
_____Total quality management (TQM)	D. Emphasizes the elimination of waste and the optimization of processes to improve efficiency and reduce errors in healthcare delivery.
_____Continuous quality improvement (CQI)	E. Emphasizes the importance of continuous improvement, customer satisfaction, and employee involvement in improving processes and outcomes.
_____Patient safety culture	F. Focuses on reducing defects and errors in processes by using statistical analysis to identify and eliminate root causes of problems.

38. The Donabedian model is a foundational concept in the field of quality improvement (QI) in health care. Developed by Dr. Avedis Donabedian, it provides a framework for evaluating health services and improving quality. The model divides quality into three interrelated categories: structure, process, and

outcome. For each category, provide a definition/description and examples specific to the work of PMHNP.

Category	Definition	Examples
Structure		
Process		
Outcome		

39. In the image below, label the Institute for Healthcare Improvement's PDSA Cycle. Provide a brief explanation of each step in the cycle.

Category	Definition	Examples
Structure		
Process		
Outcome		

40. Healthcare quality improvement (QI) includes patient safety and risk management. Risk management identifies, assesses, and prioritizes patient risks and develops ways to mitigate them, whereas patient safety prevents injury to patients throughout healthcare delivery. What are three to five ways patient safety and risk management support QI?

1. ____
____
2. ____
____
3. ____
____
4. ____
____
5. ____
____

20.5 Answers and Explanations to Chapter Activities

1. To inspire, motivate, and guide others toward a single purpose or vision is leadership. It entails leveraging one's talents, expertise, and experience to influence and steer others toward a common goal and bring out the best in people and teams.
2. Effective leaders create and communicate a vision, define goals and objectives, build and manage relationships, make decisions, and act to achieve goals. Effective leaders have good communication, interpersonal, emotional, and adaptability abilities.
3.

__D___Trait theory
__G___Behavioral theory
__A___Contingency theory
__F___Transformational leadership
__B___Situational leadership
__E___Servant leadership
__C___Authentic leadership

4.

__F___Autocratic
__H___Democratic
__D___Transformational
__A___Transactional
__G___Laissez-Faire
__J___Servant
__E___Situational
__I___Charismatic
__B___Visionary
__C___Coach-Style

5. To enhance patient engagement and facilitate the achievement of health objectives, healthcare providers employ various motivational strategies. These strategies encompass educating patients about their condition and treatment options through personalized written, video, and online resources, thus empowering them to follow their treatment plans effectively. Additionally, collaborating with patients to establish achievable and SMART (Specific, Measurable, Achievable, Relevant, Time-bound) goals helps maintain motivation and progress. Positive reinforcement, such as acknowledging and rewarding patient efforts and successes, further encourages commitment to treatment plans. Encouraging self-monitoring, whether tracking symptoms or physical activity, assists patients in staying motivated. Providing emotional and social support through empathetic interactions, active listening, and counseling is central to patient motivation. Furthermore, the integration of technology, including

telemedicine, health apps, and wearables, enables real-time feedback and support, fostering patient engagement and adherence to treatment regimens.

6. SMART goals are a framework used to set specific, measurable, achievable, relevant, and time-bound goals. Using the SMART framework to set goals can help individuals and organizations stay focused, motivated, and accountable, while also ensuring that goals are realistic and achievable within a certain timeframe.

   Here is a breakdown of what each letter in SMART stands for:

   - S—Specific: The goal should be clear and specific, and answer the questions of who, what, where, when, and why.
   - M—Measurable: The goal should be quantifiable and able to be measured in some way, either by a number, percentage, or other metric.
   - A—Achievable: The goal should be realistic and achievable within a certain timeframe, considering the resources, skills, and support available.
   - R—Relevant: The goal should be relevant to the overall purpose or mission, and aligned with other goals and priorities.
   - T—Time-bound: The goal should have a specific timeframe for completion, and include milestones or deadlines to help track progress.
   - Leadership: Good leaders recognize and prioritize issues, create tactics, and motivate others to support the cause.
   - Ethics: Advocacy should respect patient autonomy, confidentiality, and informed consent.

   Here are four examples of SMART goals:

   - Increase the number of patients who receive flu vaccinations by 20% within the next 3 months by offering free flu shot clinics at our practice every Saturday morning.
   - Reduce the average wait time for patients to see a provider by 10 min within the next 6 months by implementing a new patient scheduling system and streamlining our check-in process.
   - Improve patient satisfaction ratings by 15% within the next year by conducting patient satisfaction surveys after each appointment and using feedback to make improvements to our services.
   - Increase the number of patients who participate in our diabetes management program by 25% within the next 9 months by promoting the program through social media, email newsletters, and informational flyers in our waiting room.

7.

   __C___Maslow's hierarchy of needs
   __D___Herzberg's two-factor theory
   __A___Expectancy theory
   __E___Tuckman's stages of group development
   __B___Social learning theory

8.

__B___Forming
__E___Storming
__D___Norming
__A___Performing
__C___Adjourning

9. Maslow's hierarchy of needs is a psychological theory that categorizes human needs into five levels, with each level building upon the previous one. At the most fundamental level are physiological needs such as food, water, shelter, rest, and other basic biological requirements. Once these basic needs are met, individuals seek safety and security, encompassing personal, employment, financial, health, and property safety. The next level comprises social needs, including friendship, trust, love, and a sense of belonging within family, friends, and community. Beyond that are esteem needs, which involve self-esteem, respect from others, recognition, and a desire for accomplishment and competence. The highest level in the hierarchy is self-actualization, where individuals strive for personal growth and fulfillment by maximizing their talents, abilities, and potential. Maslow's hierarchy is often depicted as a pyramid, emphasizing that each level must be fulfilled before the individual can focus on the higher-level needs for motivation and well-being.

10.

__D___Rational decision-making model
__C___Intuitive decision-making model
__A___Problem-solving model
__B___SWOT analysis
__E___Bounded rationality model

11.

Pros	Cons
• Collaboration and buy-in: Shared governance and decision-making promote group and organization collaboration and responsibility. Better member buy-in and decision implementation can result. • Member input and diversity: Shared governance and decision-making allow for member contribution and diversity. A more imaginative and innovative approach to challenges may result. • Higher accountability and transparency: Shared governance and decision-making ensures that choices are made publicly and with member input. This can improve member trust and communication. • Enhanced morale and job satisfaction: Shared governance and decision-making give members ownership and control over their work environment, which boosts morale and job satisfaction.	• Time-consuming: Members must commit time and resources in shared governance and decision-making. • Potential for conflict and delays: If members disagree or cannot reach consensus, shared governance and decision-making can cause conflict and delays. • Risk of decision paralysis: Shared governance and decision-making can cause decision paralysis if there are too many voices and perspectives if members are afraid to make tough decisions. • Lack of expertise: Shared governance and decision-making may lead to decisions made by people without the expertise or knowledge to make them.

12.

__E___Thomas-Kilmann conflict mode instrument (TKI)
__B___Interest-based relational (IBR) approach
__C___Negotiation theory
__A___Mediation model
__D___Dual concerns model

13.

____1___Identify the issue
____2___Gather information
____3___Consider possible solutions
____4___Negotiate and find common ground
____5___Communicate effectively (4 and 5 may be interchanged)
____6___Implement the solution
____7___Evaluate the outcome

14.

__A___Conflict
__C___Conflict resolution
__F___Negotiation
__E___Mediation
__D___Arbitration
__B___Professional civility

15. Change management in health care involves planning, executing, and overseeing organizational or system changes, due to the frequent shifts in healthcare practices, laws, and technologies. Successful change management entails recognizing the need for change, anticipating challenges, and devising strategies to surmount obstacles during implementation. Nurse practitioners play a pivotal role in driving change, whether in implementing new policies, healthcare technologies, or patient care procedures. This necessitates effective leadership, communication, and problem-solving skills to identify and address barriers to transformation. Collaboration among staff, patients, and stakeholders is often essential to garner support for change initiatives. Nurse practitioners, in their pursuit of enhancing patient care, staying updated with industry advancements, and thriving within healthcare organizations, are instrumental in leading change projects and mastering the art of change management for the betterment of health care.
16. Reflective practice is a fundamental aspect of professional growth and development, particularly for mental health nurse practitioners (PMHNPs). It involves the critical examination of one's experiences and actions, leading to a deeper understanding of lessons learned and the formulation of strategies for future improvements. PMHNPs use reflective practice to assess clinical decisions, patient interactions, and personal strengths and weaknesses, which ultimately enhances their diagnosis, treatment, and communication skills. This self-reflection is particularly valuable in the emotionally challenging field of psychiatry, helping PMHNPs manage stress, burnout, and emotional responses to difficult patients. Moreover, it directly contributes to better patient care, as it enables PMHNPs to understand patients more deeply, adapt therapies, and

improve therapeutic interactions, ultimately enhancing patient outcomes. Reflective practice also upholds ethical standards and promotes interprofessional collaboration, which collectively contribute to the provision of high-quality mental health care and ongoing personal and professional growth.

17. Healthcare advocacy is an essential aspect of ensuring that patients and communities receive the care and resources they require. Nurses, including nurse practitioners, play a pivotal role as patient advocates, advocating for healthcare services, medications, equipment, and addressing patients' cultural, social, and emotional needs. This advocacy extends to interdisciplinary teams, collaborating to advocate for patient care and improved outcomes through policy creation and implementation. Effective healthcare advocacy hinges on strong communication skills, the ability to build alliances, a deep understanding of the healthcare system, and insight into the needs and priorities of patients and communities. Nurse practitioners must engage with patients, their families, and various stakeholders to gain a comprehensive understanding of their unique requirements and work collaboratively to develop solutions. By championing patient-centered care and advocating for their patients to ensure they receive the necessary care and resources, nurse practitioners can significantly enhance the quality of health care.
18.
    - Empowerment: Advocacy should empower patients and communities to make healthcare decisions.
    - Collaboration: Effective advocacy involves working with other healthcare professionals, patients, and community members to discover solutions that please everyone.
    - Professional norms and the best research and evidence should guide advocacy.
    - Cultural Competence: Advocacy should address patients' and communities' cultural, social, and linguistic needs and varied perspectives.
    - Advocacy requires active listening, effective communication, and solid relationships and alliances.
    - Leadership: Good leaders recognize and prioritize issues, create tactics, and motivate others to support the cause.
    - Ethics: Advocacy should respect patient autonomy, confidentiality, and informed consent.
19.
    - Promoting Patient-Centered Care: PMHNPs can involve patients and address their needs.
    - Addressing Stigma and Discrimination: PMHNPs can advocate for their patients by promoting mental health awareness and education.
    - PMHNPs can advocate for patients by ensuring they have access to drugs, treatment, and community resources.
    - Tackle Socioeconomic Determinants of Health: PMHNPs can help patients by addressing poverty, homelessness, and food insecurity, which can impair mental health.

- Working with Interdisciplinary Teams: PMHNPs can coordinate patient care with social workers, psychologists, and primary care doctors.
- PMHNPs can help patients manage their mental health conditions by teaching and supporting them.
- Policy Advocacy: PMHNPs can help patients by improving local, state, and national mental health policy and funding.

20. Community-based mental health treatment and special programs can improve patient advocacy by incorporating patients and community members and offering access to community services and resources. Some community-based patient advocacy programs:

    - Community Mental Health Centers: Community mental health centers provide therapy, counseling, and medication management. At these places, support groups, education, and outreach may help families understand and manage mental health conditions.
    - Mental health patients might find support via peer support programs. These programs provide a safe area for sharing stories, receiving support, and learning coping skills.
    - Assertive community treatment (ACT) delivers intensive mental health care to those with severe and persistent mental health concerns. These home and community-based programs include medication, therapy, case management, vocational, and educational support.
    - Mobile crisis response teams treat mental health crisis victims instantly. Crisis victims can receive support from these teams of mental health professionals, social workers, and law enforcement.
    - Supportive Housing Programs: Mental health patients receive safe, affordable housing, counseling, case management, and vocational and educational assistance.

21. The ACA aspires to improve health insurance quality and affordability, lower the uninsured rate by expanding public and private insurance coverage, and lower government and individual healthcare costs. The ACA extends Medicaid eligibility for low-income people, introduces subsidized health insurance exchanges, and requires most Americans to obtain health insurance. It also prohibits insurance companies from denying pre-existing disease coverage, allows young persons to stay on their parents' plans until 26, and gives subsidies to lower health insurance costs.
22. Medicare protects disabled individuals, dialysis patients, and seniors over 65, regardless of income. Medicaid aids low-income children, pregnant women, retirees, and disabled people. Key differences include: Medicaid is state-federal with state-specific coverage and eligibility requirements, unlike Medicare. Medicare covers hospital, medical, Medicare Advantage plans, and prescriptions nationwide. States offer different Medicaid coverage, some more comprehensive.

23. HIPAA (Health Insurance Portability and Accountability Act) is legislation that safeguards sensitive patient health information from unauthorized disclosure on a national level. HIPAA mandates the discrete and secure handling of protected health information (PHI) and imposes strict restrictions on the disclosure of PHI without patient consent. It upholds patients' rights, allowing them access to their medical records, the ability to correct any inaccuracies, and the right to know who has viewed their health information. Additionally, HIPAA includes penalties for privacy violations, ensuring accountability and the protection of patient confidentiality.
24. The Mental Health Parity and Addiction Equity Act (MHPAEA) has a significant impact on insurance coverage by mandating that health insurance plans provide equal coverage for mental health and substance use disorder services when compared to medical and surgical care. This means that copays, deductibles, and treatment limitations, such as the number of allowed visits, must be similar or better for mental health and addiction care compared to physical health care. MHPAEA eliminates stigma and treatment barriers associated with mental and substance use disorders, as it ensures that these conditions are treated with the same level of importance and accessibility as physical health issues. Consequently, many individuals now have improved access to and quality of mental health treatments due to the provisions of this act.
25.
    __C___Fee-for-service (FFS)
    __F___Capitation
    __A___Accountable care organizations (ACOs)
    __D___Patient-centered medical homes (PCMHs)
    __B___Telemedicine
    __E___Integrated delivery systems
26. Healthcare accreditation serves as a vital mechanism for ensuring the quality and safety of healthcare organizations and their activities. Accredited entities assess compliance with established benchmarks, aiming to enhance patient outcomes, professional practices, and regulatory adherence. Accreditation provides reassurance to patients, providers, and stakeholders, signifying the effectiveness and safety of healthcare services. In the field of psychiatric-mental health nursing, several accrediting bodies play key roles: The Joint Commission evaluates and certifies healthcare providers, focusing on patient safety and quality. It assesses various aspects of psychiatric-mental health facilities, including treatment, services, treatment environment, patient safety, patient rights, education, and staff certifications. Commission on Accreditation of Rehabilitation Facilities (CARF) accredits mental health services based on outcomes and value. Its evaluation covers leadership, staff credentials, care continuity, patient satisfaction, and treatment effectiveness. The ANCC (American Nurses Credentialing Center) certifies psychiatric-mental health nurses, ensuring they meet rigorous knowledge and expertise standards. While not a facility accreditor, ANCC certification contributes to raising the overall quality of health care by certifying practitioners. COA (Council on Accreditation) accredits many

social and behavioral health services, including mental health and substance use therapy. COA's assessment focuses on organizational performance, service delivery, administration, and management, with an emphasis on respecting cultural diversity and generating positive outcomes.

27. Licensure is essential for psychiatric-mental health nurse practitioners (PMHNPs) to ensure competency, protect patient safety, and grant legal recognition. Licensure requirements can vary between states and countries but generally include completing accredited education, obtaining national certification, accumulating clinical hours, passing state-specific licensure exams, and engaging in continuing education. PMHNPs' licensure guarantees their ability to provide mental health and psychiatric care within their scope of practice, receive reimbursement for services, and maintain professional credibility, ultimately upholding the highest standards of care and ensuring patient well-being.
28. Certification in health care refers to the process of validating an individual's expertise and competence in a specific field or specialty through standardized assessments and examinations. It holds paramount importance as it assures patients, employers, and healthcare organizations that a healthcare provider possesses the necessary knowledge, skills, and qualifications to deliver high-quality care. In the field of psychiatry-mental health, certification is particularly vital, as it demonstrates a practitioner's proficiency in diagnosing and treating complex mental health conditions. For example, certification as a psychiatric-mental health nurse practitioner (PMHNP) ensures that the practitioner has met rigorous educational and clinical standards, thereby safeguarding patient well-being and promoting trust among patients and interdisciplinary healthcare teams. Certification in this context signifies a commitment to excellence in mental health care and enhances the overall quality of psychiatric services.
29. In psychiatry-mental health, three essential patient safety regulations or guidelines contribute significantly to patient well-being. First, the strict protocols governing the use of seclusion and restraint techniques help prevent physical or psychological harm to patients while maintaining their privacy and dignity. Second, robust suicide risk assessment and continuous monitoring ensure the early identification of individuals at risk of self-harm or suicide, facilitating prompt interventions and providing vital support during crises. Lastly, prescription management guidelines for psychiatric medications focus on reducing errors, adverse effects, and interactions, thereby enhancing patient safety by ensuring that medications are prescribed, dispensed, and monitored with precision, effectively addressing mental health conditions while minimizing potential risks. These guidelines collectively prioritize patient safety, protect their rights, and promote the overall quality of psychiatric care.
30. Quality improvement initiatives in psychiatric-mental health care refer to systematic efforts aimed at enhancing the overall quality and safety of mental health services through continuous assessment, analysis, and improvement of care processes and outcomes. These initiatives are of paramount significance as they promote better patient outcomes, improved treatment effectiveness, and enhanced patient safety in the field of psychiatric-mental health. By identifying

areas for improvement, implementing evidence-based practices, and monitoring progress, quality improvement initiatives help reduce errors, enhance treatment strategies, and ensure that individuals receiving mental health care experience the highest standards of care, ultimately fostering trust and confidence in the mental health system.

31. Electronic health record (EHR) laws play a pivotal role in psychiatry and mental health by establishing standards for the adoption and utilization of EHR systems, ensuring the safeguarding, simplification, and enhancement of patient health information management. These regulations offer significant benefits to patient safety and care. They standardize data recording and exchange, facilitating comprehensive and coordinated care, which is foundational in psychiatry where patients often consult multiple healthcare providers. Enhanced privacy and protection measures are enforced to safeguard sensitive psychiatric-mental health data through restricted access and encryption. EHRs contribute to more accurate and clear documentation, for continuity of care and error reduction, especially in the complex landscape of mental health treatment. Additionally, EHRs offer clinical decision support capabilities, aiding clinicians in managing complex mental health cases with multiple medications and comorbidities. Patients are empowered to participate in their care through access to their health records, positively impacting mental health outcomes. Furthermore, EHRs provide valuable data for quality monitoring and research, enabling the identification of trends, treatment modifications, and overall improvement in psychiatric care.
32. Psychiatry-mental health evidence-based practice guidelines are informed by a variety of research methodologies, including randomized controlled trials (RCTs), cohort studies, case-control studies, and qualitative research. These studies generate the empirical foundation upon which guidelines are constructed. Systematic reviews and meta-analyses are essential tools for summarizing and synthesizing this evidence, providing a comprehensive overview of the available data. To ensure the quality and relevance of the evidence, the Grading of Recommendations, Assessment, Development, and Evaluation (GRADE) approach is employed, which assesses factors such as study design, consistency of outcomes, directness of evidence, precision, and potential bias. By rigorously evaluating these criteria, GRADE helps ensure that the resulting guidelines are based on the highest quality evidence and are directly applicable to clinical practice in the field of psychiatry-mental health, ultimately promot ing the delivery of effective and evidence-based care to individuals with mental health conditions.
33. Psychiatrists, clinical psychologists, mental health nurses, social workers, and sometimes patients or patient advocates create evidence-based practice guidelines. Pharmacologists, neurologists, and occupational therapists may be involved depending on the guideline. Since mental health patients' requirements are complex, multidisciplinary advice ensures a wide range of perspectives and knowledge. It helps generate complete, practical guidelines.

34. A transparent guideline development process in psychiatry-mental health means that the entire process, from evidence assessment to recommendation formulation, is open, clear, and accessible to all stakeholders involved, including clinicians and patients. Transparency entails clearly documenting the methods used, disclosing potential conflicts of interest, and making all relevant evidence and decisions publicly available. This transparency benefits clinicians and patients by instilling confidence in the guidelines' credibility, ensuring that recommendations are based on rigorous evidence rather than biases or undisclosed interests. Clinicians can trust that the guidelines are developed through a fair and impartial process, enhancing their confidence in implementing recommended practices. Patients, on the other hand, gain transparency into the rationale behind their treatment options, enabling them to make more informed decisions about their mental health care and fostering a sense of shared decision-making between patients and clinicians, ultimately leading to improved outcomes and patient satisfaction.
35. The consensus-building process in developing practice guidelines for psychiatry-mental health involves the collaboration of a diverse group of experts, including clinicians, researchers, and stakeholders, to establish evidence-based recommendations. This process includes rigorous evidence review, extensive discussions, and external input to ensure that guidelines are comprehensive, well-informed, and relevant to the evolving field of mental health. It is paramount to integrate various expert perspectives in psychiatry-mental health because the discipline encompasses a wide range of conditions and treatments, each requiring a nuanced understanding. The inclusion of diverse perspectives promotes a holistic and evidence-driven approach to mental health care, ultimately benefiting patients by enhancing the quality and effectiveness of clinical practice.
36. In psychiatry-mental health, dynamic practice guidelines refer to guidelines that are flexible and capable of adapting to evolving evidence, new research findings, and changes in clinical practice over time. Unlike static guidelines that remain fixed, dynamic guidelines are designed to be regularly updated to reflect the latest scientific knowledge and best practices. The frequency of updates for evidence-based practice guidelines can vary but should generally occur every few years or when significant new evidence emerges. This regular updating is essential because the field of mental health is continually evolving, with ongoing research and developments in treatments, interventions, and understanding of mental health conditions. By staying current, dynamic guidelines ensure that clinicians have access to the most up-to-date recommendations, ultimately promoting the delivery of high-quality, evidence-based care to individuals with mental health issues and improving patient outcomes.
37.

__D___Lean management
__F___Six Sigma
__A___Plan-Do-Study-Act (PDSA)

__E___Total quality management (TQM)
__C___Continuous quality improvement (CQI)
__B___Patient safety culture

38.

Category	Definition	Examples
Structure	Attributes of the settings where care occurs, including physical and organizational environment, facilities, equipment, and human resources.	Availability of private counseling rooms, access to psychiatric resources, ratio of PMHNPs to patients, secure and confidential record-keeping systems.
Process	Methods and procedures used in delivering health care, encompassing all actions taken by healthcare professionals and patients.	Use of evidence-based therapy techniques, medication management, regular patient follow-ups, coordination with other healthcare providers.
Outcome	Effects of health care on the health status of patients and populations, including the end results of all healthcare activities.	Improvement in patient mental health symptoms, patient satisfaction with care, adherence to treatment plans, reduction in hospital readmissions.

39. The Plan-Do-Study-Act (PDSA) Cycle manages process and product improvements in a continuous loop. Iterative cycles allow for ongoing improvement and refinement by returning to planning after each cycle. A brief explanation of each cycle stage follows:

- Plan: Set goals and plan how to achieve them. This step comprises identifying the issue or opportunity for improvement, understanding the current process, and hypothesizing about how to improve.
- Do: This phase implements the plan. Small adjustments are implemented and their effects are measured. This phase tests the hypothesis from planning.
- Study: Data are analyzed to determine change efficacy. This step involves comparing data to expected results and analyzing differences. Learning from the outcomes and testing the hypothesis is the goal.
- Act: Study analysis determines next steps. If the tweak worked, it may be expanded. If it fails, lessons learned are used to plan a new cycle with alternative improvements.

40.

- Error and Adverse Event Prevention: Patient safety and risk management aid healthcare companies in preventing harm to patients. Healthcare organizations can reduce errors and adverse occurrences by employing safety practices including medication reconciliation and patient identification.
- Improving Communication and Teamwork: Patient safety and risk management can improve healthcare professional communication and teamwork, improving patient outcomes. Healthcare organizations can detect and mitigate patient hazards by fostering provider communication and collaboration.

- Incident Analysis: Patient safety and risk management use occurrences and near-misses to find improvements. Healthcare institutions can prevent such mishaps by conducting root cause analysis and implementing corrective action plans.
- Staff and Patient Education: Patient safety and risk management require teaching healthcare providers and patients about safety risks and mitigation techniques. Healthcare organizations may foster a culture of safety and empower professionals and patients to promote patient safety through education and training.
- Improving Outcomes: Patient safety and risk management reduce adverse occurrences and improve care. Healthcare businesses can increase patient satisfaction and health outcomes by prioritizing patient safety and risk management.

References and Resources

American Association of Nurse Practitioners. All about NPs. 2021. https://www.aanp.org/about/all-about-nps.

American Association of Nurse Practitioners. Advocacy. 2023. https://www.aanp.org/advocacy.

American Nurses Association. Advanced practice registered nurses. 2021. https://www.nursingworld.org/practice-policy/workforce/what-is-nursing/aprn/.

American Psychiatric Association, editor. Diagnostic and statistical manual of mental disorders: DSM-5-TR. 5th ed., text revision. American Psychiatric Association Publishing; 2022.

Anderson C. Exploring the role of advanced nurse practitioners in leadership. Nurs Stand (R Coll Nurs (Great Britain): 1987). 2018;33(2):29–33. https://doi.org/10.7748/ns.2018.e11044.

Baggs JG. Leadership and the advanced practice nurse. In: Fitzpatrick JJ, Wallace AM, editors. Advanced practice nursing: essential knowledge for the profession. 4th ed. Jones & Bartlett Learning; 2018. p. 287–98.

Birch K, Ling A, Phoenix B. Psychiatric nurse practitioners as leaders in behavioral health integration. J Nurse Pract. 2021;17(1):112–5. https://doi.org/10.1016/j.nurpra.2020.09.001.

Cleary M, Horsfall J, Deacon M, Jackson D. Leadership and mental health nursing. Issues Ment Health Nurs. 2011;32(10):632–9. https://doi.org/10.3109/01612840.2011.584362.

Evans N. Leading change, adding value. Nurs Manag (Harrow). 2016;23(4):10. https://doi.org/10.7748/nm.23.4.10.s9.

Fitzpatrick JJ, Alfes CM. Nurse leadership and management: foundations for effective administration. Springer; 2022.

Heinen M, van Oostveen C, Peters J, Vermeulen H, Huis A. An integrative review of leadership competencies and attributes in advanced nursing practice. J Adv Nurs. 2019;75(11):2378–92. https://doi.org/10.1111/jan.14092.

Institute for Healthcare Improvement. Quality improvement. 2023. https://www.ihi.org/topics/quality-improvement/.

Johnson K, Vanderhoef D, Magrath N. Psychiatric-mental health nurse practitioner review and resource manual. American Nurses Credentialing Center, American Nurses Association; 2020.

Kelly RJ, Hearld LR. Burnout and leadership style in behavioral health care: a literature review. J Behav Health Serv Res. 2020;47(4):581–600. https://doi.org/10.1007/s11414-019-09679-z.

National Association of Clinical Nurse Specialists. Advocacy & policy. 2023. https://nacns.org/advocacy-policy/.

Sundberg K, Vistrand C, Sjöström K, Örmon K. Nurses' leadership in psychiatric care: a qualitative interview study of nurses' experience of leadership in an adult psychiatric inpatient care setting. J Psychiatr Ment Health Nurs. 2022;29(5):732–43. https://doi.org/10.1111/jpm.12751.

Weber M, Delaney KR, McCoy KT, Snow D, Scharf MR, Brackley MH. Quality and safety graduate competencies in psychiatric mental health nurse practitioner education. Arch Psychiatr Nurs. 2012;26(5):350–7. https://doi.org/10.1016/j.apnu.2012.06.005.

Weberg D, Mangold K. Leadership in nursing practice: the intersection of innovation and teamwork in healthcare systems. 4th ed. Jones & Bartlett Learning; 2022.

Weberg D, Mangold K, Porter-O'Grady T, Malloch K. Leadership in nursing practice: changing the landscape of health care. 3rd ed. Jones & Bartlett Learning; 2018.

Zakhari R. The psychiatric-mental health nurse practitioner certification review manual. Springer Publishing Company; 2021.

Notes:

Notes:

Appendix A: Crunch Time Review

It's "Crunch Time"! If you're reading this, you're probably stressed about the upcoming exam and looking for ways to cram in the last bits of important information at the last minute. Don't be concerned; you're not alone. Many psychiatric-mental health nurse practitioner (PMHNP) candidates find themselves in this situation at some point, and it's completely normal to be nervous. But don't let your stress get the best of you! As they say, a little bit of anxiety can be beneficial because it can motivate you to study and do your best.

The good news is that it's never too late to go over the material again and increase your chances of passing the exam. This chapter will go over the unusual content that you may encounter on the exam. These are the topics that may not have received as much attention in your lectures or textbooks. But that doesn't mean they're unimportant! In fact, these unusual topics might be just what you need to stand out from the crowd and get a higher score. In addition to unusual content, we'll go over tried-and-true concepts. These are the fundamental ideas and principles that frequently appear on exams. It's critical to understand these concepts because they serve as the foundation of your knowledge in your field.

Finally, we'll review some key points for clinical practice. These are the practical skills and techniques you'll need to master if you want to advance in your career. You can ensure that you have a thorough understanding of the material and are well-prepared for the exam by focusing on these areas. And if you come across a question that stumps you, don't freak out! Simply take a deep breath, relax, and do your best to respond. You never know, it could be one of those "trick" questions that examiners like to include to keep things interesting.

You should feel more confident and prepared to take the exam by the end of this chapter. Remember that even if you only have a short time to study, you can still have a significant impact on your performance. You can make the most of your time and increase your chances of success by taking the right approach. Remember, you've got this—you're an excellent student who is more than capable of performing well on this exam. So don't let something as minor as last-minute studying get

T. Stewart, *Psychiatric-Mental Health Nurse Practitioner Program Companion and Board Certification Exam Review Workbook*,
https://doi.org/10.1007/978-3-031-60894-0

in your way. You'll be able to breeze through that exam and come out on top with a little bit of focus and determination.

To you, my future colleague, *Good Luck*!

1.1 Practice Activities

1. To reduce a patient's chance of developing extrapyramidal symptoms during their first psychotic episode, a PMHNP should consider giving what type of antipsychotic? Why?

2. A PMHNP is working with a patient from a different cultural background. How might the PMHNP determine if they should interpret the signs and symptoms? If there is cultural support, then what are next steps?

3. A 28-year-old woman has been feeling depressed, paranoid, and not sleeping well since she got married 4 months ago. What labs should the PMHNP make sure to include before diagnosing a psychiatric disorder and prescribing medication?

4. What is a general lithium serum level to denote toxicity?

5. Which of the following is false about lithium? Select all that apply.
   __________naturally occurring element
   __________neuroprotective
   __________best for a bipolar depressive episode
   __________decreases suicidal ideation

6. Which of the following will not increase lithium levels? Select all that apply and explain why.
   __________NSAID
   __________hyperkalemia
   __________hypernatremia
   __________thiazides
   __________ACEI
   __________hyponatremia

7. When should a PMHNP refer out the care of a patient to another member of the interprofessional team?

8. A PMHNP is seeing a patient referred by a neuropsychologist after they were diagnosed with ADHD. Which non-stimulant medications are good options for the patient? What is the mechanism of action of these medications?

9. An adolescent patient with ADHD has developed a tic. What might be the etiology of this new tic? How can the PMHNP intervene?

10. A 21-year-old male patient with Bipolar 1 disorder was started on a new medication after a manic episode several months ago. He recently was admitted to the medical floor of the hospital for fever, bleeding gums, fatigue, and pallor. What was his diagnosis? Which medication was he probably started on for his Bipolar 1?

11. Which two mood stabilizers have been documented to cause Stevens-Johnson syndrome? In which populations?

12. Differentiate Oppositional Defiant Disorder and Conduct Disorder in pediatric populations.

ODD	CD

13. A new pediatric patient comes to establish care. He has been diagnosed with Reactive Attachment Disorder. What signs and symptoms would you expect to see in his medical notes and behavior during your meetings?

14. A 52-year-old patient makes an appointment with a PMHNP for anxiety and insomnia. She takes no prescription medications. Labs show elevated liver enzymes, and UA shows dark urine. What might be the cause?

15. Joseph is 48 years old with a history of cirrhosis. He has struggled with depression for years and is seeking a new medication after he has failed several SSRI and SNRI medications. What TCA should his PMHNP avoid?

16. Distinguish tic syndrome from Tourette's.

17. Which three medications are FDA approved to treat Tourette's?

18. Write the neuroanatomical structure(s) where each of the following neurotransmitters is made.

Dopamine	
Norepinephrine	
Acetylcholine	
Serotonin	

19. A patient with schizophrenia presents with newly developed extrapyramidal symptoms. Which dopamine pathway is likely implicated?

20. A patient with schizophrenia presents with galactorrhea. Labs show an elevated prolactin level. Which dopamine pathway is likely implicated?

21. What are the goals of community education programs with regard to mental illness? What makes it an example of a good primary prevention method?

22. You are seeing a pediatric patient and suspect they are being abused. What steps should you take during the appointment time?

23. A foster parent brings in her foster child for a court-required therapy session with the PMHNP. During play therapy, your pediatric patient is engaging in sexual play with the toys. What should you do first? And, what should you not do?

24. You are meeting with a teen patient and are conscious about building trust and rapport. What should you tell the patient about confidentiality?

25. Which ethnic group has the highest rate of suicide in the USA? How might the PMHNP approach working with this population?

26. A Native American patient has been involuntarily hospitalized. He requests to have a carved stick noted for its healing properties in his room. As his PMHNP, what would you decide?

27. While each lab may have its own normal lab values/ranges, what is a normal range of TSH?

28. For hyperthyroid and hypothyroid, identify if the T4, T3, and TSH levels are high or low, and list the key signs and symptoms associated with each.

	T3	T4	TSH	Sx
Hypothyroid				
Hyperthyroid				

29. A patient with Bipolar 1 disorder is on Depakote. Labs show his Depakote level is 157. What does this value tell us? What signs or symptoms, if any, should we expect? What intervention should the PMHNP take?

30. During her pregnancy, Jalissa took Depakote for her Bipolar 1 disorder. Before deciding to stay on this medication, her PMHNP discussed that Depakote is linked to increased risk for ______________________________ in newborns.
31. Kava Kava should not be combined with which types of medications? Why?

32. A patient with Bipolar 1 disorder would like to start a mood stabilizer, but is concerned about weight gain. Which medication might the PMHNP recommend?

33. A patient with schizophrenia would like to switch to an antipsychotic that has lower risk of metabolic effects and sedation. Which medication(s) might the PMHNP recommend?

34. Which values should be tested intermittently in a patient on ziprasidone?

35. A PMHNP has a patient on Clozaril. For each of the following ANC levels, what should the PMHNP's action be?

2500–1501 neutrophils/microL	
1500–1001 neutrophils/microL	
1000–501 neutrophils/microL	
<500 neutrophils/microL	

36. Which labs should be checked before starting a patient on lithium?

37. What teratogenic effect is associated with lithium use during the first trimester?

38. Which symptoms are common negative effects from lithium use?

39. Which symptoms are commonly seen in lithium toxicity?

40. One of your patients with schizophrenia presents to the ED complaining of muscle rigidity, fever, tachycardia, diaphoresis, and confusion. What is diagnosis? What lab values might be expected? How do you treat it?

41. A patient's prescription for Sertraline was recently increased by her PMHNP. The patient took a nap and woke up with a migraine. She then took Sumatriptan. A couple of hours later the patient noted myoclonic jerks and hyperreflexia. What order would you give in the ED?

42. Before switching a patient from an SSRI to an MAOI, a PMHNP should wait at least _______________ days. If the patient was on fluoxetine, then the wait should be at least _______________________ weeks. However, if the patient will switch from an MAOI to fluoxetine, then the wait is just _____________________ weeks.

43. Maria, a 40-year-old Latina, was diagnosed with ovarian cancer. As a result, her depression worsened. She is asking for an antidepressant to help her through this tough time. Which SSRI would be the PMHNP's first-line choice?

44. If a patient is depressed and complains of low energy/fatigue, and have not had luck on SSRIs, which medication may be of particular use? Patients with which medical histories should avoid this medication, however?

45. Casey, a 23-year-old nursing student, endorses unipolar depression and pain. Which medication may be a good choice for her?

46. A PMHNP starting a 12-year-old client on fluoxetine for depression. What information should the PMHNP be sure to share with the client's parents?

47. Why is research on children with depression limited?
    A. Parents don't want their children in research because of the chance they may get placebo.
    B. Children's metabolism is too high and can skew data.
    C. They drop out because they don't want to come to appointments.
    D. Children undergo too many bodily changes and hormone fluctuation.

48. Which psychiatric diagnosis has the highest risk of homicidal behavior?

49. What neuroanatomical structure(s) is often enlarged on MRI imaging studies in persons with schizophrenia?

50. Aggression and impulsivity in patients with schizophrenia are associated with which areas of the brain?

51. For each of the following, identify if it is associated with the amygdala (A), hippocampus (H), or both (B).
__________fear
__________stress
__________anxiety
__________aggression
__________learning
__________emotions
__________memory

52. Which of the following prescription medications could potentiate positive symptoms of schizophrenia? (Select all that apply.)
A. Methylphenidate
B. Lorazepam
C. Amantadine
D. Trazodone

53. One of your patients with schizophrenia has had numerous involuntary hospitalizations over the past 2 years. The patient does not adhere to their medication schedule? What is ACT, and why might this be a plausible option for this patient?

54. Nursing students organize a social skills training for patients with schizophrenia. They learn proper greetings, conversation skills, and culturally appropriate ways to ask for help. Would this be considered primary, secondary, or tertiary prevention? Why?

55. Explain how to calculate long-term antipsychotic injections doses.

56. A patient may not receive more than __________________ of Haldol at once. They would need to come back in a week to receive the remaining dose.

57. Mirtazapine and venlafaxine are least likely to cause __________________ __________________________________.

58. Explain the differences between thought content and thought processes.

59. Label each of the following examples as linear (L), tangential (T), or circumstantial(C) thought process.

__________ "I went shopping for milk and then came home."

__________ "I was thinking about going to the store and then I saw a bird outside and it reminded me of the time I went on a hike and saw a bird like that. Oh, and I need to get some milk."

__________ "I was thinking about going to the store. I mean, I need milk, but it's a long way away. And traffic can be horrendous. Perhaps I should simply order it online. However, I would have to wait for it to be delivered. Oh, I'm not sure. "How do you think I should proceed?"

__________ "I was walking to the store the other day when I noticed this dog by the side of the road. And then I remembered how I used to have a dog when I was a kid, and how much fun it was. Then I realized how much I miss having a dog now and how I should probably get another one. But then I wondered if I'd have enough time to care for a dog, or if I could even afford one. Then I remembered how much I miss my old dog and how much I wish I could have it back. And then I realized I was already at the store and hadn't realized it."

_________ "I was just thinking about going to the store, but then I remembered that I didn't have my keys. So I had to return inside to retrieve them. Then I saw a commercial on TV for a new brand of chips. They looked fantastic. Have you given them a shot yet? Oh, and then I noticed this cat outside, which reminded me of a pet I had as a child. She was so fluffy and amusing. I used to have a lot of fun playing with her. What was I on about, again?"

__________ "I was thinking we should go to that new Italian restaurant downtown. At 7:00, we could meet there." "What are your thoughts?"

60. Another name for the Mini Mental Status exam is the ________________________ Scale.

61. The clock drawing test is a screen for neurological problems and takes only 1–2 min. If done incorrectly, the patient may have damage to the right __________________________ lobe.

62. A patient gets an infection. He is currently taking atorvastatin, carbamazepine, and levothyroxine. Which antibiotics should the prescriber avoid?

63. In the table below, list medications that may cause mania or depression.

Mania	Depression

64. Which medication may be linked to the onset of mania in bipolar patients?
   A. Ibuprofen
   B. Interferon

C. Isoniazid
D. Isotretinoin

65. If a patient is taking an inducer medication and an inhibitor medication, the prescriber should make changes based on the ______________________ __________.

66. A patient is on olanzapine. He also is a smoker. During a recent visit, the patient mentions that he stopped smoking a month ago. What changes, if any, should be made to his olanzapine prescription?

67. Normal prolactin levels for men is ________________ and for women is __________________. Long-term high levels of prolactin has been associated with the development of ____________________________________.

68. Victor, a 35-year-old Russian patient with well-managed schizophrenia, visits your clinic to establish care. He reports sexual dysfunction and gynecomastia. Labs show his prolactin level is 27 ng/mL. Which antipsychotic medication is Victor likely taking? Why does this medication cause these side effects?

69. Which of the dopamine pathways is associated with positive symptoms of schizophrenia?

70. Why does a reduction in dopamine levels in the nigrostriatal pathway cause motor movement dysfunction?

71. ______________________________ for nausea and vomiting increases the risk for tardive dyskinesia.

72. What are common symptoms of tardive dyskinesia?

73. Which pair of neurotransmitters is most associated with addiction?
    A. Serotonin and norepinephrine
    B. Dopamine and acetylcholine
    C. GABA and dopamine
    D. GABA and glutamate

74. Parents bring in their 16-year-old daughter to the ED. Their daughter is endorsing insomnia, tremors, irritability, agitation, and mood swings. Which substance is the teenager most likely abusing?

75. Which medication is not linked to delayed gastric emptying?
    A. Semaglutide
    B. Famotidine
    C. Omeprazole
    D. Aripiprazole

76. A 17-year-old ice skater comes to the ED after fainting. He is 70″ tall and weighs 134 lbs. What signs and symptoms might the PMHNP expect to see on examination? What diagnosis might be likely?

77. Proton pump inhibitors (e.g., pantoprazole) can decrease the absorption of other medications. Therefore, patients should be educated to wait ______________ hours before taking their psychiatric medications.

78. Geriatric patients on SSRIs should be monitored for increased ____________ __________________________.

79. What is apoptosis?

80. If a patient older than 45 years is diagnosed with bipolar disorder, the etiology of this disorder may be due to a(n)________________________________.

81. In addition to a lack of sleep, what signs and symptoms may present during a manic episode? Use the DIGFAST mnemonic.

D	
I	
G	
F	
A	
S	
T	

82. Individuals with Borderline Personality Disorder often exhibit recurrent ______________________ behavior. Marsha Linehan's ________________ ______________________ therapy has been shown to decrease episodes of this behavior.

83. If a patient with Borderline Personality Disorder endorses depressed mood and emotional lability, ________________________________ is the recommended mood stabilizer to prescribe.

84. What is conversion disorder? What is its etiology? Provide an example.

85. The parents of a 6-year-old boy bring their son in for an appointment. The child has been crying, experiencing insomnia, having peer conflicts at school, and arguing with siblings and parents. His family moved a couple of months ago right before the start of the school year. What diagnoses might the PMHNP consider?

86. In the table below, differentiate factitious disorder from malingering.

Factitious disorder	Malingering

87. Acute stress disorder can be diagnosed if the symptoms are present for less than ____________ month(s). If symptoms are present for longer, then a diagnosis of ____________________________________ should be considered.

88. What therapeutic interventions are useful for patients with PTSD who are experiencing hyperarousal, flashbacks, and nightmares?

89. Individuals with panic disorder experience episodes of impending doom. First-line medications to treat panic attacks and panic disorder may include ______________________________ and ______________________________.

90. Individuals with what respiratory element should not be prescribed β-blockers? Why?

91. What medications may be useful for patients who experience performance anxiety?

92. What neurotransmitters are implicated in ADHD? How do each of these manifest in signs or symptoms associated with ADHD?

93. The ________________________________ is the site of executive function in the brain. Signals for attention, cognitive processing, working memory, and problem-solving are centered here.

94. When should aftercare planning begin?

95. A 10-year-old is recovering from a strep throat infection. What behaviors should the parents watch for after the strep infection clears?

96. The neurotransmitters ______________________________ and ______________________ are implicated in Obsessive-Compulsive Disorder. For this reason, clomipramine may be useful.

97. A patient who endorses nightmares should be asked if any nuclear family members have a history of nightmares.
TRUE FALSE

98. Generalized Anxiety Disorder is characterized by excessive worry, fear, or apprehension lasting at least __________ months.

99. Explain the Broken Mirror Theory of Autism Spectrum Disorder.

100. Which neurotransmitters are implicated in Autism Spectrum Disorder?

101. Parents bring in their young child because they are concerned that he may have Autism Spectrum Disorder. What behaviors of concern might the parents tell the PMHNP that they are noticing? When the child is playing with toys in the PMHNP's office, what actions might the child do with the toys?

102. For each of the following, label if the behavior or description is more associated with delirium (Dl), dementia (Dm), or both (B).
    ___________Acute onset, disturbance of consciousness and cognition
    ___________Inattention
    ___________Meds = haldol if agitation, psychosis
    ___________Avoid benzos
    ___________Do urinalysis with culture and sensitivity, esp. in older female patients
    ___________Progressive, chronic
    ___________Irritable
    ___________Personality changes
    ___________Check folic acid and B12
    ___________Will try to answer, laugh, or confabulate by making up answer

103. Subcortical dementia is associated with ________________________ infection. Patients will exhibit motor and behavioral abnormalities, decline in concentration, and lack of coordination. Antiretroviral therapy is the treatment.

104. What is pseudodementia? How does it present? In which population?

105. Individuals with ______________________________ will endorse visual hallucinations and Parkinson-like symptoms simultaneously.

106. Another name for Frontotemporal Dementia is ______________________________. It is more often seen in men, who show changes in ______________________________, ______________________________, and ______________________________.

107. The PMHNP receives lab results for a pediatric patient who lives in a rural area. The patient has elevated lead levels. What signs and symptoms might be expected in this child?

108. What are risk factors for osteoporosis?

109. The PMHNP is working on the Consultant Liaison service in the hospital. She is called to Labor and Delivery because a newborn was born prematurely and is not expected to live much longer. The team would like to provide support to the parents during this tragic time. The PMHNP arrives and asks where the parents and newborn are located. The newborn is in an incubator adjacent to the mother's room. The nurses tell the PMHNP that the baby may have less than an hour to live. What actions should the PMHNP take?

110. Grief follows a fairly linear trajectory for most individuals.

TRUE FALSE

111. Provide a brief explanation and examples of techniques for each of the following therapies.

Therapy	Explanation	Techniques
Cognitive therapy		
Behavioral therapy		
Cognitive-behavioral therapy		

Therapy	Explanation	Techniques
Humanistic therapy		
Multisystemic family therapy		
Interpersonal therapy		
Strategic therapy		
Solution-focused therapy		
Family systems therapy		
Structural family therapy		

112. What are the psychological benefits to children engaging in physical activity?

113. A PMHNP has a patient who is moving out of state. What steps should the provider take to ease the patient's transition?

114. Parents are concerned that their 4-year-old son often plays with his penis. What might the PMHNP tell the parents?

115. During an appointment, an 11-year-old boy confides to the PMHNP that he is "growing boobs" and that they are sore. How should the PMHNP react?

116. Why are women more likely to get drunk and develop alcohol-related liver problems than men who drink the same amount and type of alcohol?

117. Babies will have a palmar grasp and startle reflex until ____________ month(s). Babinski fanning of their toes will be present until a maximum of ____________________ year(s), however.

118. What are phosphodiesterase-5 inhibitors used for? What is the mechanism of action? Give examples of this medication and of any medications which should be avoided while taking a PDE-5 inhibitor.

119. A patient has a BMI of 21, yet she is diagnosed with an eating disorder. Which eating disorder is most likely her diagnosis and why?

120. The legal principle of ______________________________ protects individuals against unlawful hospitalization.

121. Before educating on medication, a provider should first assess what a patient knows or believes about the medication.

TRUE FALSE

122. The labs for a patient with an autoimmune disease would most likely show an (increased/decreased) cytokine level.

123. A PMHNP refers an adult patient with enuresis to their primary care provider. What medication might the PMHNP expect the PCP to prescribe for the patient if the patient cannot take anticholinergic medications? Why?

124. Psychiatric nurses on the night shift admit a patient who claims to be a famous Nigerian rapper. They look up the patient on social media to confirm his story. Is this allowed? Why/why not?

125. A patient goes to pick up their medication from the pharmacy. The pharmacist tells them that a new black box warning has been issued on this medication. The patient is concerned and calls her PMHNP. What should the PMHNP do?

126. Psychiatric medication prescribers often use medications off label. What should a prescriber tell the patient when prescribing a medication off label?

127. What is the goal of reflective practice for a PMHNP? What are some forms of reflective practice that hospital-based healthcare teams can engage in?

128. For each of the following scales, provide the total possible score range, and then how the score breaks down for each level.

Mental status

MMSE (________)	SLUM (________)
Normal = ________ Mild = ________ Moderate = ________ Severe = ________	Normal = ________ Mild = ________ Dementia = ________

Depression

HAM D (0–76)	PHQ-9 (0–27)	Beck (0–63)
Normal = ________ Mild = ________ Moderate = ________ Severe = ________ Very severe = ________	Normal = ________ Mild = ________ Moderate = ________ Moderate to severe = ________ Severe = ________	Normal = ________ Mild = ________ Moderate = ________ Severe = ________

Anxiety

HAM A (________)	GAD (________)
Mild = ________ Moderate = ________ Severe = ________	Normal = ________ Mild = ________ Moderate = ________ Severe = ________

Withdrawal

COWS (opioid)	CIWA (alcohol)
Normal = ________ Mild = ________ Moderate = ________ Moderate to severe = ________ Severe = ________ Start treatment at score > ________	Normal = ________ Mild = ________ Moderate = ________ Severe = ________ Start treatment at score > ________

129. Arrhythmias can be caused by ________________________, which is used to treat opioid addiction.

130. If a patient scores "moderate" on the COWS scale, it is recommended that they be started on ________________________.

131. For the COWS and CIWA assessments, provide a list of signs and symptoms that the rater will be looking for.

COWS	CIWA

132. Which medication used for alcohol use disorder is not metabolized in the liver?

133. What is appreciative inquiry?

134. What are the key components to Yalom's therapy model?

135. What are some rights of patients?

136. A patient presents to the ED in an acute psychotic episode. This is their first psychotic event. What are three medications that might be the best choices for this patient? Why?

137. Explain the Recovery Model and how its emphasis may differ from other models.

138. The four-point Quality Improvement model is comprised of ________, ________, ________, and ________. QI aims to improve systems, decrease costs, and improve productivity in general.

139. What is SBIRT?

140. During a clinic visit, a patient threatens to kill his ex-wife for asking for more child support. What action should the PMHNP take? Why?

141. An involuntarily committed patient who has not been found incompetent, absent an emergency, has a qualified right to refuse psychotropic medication as upheld in the court case ______________________________ __________.

142. The court case ______________________________ ruled that if an individual is not posing a danger to self or others and is capable of living without state supervision, the state has no right to commit the individual to a facility against his or her will.

143. Piaget's ____________________ stage is associated with magical thinking. It is seen in children aged 2–7.

144. Evelyn is a senior in high school. She is enrolled in AP classes and won the science fair. Her teachers are amazed by her logic, ability to test hypotheses, and abstract thinking. Evelyn would be considered in Piaget's __________ ____________________ stage.

145. A fifth grader constantly questions his competence when comparing himself to his classmates. His struggles evidence the crises that school-aged children undergo in Erikson's ______________________________ ___ stage.

146. List as many risk factors and protective factors for suicide that you can.

Risk factors	Protective factors

1.2 Answers to Practice Activities

1. A PMHNP may prescribe a low-potency or atypical antipsychotic to reduce extrapyramidal symptoms (EPS) in a first psychotic episode. These antipsychotics cause fewer extrapyramidal effects than high-potency or typical ones. Antipsychotics can generate extrapyramidal effects. Muscle spasms, tremors, rigidity, and unusual motions occur. All antipsychotics can cause EPS although high-potency or typical ones are more common. Low-potency or atypical antipsychotics are better tolerated and less likely to induce side effects.

2. PMHNPs should question patients from other cultures to interpret their symptoms or explain their meaning. This helps the PMHNP rule out mental illness and assess culturally typical symptoms. If the patient's symptoms are cultural, the PMHNP should provide brief supportive therapy, use the Cultural Formulation Interview (CFI) to clarify the patient's illness or condition, contextualize it in the local culture and surroundings, and empower the patient to participate in their care.
3. The PMHNP should order the following labs before diagnosing and prescribing medication for a 28-year-old woman with depression, paranoia, and sleep disorders since getting married 4 months ago:
   - Complete blood count: This test counts red, white, and platelets.
   - Blood thyroid hormones and TSH are tested for thyroid function.
   - Enzyme and protein tests assess liver function.
   - The PMHNP should order a pregnancy test for reproductive-age patients.
4. Lithium often treats bipolar disorder. It lowers suicide risk and mood swings. Toxic lithium levels often exceed 1.5 mEq/L. PMHNPs may order lithium blood tests. The toxicity of lithium depends on age, weight, kidney function, and concomitant medicines. To minimize more complications, the PMHNP should quickly lower lithium levels if they sense risk. Lithium may be reduced, stopped, or patients given IV fluids.
5. Lithium works better for manic or hypomanic bipolar illness episodes than depression.
6. Too much salt can hinder lithium absorption and efficiency. Kidneys filter lithium from the small intestine and excrete it in urine. Sodium aids lithium absorption and excretion. High salt limits renal lithium reabsorption, increasing lithium clearance.
7. If the patient has a complex or severe mental health issue that requires additional therapy, the PMHNP may recommend them to a psychiatrist or psychologist. Patients may also need to see a primary care physician and/or social worker if comorbid medical conditions or social issues are complicating mental health concern. Referrals to an interprofessional team member may be warranted if a different perspective would be useful.
8. Non-stimulant medicines may help neuropsychologist-referred ADHD patients. A few examples:
   - SNRI atomoxetine addresses ADHD in children and adults. Increased brain norepinephrine increases focus.
   - Blood pressure medication clonidine decreases ADHD impulsivity and hyperactivity. Active brain alpha-2 adrenergic receptors reduce ADHD symptoms and neurotransmitter activity.
   - Guanfacine relieves hypertension like clonidine. It lowers ADHD hyperactivity and impulsivity. Active brain alpha-2 adrenergic receptors reduce ADHD symptoms and neurotransmitter activity.
9. Teen ADHD tics are often ambiguous. Tics are involuntary, repetitive movements or sounds caused by several factors. The tic can be inherited or can result from dopamine and serotonin abnormalities. Tics can also result from stress and medicines. To evaluate if ADHD teenagers' tics are causing

considerable impairment or distress, the PMHNP should examine their intensity and frequency. The PMHNP may refer the patient to a specialist for further evaluation and treatment if the tic causes serious disability or suffering. The PMHNP can teach patients and families how to manage tics. PMHNPs can also help patients identify and control tic triggers like stress and medicine side effects. PMHNPs may need to change patients' treatment plans or refer them to other doctors.

10. Bipolar disorder and seizures are treated with carbamazepine. It inhibits brain ion channels and neurotransmitter release. Aplastic anemia is rare and severe when the bone marrow fails to produce enough blood cells. Drugs, infections, and autoimmune diseases can cause it. Aplastic anemia symptoms include tiredness, shortness of breath, and easy bruising or bleeding require medical attention.
11. Rare yet dangerous skin and mucous membrane condition Stevens-Johnson syndrome is a blistering red rash that kills and sheds the top layer of skin. Carbamazepine is particularly risky for Asians with HLAB*1502 allele. Lamictal may be risky for all groups if titrated too quickly.
12. Kids can have ODD/CD. ODD and CD involve disruptive and aggressive behavior, but there are key differences. Defiance, arguing, and noncooperation are ODD symptoms. ODD kids oppose authority, disobey rules, and defy convention. They may be irritated and angry. Little aggression is present. Most ODD cases are in 6–18-year-olds. Family therapy is the first defense. Practice child control, positive reinforcement, and boundaries. A more serious condition, CD is aggressive and destructive. Some suspect ODD progression. Combative, violent, and vandalous CD youths may conduct other crimes. Others may be indifferent to their behavior. Children over 10 are diagnosed with CD most often. Treatments for mood and aggression include medication and therapy.
13. Reactive Attachment Disorder can result from early caregiver disturbances including abuse, neglect, or several caregivers (e.g., foster children). Friendships may be difficult for RAD kids. Shy, avoidant kids may be inhibited RAD. Disinhibited RAD kids may act erratically and have impulse control issues. PMHNPs may identify certain symptoms in new pediatric RAD patients' medical notes and meetings. Possible RAD symptoms:
    - Building and maintaining strong relationships is hard
    - Social apathy
    - Trouble showing emotion
    - Lacking self-control and patience
    - Trouble obeying rules misconduct or aggression
    - Trouble connecting
14. For many causes, a 52-year-old anxiety and insomnia patient without medicines may have elevated liver enzymes and dark urine. Causes may include:
    - High liver enzymes may indicate cirrhosis, hepatitis, or fatty liver.
    - Dark urine may suggest dehydration.

- In high doses, over-the-counter acetaminophen can damage the liver and elevate liver enzymes.
- Over-the-counter anxiety and insomnia medications may elevate liver enzymes and discolor urine. Kava is a popular OTC psychiatric medication.
- Alcohol misuse raises liver enzymes and damages the liver.

15. Tricyclic antidepressants (TCAs) treat mood disorders like depression. They inhibit serotonin and norepinephrine reuptake. The PMHNP should not give amitriptyline to Joseph, a 48-year-old depressive patient who has failed various SSRI and SNRI medicines. Taking amitriptyline can damage the liver.
16. Tic syndrome and Tourette's syndrome cause involuntary movements and sounds. These conditions differ greatly. Non-medical tics define tic syndrome. Tic syndrome can develop at any age and usually resolves. Tic syndrome rarely affects cognition or behavior. Tourette's syndrome is neurodevelopmental and causes motor and vocal tics. In childhood, Tourette's syndrome is connected to ADHD and OCD. Tourette's demands long-term treatment.
17. Many Tourette's medicines are FDA approved. Some medication options include:
    - Haloperidol lowers Tourette's tics.
    - Tourette's tics are reduced by pimozide.
    - Fluphenazine lowers Tourette's tics.
    - Atypical antipsychotic aripiprazole affects dopamine and serotonin.
18.

Dopamine	Substantia nigra and ventral tegmental area
Norepinephrine	Locus coeruleus
Acetylcholine	Nucleus of Meynert
Serotonin	Raphe nuclei
GABA	Hippocampus and amygdala

19. Antipsychotics may cause EPS. Tremors, rigidity, akathisia, and dystonia appear in EPS. Through the nigrostriatal pathway, dopamine travels from the substantia nigra to the basal ganglia. Dysregulated nigrostriatal systems cause EPS tremors and stiffness.
20. Prolactin increases breast milk production. Dopamine controls prolactin. The hypothalamus sends dopamine to the pituitary gland via the tuberoinfundibular canal. The tuberoinfundibular pathway dysregulation causes galactorrhea by increasing prolactin.
21. Community education projects reduce stigma and increasing awareness of mental health issues and their treatment. By providing realistic information, these initiatives help communities recognize the signs of mental illness, promote early diagnosis, and connect individuals with local resources for support and treatment. Additionally, community education helps individuals and families manage mental health conditions effectively, improving their overall quality of life. These projects serve as primary prevention methods, focusing on avoiding mental health issues and reducing their impact through early

detection and education, ultimately reaching a broader audience and benefiting both individuals and communities.

22. During a pediatric appointment when there is suspicion of abuse, several important steps should be taken. First, it is crucial to create a safe and comfortable environment for the patient, considering their emotional well-being. Obtain informed consent from the patient if they are capable of understanding, and follow your state's child abuse evaluation requirements if they cannot consent. Document any findings related to abuse, including injuries such as bruises or wounds, specifying their location, size, and characteristics. Engage in non-judgmental questioning to gather information about the patient's situation, paying close attention to their directives. It is mandatory to report suspected abuse to the appropriate authorities in accordance with your state's laws, prioritizing the safety and well-being of the patient. After interviewing the child and caregiver, consider making inquiries with Child Protective Services (CPS) to ensure the child's protection and support.
23. If a child engages with toys sexually during treatment, do these steps:
    - Relax and don't overreact to behavior. This will make patients feel comfortable and supported.
    - Discover behavior meaning: Question the patient about sexual play. Approach the action from the patient's perspective rather than assuming its interpretation.
    - Talk about these limits: Discuss patient behavior and boundaries. Inappropriate touching and sexual misconduct are unacceptable.
    - Behavior tracking: Keep track of the play, patient ideas and feelings, and interventions and conversations.
    - Ignoring the behavior may send the message that it's OK or discourage the patient from talking about their feelings. Reacting too much may embarrass or misunderstand the patient, hurting the therapeutic interaction. Do not assume patient motivations or behavior. Be receptive to the patient's behavior. Avoid touching the child, urging them to stop, reading and taking notes, and talking to caretakers.
24. Maintaining a safe and supportive therapeutic relationship with young patients hinges on establishing trust and open communication regarding confidentiality. Healthcare professionals should clearly define the boundaries of patient confidentiality, emphasizing that it is upheld unless there is a risk of imminent harm or abuse. It's crucial to discuss the limitations of confidentiality, especially in cases where a patient's safety or the safety of others is at stake. By explaining the significance of confidentiality in therapy and its role in building trust, healthcare providers can enhance the therapeutic alliance. Additionally, honesty is vital in explaining any exceptions to confidentiality and clarifying what information can and cannot be shared with the patient.
25. American Indian/Alaska Native (AI/AN) populations experience alarmingly high suicide rates, which are twice as high as the general population, as reported by the CDC. Several factors contribute to these rates, including historical trauma resulting from forced migration, cultural genocide, and racism,

which can have long-lasting effects on AI/AN mental health. Geographical isolation of AI/AN communities can lead to feelings of loneliness and detachment from necessary support systems, while cultural barriers and a shortage of mental health professionals can limit access to mental healthcare. To address these challenges, psychiatric-mental health nurse practitioners (PMHNPs) should provide culturally sensitive care, respecting AI/AN customs and potentially collaborating with indigenous representatives or cultural liaisons. Trauma-informed treatment is essential for many AI/AN individuals, recognizing the mental health impact of trauma and offering safe and supportive care. Active engagement with AI/AN populations through community-based initiatives may be more effective than traditional treatment approaches, and PMHNPs should seek informed consent when considering involving patient-culture shamans or healers in the care process.

26. When dealing with involuntarily hospitalized Native American patients, PMHNPs should take into account their cultural and spiritual practices, including the use of a healing-infused carved stick. The selection of such a tool involves careful considerations. Patient and public safety must be a top priority, and any sharp or potentially dangerous carved sticks should not be allowed in the room. The therapeutic value of the carved stick should also be assessed, as it may contribute to calming the patient. Additionally, it is essential to respect the patient's cultural, spiritual, and carved stick preferences to demonstrate cultural awareness and respect for their traditions.
27. TSH is normalized differently by lab and test. The usual TSH range is 0.4–4.0 mU/L. Since test laboratories have varied normal ranges.
28.

	T3	T4	TSH	Sx
Hypothyroid	Low	Low	High	Cold, lethargic, weight gain, decreased libido, depression, goiter, constipation
Hyperthyroid	High	High	Low	Hot, agitated, anxious, irritable, achy, mood swings, weight loss, manic, goiter

29. >150 mcg/mL is a toxic Depakote level (normal range is 50–125 mcg/mL); the patient may experience disorientation, lethargy, respiratory depression, nausea, vomiting, elevated AST/ALT, RUQ pain, jaundice, and dark urine. The PMHNP should discontinue the medication, check for interactions with other medications, and monitor liver function tests and ammonia levels.
30. Spina Bifida (neural tube defects).
31. Kava kava has potential interactions with several drugs that should be avoided. It may enhance the sedative effects of benzodiazepines and alcohol, leading to drowsiness. Additionally, kava kava can impair the effectiveness of antipsychotic medications and interact with TCAs and selective serotonin reuptake inhibitors (SSRIs), possibly increasing side effects or toxicity. Furthermore, it may augment the sedation caused by hypnotic or Z-drug medications, potentially resulting in excessive sleepiness and respiratory depression.

32. Lamotrigine may not induce weight gain (Lamictal). Patients with Bipolar 1 disorder often take lamotrigine as a mood stabilizer. Clinical investigations have indicated that lamotrigine causes less weight gain than valproate (Depakote) or lithium. Lamotrigine may still cause weight gain in some patients, so it's crucial to discuss the risks and benefits with a doctor before starting it.
33. Aripiprazole, clozapine, and lurasidone have reduced weight gain and sedation.
34. Ziprasidone (Geodon) is prescribed for the treatment of conditions like schizophrenia and bipolar disorder, and it requires careful monitoring of specific parameters to ensure patient safety. The monitoring needs and healthcare provider's recommendations will determine which values should be periodically evaluated. These include regular checks of blood pressure and heart rate due to potential increases caused by ziprasidone. Additionally, monitoring cholesterol and triglyceride levels is essential since ziprasidone may elevate them. Regular blood sugar testing is also necessary because ziprasidone can affect blood glucose levels. Lastly, due to its potential impact on heart electrical activity, particularly the QTc interval, ECG (electrocardiogram) checks should be performed regularly to ensure the patient's well-being and safety.
35.

2500–1501	This is considered normal, and the PMHNP should continue with the current therapy.
1500–1001	The PMHNP should check the ANC again in a few days, closely monitor the patient, and consider adjusting the Clozaril dose as needed.
1000–501	The PMHNP should discontinue the medication, monitor the ANC until it is greater than 1500, and then resume the medication as if it were a new prescription, gradually increasing the dose as needed.
<500	The patient should be admitted to the hospital for further evaluation and management by the PMHNP.

36. CBC, electrolytes, TSH, T3/T4, creatinine, BUN, and HCG if applicable.
37. Lithium consumption in the first trimester can cause Ebstein's anomaly. Rare congenital cardiac condition, Ebstein's abnormality affects the tricuspid valve.
38. Hypothyroidism, tremors, rash, T wave inversions, GI distress, polydipsia, polyuria, diabetes insipidus, leukocytosis, and sleepiness.
39. A lithium level >1.5 causes nausea, vomiting, diarrhea, disorientation, tremors, tiredness, muscle weakness, heart palpitations, unsteadiness, seizures, and coma.
40. Clients on antipsychotics with muscle rigidity, fever, tachycardia, diaphoresis, and confusion are likely to have neuroleptic malignant syndrome (NMS) in the ER. NMS is rare but deadly and can result from side effects of antipsychotics. Creatine kinase increase, myoglobinuria, leukocytosis, and raised liver function tests; cease offending medicine and give Bromocriptine (D2 agonist) and Dantrolene.
41. Sertraline (an SSRI) users who experience myoclonic jerks and hyperreflexia after taking sumatriptan (a migraine drug) may have serotonin syndrome.

High serotonin levels can cause serotonin syndrome, a deadly illness. Orders may include:

- Stopping serotonin-raising medications: In this instance, the doctor may reduce or alter sertraline and also stop the migraine medication.
- Fluids and drugs may be given to treat fever, muscle rigidity, and other serotonin syndrome symptoms.
- Your doctor may prescribe cyproheptadine or chlorpromazine to reduce serotonin levels and treat serotonin syndrome.

42. 14 days; 5–6 weeks; 2 weeks.
43. Drug interactions are lower with (es-)citalopram. They may be an excellent alternative for cancer patients because they rarely interact with other cancer drugs. For cancer patients who need to stay attentive and functional, SSRIs do not cause drowsiness or cognitive impairment like other antidepressants.
44. Bupropion is an NDRI. It promotes energy without sexual negative effects like other antidepressants. This medicine reduces the seizure threshold, thus patients with a history of seizures and eating disorders should avoid it.
45. Cymbalta (duloxetine) helps depression and pain. Blocking brain serotonin and norepinephrine reuptake improves mood and reduces depression.
46. When initiating a child or adolescent on fluoxetine (or any other depression medication), the PMHNP must inform the parents about several crucial points. First, they should explain the reason for starting fluoxetine, ensuring parents understand how it will treat depression. The PMHNP should also discuss the benefits of fluoxetine, such as its potential to enhance mood and functioning, while also addressing its potential dangers and side effects, including common ones like nausea, diarrhea, and headache, as well as rare but serious adverse effects like suicidal thoughts or acts. Parents should be informed about the need for monitoring and follow-up appointments, as fluoxetine may take weeks to work, and the child's symptoms and behavior need continuous assessment. Finally, any additional concerns or questions parents have regarding their child's medication, including diet, other medications, and potential interactions or contraindications, should be discussed. Additionally, it's important to note that during the first month of medication, all antidepressants can increase pediatric suicidal thoughts, and fluoxetine, in particular, may cause insomnia if taken at night, so parents should administer it in the morning with breakfast. Parents should also monitor the child for alcohol use, which can exacerbate depression and interfere with medications.
47. (A) Parents don't want their children in research because of the chance they may get placebo. Other reasons include stigma, restricted access, diagnostic difficulty, and ethics.
48. Most people with psychiatric disorders are not violent or dangerous. Antisocial personality disorder (sociopathy or psychopathy) is a psychiatric condition characterized by disrespect for others' rights and a lack of remorse or empathy. Not all people with antisocial personality disorder commit violent or homicidal acts although they are more prone to do so. Substance addiction, a history of violence, and access to firearms are other risk factors for violent

conduct in people with antisocial personality disorder or other psychiatric problems.

49. Schizophrenia often enlarges the brain's lateral ventricles, which produce and circulate cerebrospinal fluid. Lateral ventricle enlargement is present in up to 75% of schizophrenia patients and may indicate aberrant brain development. The amygdala, which processes emotions, and the hippocampus, which stores memories and navigates space, may also be enlarged in schizophrenia. These brain abnormalities may cause schizophrenia's cognitive, emotional, and behavioral symptoms.
50. Schizophrenia may enhance aggression and impulsivity due to amygdala dysfunction. The prefrontal cortex, which regulates emotion and behavior, and the basal ganglia, which control movement and decision-making, are also linked to aggression and impulsivity in schizophrenia patients.
51.
    __A__ Fear
    __B__ Stress
    __B__ Anxiety
    __B__ Aggression
    __A__ Learning
    __A__ Emotions
    __H__ Memory
52. (A and C) Methylphenidate may worsen schizophrenia symptoms. It boosts brain chemicals like dopamine. Positive symptoms like hallucinations and delusions may worsen in schizophrenia patients with high dopamine levels. Amantadine, an antiviral, can treat Parkinson's disease. It boosts brain dopamine. Positive symptoms may worsen in schizophrenia patients with high dopamine levels.
53. Assertive Community Treatment (ACT) is intense community-based mental health treatment for severe mental diseases like schizophrenia. ACT teams often include psychiatrists, nurses, social workers, and peer support specialists. These professionals work with the patient to create a customized treatment plan. ACT teams help with medication management, therapy, social skills training, and daily living chores like budgeting and housing. ACT may help patients who have undergone many involuntary hospitalizations due to medication nonadherence.
54. Patients need social skills training for tertiary prevention. Tertiary prevention minimizes disease or condition effects. It involves interventions to help people with persistent or chronic problems maintain or improve their quality of life. Schizophrenia patients receive social skills training to improve their community functioning and interpersonal abilities. This can reduce the harmful effects of schizophrenia on their daily lives and improve their quality of life.
55. Determine how much oral medication the patient takes daily. Multiply by 20 for high risk. A patient taking 10 mg/day × 20 would receive a 200 mg

injection at the month's start. Once you've reached maintenance, multiply daily dose by 10–15. Thus, the monthly dose would be 100–150 mg.

56. 100 mg.
57. Sexual dysfunction, SIADH/hyponatremia.
58. Thought content is what someone is thinking about. They perceive, believe, and interpret events and situations. How a person thinks and arranges their thoughts is called thought processes. This involves thinking logic, coherence, and clarity. Thus, thought content is what someone thinks about and thought processes are how they think about it. In schizophrenia, depression, and anxiety disorders, either can be dysfunctional.
59.

_____L_______ "I went shopping for milk and then came home."

_____T_____ "I was thinking about going to the store and then I saw a bird outside and it reminded me of the time I went on a hike and saw a bird like that. Oh, and I need to get some milk."

_____C_____ "I was thinking about going to the store. I mean, I need milk, but it's a long way away. And traffic can be horrendous. Perhaps I should simply order it online. However, I would have to wait for it to be delivered. Oh, I'm not sure. "How do you think I should proceed?"

_____C_____ "I was walking to the store the other day when I noticed this dog by the side of the road. And then I remembered how I used to have a dog when I was a kid, and how much fun it was. Then I realized how much I miss having a dog now and how I should probably get another one. But then I wondered if I'd have enough time to care for a dog, or if I could even afford one. Then I remembered how much I miss my old dog and how much I wish I could have it back. And then I realized I was already at the store and hadn't realized it."

____T_____ "I was just thinking about going to the store, but then I remembered that I didn't have my keys. So I had to return inside to retrieve them. Then I saw a commercial on TV for a new brand of chips. They looked fantastic. Have you given them a shot yet? Oh, and then I noticed this cat outside, which reminded me of a pet I had as a child. She was so fluffy and amusing. I used to have a lot of fun playing with her. What was I on about, again?."

____L_______" "I was thinking we should go to that new Italian restaurant downtown. At 7:00, we could meet there. "What are your thoughts?"

60. Folstein Scale/Test.
61. The clock drawing exam evaluates neurological function by drawing a clock face with the numbers in the correct placements. This may indicate right parietal lobe injury if done incorrectly. The parietal lobe processes spatial information and orients people.
62. Clarithromycin and erythromycin are inhibitors and may boost carbamazepine levels, thus the prescriber should avoid these. This can cause aplastic anemia and agranulocytosis. The prescriber must discuss safer antibiotics with the patient.

63.

Mania	Depression
Steroids (including nasal sprays)	Steroids (can cause psychosis)
Disulfiram	Beta-blockers
Isoniazid	Interferon
SSRIs	Isotretinoin (Accutane)
	Retrovirals
	Antineoplastics
	Benzodiazepines
	Progesterone

64. (C) Isoniazid may be linked to the onset of mania in bipolar patients.
65. The prescriber should make changes based on the inhibitor because it may raise the level of the inducer medication in the body, potentially leading to overdose or negative side effects.
66. Reduce the olanzapine dose because he is no longer using nicotine, which is an inducer.
67. Normal prolactin levels for men are typically less than 20 ng/mL, while normal levels for women are typically less than 25 ng/mL. Long-term prolactin levels have been linked to the development of galactorrhea, osteoporosis, breast cysts, Parkinson's disease, and ovarian cancer.
68. The tuberoinfundibular pathway is influenced by risperidone. Although paliperidone and olanzapine may also have this effect, risperidone is the most commonly associated with it.
69. Positive symptoms of schizophrenia, such as hallucinations and delusions, are associated with the mesolimbic pathway. The mesolimbic pathway connects the ventral tegmental area (VTA) to the nucleus accumbens in the brain.
70. Parkinson's disease can develop from nigrostriatal dopamine insufficiency, which increases acetylcholine activity. Because dopamine inhibits the nigrostriatal pathway, low dopamine levels increase cholinergic activity, affecting movement control.
71. Metoclopramide, a common nausea and vomiting drug, has been associated to tardive dyskinesia, a movement disease characterized by involuntary, repetitive facial, lip, tongue, and limb movements.
72. Neurological condition tardive dyskinesia causes involuntary facial, tongue, and limb movements. Common tardive dyskinesia symptoms:
    - Face movements including grimacing, tongue protrusion, and lip smacking are involuntary.
    - Choreiform and athetotic motions are involuntary limb movements.
    - Involuntary pelvic and trunk motions.
    - Stiffness at the neck.
    - Speech or swallowing issues.
    - Uncontrollable eye motions
73. (C) GABA and dopamine.
74. Stimulants.

75. Aripiprazole (D).
76. Anorexia nervosa is characterized by extremely low body weight, which is frequently significantly below the normal range for age and height.
    - Fear of gaining weight or becoming obese
    - Body image distortion and/or denial of being underweight
    - Obsessive obsession with weight, food, and/or exercise
    - Extremely limited eating habits, such as avoiding entire food groups or consuming only very low calorie foods
    - Chronic fatigue and/or a lack of energy
    - Women's amenorrhea (absence of menstrual periods)
    - Cold sensitivity
    - Dry skin and hair, as well as brittle nails
    - Constipation
    - Mood swings, such as irritability and anxiety
    - Concentration issues
77. At least one, but preferably two.
78. Anxiety, risk of falling.
79. Apoptosis is programmed cell death that happens during development and in reaction to stress or damage. It involves structured, systematic destruction of cell components, unlike necrosis, which is more chaotic. Maintaining cell growth and death requires apoptosis, which is activated by a complex network of signaling channels in response to numerous stimuli. Apoptosis has been examined in psychiatry for its role in depression, schizophrenia, and Alzheimer's disease. Some treatments for various illnesses may modulate apoptosis, which may contribute to their development.
80. Medical condition.
81.

D	Distractibility
I	Impulsivity, irresponsibility, irritability
G	Grandiosity
F	Frustration, flight of ideas
A	Activity increased
S	Sleep deficit
T	Talkativeness

82. Dialectical Behavior Therapy (DBT) by Marsha M. Linehan reduces suicidal behavior in Borderline Personality Disorder patients. The cognitive-behavioral treatment DBT improves emotion control and reduces impulsivity and self-harm.
83. Valproic acid (Depakote).
84. Conversion disorder is a psychological disorder distinguished by the presence of physical symptoms that are not explained by a medical condition or the direct effects of a substance. These symptoms, which can include numbness, paralysis, blindness, or other sensory or motor disturbances, are frequently brought on by emotional conflicts or stressors. Although the exact cause of

conversion disorder is unknown, it is thought to be related to psychological factors such as unconscious conflicts or repressed emotions. These conflicts or emotions may be triggered by traumatic experiences in the past or by current stressors, and they may manifest as physical symptoms as a way of coping with or avoiding these psychological issues.

85. Adjustment disorder: If the child's symptoms began around the time of the family's move and are causing significant distress or impairment in functioning, this diagnosis may be considered. Adjustment disorder is a short-term condition that occurs as a result of a specific stressor (such as a move) and typically resolves within 6 months. Acute stress disorder (ASD) may also be on the differential.

    Separation anxiety disorder: If the child's symptoms are primarily related to separation from caregivers and are causing significant distress or impairment in functioning, this diagnosis may be considered. When separated from caregivers, children with separation anxiety disorder may experience crying, insomnia, and difficulty in social situations.

86.

Factitious disorder	Malingering
• Psychological disorder characterized by the intentional induction or feigning of physical or psychological symptoms in order to play the sick role • May seek medical treatment or be hospitalized • May exaggerate or invent symptoms in order to gain attention or sympathy • Do not intentionally harm themselves • Do not necessarily benefit financially from their illness	• Deliberate creation of false or exaggerated physical or psychological symptoms • To obtain some external benefit, such as financial compensation or the avoidance of work or military duty • May purposefully injure themselves or fabricate symptoms in order to achieve their goal • DSM does not include malingering

87. Traumatic events might cause ASD. It is characterized by dissociation, avoidance, and bad mood or cognition within 1 month of the trauma. If symptoms last shorter than a month, ASD may be diagnosed. PTSD should be addressed if symptoms last more than a month. After experiencing a horrific occurrence, PTSD can include reliving, avoiding reminders, bad mood or cognition, and hyperarousal. ASD and PTSD can be treated with antidepressants and cognitive-behavioral therapy (CBT).
88. CBT is a therapeutic approach that focuses on identifying and changing negative thought patterns and behaviors contributing to symptoms, including in cases of PTSD. CBT for PTSD may involve exposure therapy to gradually confront and process traumatic memories and cognitive restructuring to challenge and modify negative thoughts related to the trauma. Eye Movement Desensitization and Reprocessing (EMDR) is another therapy that helps individuals process traumatic memories using bilateral stimulation techniques, such as eye movements or tapping, which can be beneficial for PTSD-related symptoms like flashbacks and nightmares. Image Rehearsal Therapy (IRT) is a CBT aimed at reducing the frequency and intensity of nightmares in PTSD

patients by identifying nightmare themes, creating positive alternative endings, and practicing new endings mentally. Additionally, techniques like deep breathing, progressive muscle relaxation, and mindfulness meditation can assist PTSD sufferers in managing arousal and coping with triggers that may lead to flashbacks or nightmares.

89. β-blockers and benzodiazepines relieve hypertension and tachycardia. By blocking adrenaline, β-blockers may help alleviate physical panic episodes. Benzodiazepines increase brain GABA, which reduces anxiety and relaxes. Benzodiazepines are often used to treat panic attacks because they lessen symptoms immediately.
90. Asthmatics and COPD patients should not take β-blockers. β-blockers can aggravate airway tightness and respiratory symptoms in those with them. A β-blocker with a lower affinity for the β-2 receptors in the lungs, such as atenolol or metoprolol, or a bronchodilator medication may be needed to prevent bronchospasm.
91. β-blockers, hydroxyzine, and SSRIs may help performance anxiety patients. Hypertension and heart disease are treated with propranolol and other β-blockers. Adrenaline inhibition lowers heart rate and blood pressure. β-blockers may help reduce physical symptoms of anxiety such tremors, palpitations, and sweating, especially in persons with performance anxiety. Hydroxyzine, an antihistamine, may relieve anxiety. Histamine, a stress molecule, is inhibited by it. Hydroxyzine may relieve anxiety, irritability, and sleep issues. Treatment of anxiety disorders often involves SSRIs. They inhibit serotonin reuptake, which regulates mood and anxiety. SSRIs may reduce worry, compulsive thinking, and concentration issues.
92. Dopamine regulates locomotion, motivation, and reward. Low dopamine levels in certain brain regions are connected to ADHD. Attention, arousal, and stress are regulated by norepinephrine. Low norepinephrine levels in certain brain regions are connected to ADHD. Serotonin regulates mood, sleep, and appetite. Low serotonin levels in certain brain regions are connected to ADHD.
93. The dorsolateral prefrontal cortex (DLPFC) is behind the forehead in the frontal lobe. It performs executive activities like attention, cognitive processing, working memory, and problem-solving. Behavior regulation and complicated cognitive task planning are hypothesized to include the DLPFC. Emotion control and inappropriate reaction suppression are also its functions. ADHD, schizophrenia, and depression have been linked to the DLPFC.
94. Early aftercare planning is essential. Aftercare planning involves arranging for continued care and assistance after hospitalization or intensive outpatient therapy. Aftercare planning should begin when the patient is stable and agreeable. This may happen early in treatment or later, depending on the patient's needs and progress. It's important to include the individual and any relevant family members or caregivers in aftercare planning to ensure it meets their requirements and preferences. Aftercare plans may involve medication management, individual treatment, group therapy, and family or social support.
95. After strep throat, parents should watch for changes in their child's behavior or mental state. A strep infection can cause pediatric autoimmune

neuropsychiatric disorders associated with streptococcal infections (PANDAS). PANDAS is an uncommon illness that causes OCD or tic disorders like Tourette syndrome after a strep infection. Early management with drugs and behavioral therapy may avert long-term consequences in PANDAS. Most children with strep infections do not develop PANDAS.

96. Serotonin and norepinephrine are connected to OCD. Low serotonin levels in particular brain regions have been related to OCD. Serotonin governs mood, sleep, and hunger. Low brain norepinephrine levels may cause OCD. Norepinephrine controls attention, arousal, and stress. Tricyclic antidepressants like clomipramine limit serotonin and norepinephrine reuptake, which can boost brain neurotransmitters and treat OCD.
97. TRUE. Nightmares have genetic links; therefore, persons with a family history may have them too.
98. 6 months.
99. Broken Mirror Theory of ASD discusses ASD's social and communication issues. This theory claims that ASD sufferers have a "broken mirror" in the brain that affects their ability to read social and emotional cues. According to the notion, people with ASD cannot "mirror" others' facial expressions, gestures, and other nonverbal actions, which is crucial to social communication. This deficit in social mirroring may make it hard to recognize and interpret others' intentions and feelings and start and maintain social connections. The amygdala and fusiform gyrus, which process social and emotional stimuli, are dysfunctional in ASD patients. ASD's exact causes are unknown although a complex mix of genetic, environmental, and neurological factors is likely to cause it.
100. In individuals with Autism Spectrum Disorder (ASD), there are associations with neurotransmitter imbalances in specific brain regions. Low serotonin levels in certain areas of the brain have been linked to ASD, and serotonin plays a role in regulating mood, sleep, and appetite. Dopamine levels in specific brain regions can also be aberrant in individuals with ASD, affecting functions such as movement, motivation, and reward. Additionally, low norepinephrine levels in certain brain regions have been associated with ASD, and norepinephrine is involved in attention, arousal, and stress regulation. Furthermore, aberrations in glutamate levels in specific brain regions, which influence learning and memory, have also been linked to ASD.
101. These may include challenges in social interaction and communication, such as difficulty maintaining eye contact, a lack of interest in social activities, trouble initiating or sustaining conversations, engagement in specific habits or hobbies, and difficulties with processing sensory information (e.g., visual, auditory, or tactile issues). During playtime at the PMHNP's office, children with ASD may display various behaviors, including engaging in toy rituals such as lining objects up or turning them, hyper-focusing on one specific toy or its components (e.g., obsessively spinning vehicle wheels), demonstrating disinterest in toys or peers, and struggling with imaginative play, such as not pretending that toys represent people or objects.

102.

____Dl______Acute onset, disturbance of consciousness and cognition
____Dl______Inattention
____Dl______Meds = haldol if agitation, psychosis
____B_______Avoid benzos
____Dl______Do urinalysis with culture and sensitivity, esp. in older female patients
____Dm_____Progressive, chronic
____B_______Irritable
____B_______Personality changes
____Dm_____Check folic acid and B12
____Dm_____Will try to answer, laugh, or confabulate by making up answer

103. HIV infection may induce subcortical dementia. HIV-related subcortical dementia can include motor and behavioral problems, focus loss, and coordination issues. Antiretroviral therapy is the main treatment for HIV-related subcortical dementia. Antiretroviral therapy slows disease development and prevents brain damage.
104. Cognitive symptoms that resemble dementia but are caused by a different ailment or event are called pseudodementia. Depression, anxiety, and substance misuse can cause pseudodementia. Cognitive symptoms of pseudodementia include memory loss, trouble concentrating and making decisions, and executive function impairment. Treatment of the underlying illness frequently reverses these symptoms. In contrast, dementia is an irreversible cognitive loss caused by brain injury. While pseudodementia can affect anybody, it is more common in older adults and those with a history of mood problems or substance addiction. Note that pseudodementia is a description of dementia-like symptoms, not a diagnosis.
105. Lewy Body Dementia (LBD) is a neurodegenerative disorder characterized by the presence of abnormal protein deposits in the brain known as Lewy bodies. This condition leads to a range of symptoms, including cognitive decline, visual hallucinations, and motor symptoms similar to those seen in Parkinson's disease, such as tremors, stiffness, and difficulties with movement. LBD is unique in that it often presents with prominent visual hallucinations and fluctuating cognitive abilities, which can be challenging for both individuals with the condition and their caregivers to manage.
106. Pick's disease is frontotemporal dementia. Language, conduct, and decision-making are affected by brain damage to the frontal and temporal lobes in this dementia. Men are more likely to develop frontotemporal dementia, which alters personality, conduct, and language. Frontotemporal dementia can cause changes in social behavior, vocabulary, and decision-making. Progressive frontotemporal dementia worsens over time.
107. Lead poisoning in children can cause the following signs and symptoms:
    - Delays in development or learning difficulties
    - Irritability or behavioral modifications
    - Appetite loss
    - Weight reduction
    - Hearing impairment

- Pain in the abdomen
- Constipation
- Vomiting
- Tiredness or lethargy

108. Osteoporosis is a condition characterized by weakened bones that are more prone to fractures, and several risk factors contribute to its development. These risk factors include age, with older individuals, especially postmenopausal women, being more susceptible to osteoporosis. Additionally, a family history of the condition can increase one's risk, as can having low bone mass or density. Underweight individuals may also be at greater risk due to their lower bone density. Certain medications, such as corticosteroids and cancer treatments, can elevate the risk of osteoporosis, as can several medical conditions like rheumatoid arthritis, Crohn's disease, and celiac disease. Lifestyle factors like physical inactivity, a diet lacking in calcium and vitamin D, as well as smoking and excessive caffeine consumption, are also associated with an increased risk of osteoporosis.
109. The PMHNP may do the following:
    - The PMHNP should listen to the parents' concerns and offer emotional support during this tough period. Parents feel supported and less alone when the PMHNP comforts, encourages, and understands them.
    - The PMHNP can tell parents of what to expect in the coming hours, including the potential of the newborn dying. After a baby dies, the PMHNP can help parents arrange a funeral and get grief assistance.
    - The PMHNP can help parents communicate with the healthcare team and understand medical information. The PMHNP can help parents express their feelings and communicate.
    - The PMHNP can help parents create a memory box or take photos of their infant. The PMHNP can help parents plan a memorial for their newborn.
    - Let parents hold a dying baby to grieve.
110. FALSE. Grief is multifaceted and individual, thus there is no "one size fits all" strategy. Some grieve linearly, embracing the loss over time, while others experience severe and changing emotions. Grief can produce sadness, anger, guilt, and anxiety. As you adjust to the loss, you may have good and terrible days and feel different emotions. Grief can also affect physical, cognitive, and behavioral health.
111.

Therapy	Explanation	Techniques
Cognitive therapy	• Focuses on changing negative or distorted thoughts and beliefs that contribute to emotional distress	• Identifying and challenging negative thoughts, developing more realistic and positive beliefs, problem-solving and decision-making skills
Behavioral therapy	• Focuses on changing maladaptive behaviors by reinforcing positive behaviors and extinguishing negative behaviors	• Reward systems, exposure therapy, contingency management

Therapy	Explanation	Techniques
Cognitive-behavioral therapy	• Combines cognitive therapy and behavioral therapy to address negative thoughts, beliefs, and behaviors that contribute to emotional distress	• Identifying and challenging negative thoughts and beliefs, reinforcing positive behaviors, exposure therapy
Humanistic therapy	• Focuses on the individual's personal growth, self-awareness, and self-actualization	• Empathy, non-judgmental attitude, reflective listening, person-centered counseling
Multisystemic family therapy	• Focuses on the interactions and dynamics within a family system, as well as the individual's relationships and interactions with other systems (e.g., school, community)	• Family meetings, communication skills training, problem-solving skills training
Interpersonal therapy	• Focuses on the individual's relationships with others and how those relationships may contribute to emotional distress	• Communication skills training, identifying and addressing relationship patterns, social skills training
Strategic therapy	• Focuses on changing the individual's behavior by addressing the underlying goals and motivations behind the behavior	• Role-playing, reframing, paradoxical interventions
Solution-focused therapy	• Focuses on finding solutions to problems and helping the individual to move forward, rather than dwelling on the past	• Goal-setting, focusing on strengths and resources, identifying and building upon small steps towards change
Family systems therapy	• Focuses on the interactions and dynamics within a family system, and how those dynamics may contribute to emotional distress	• Family meetings, communication skills training, problem-solving skills training
Structural family therapy	• Focuses on the roles and boundaries within a family system, and how those roles and boundaries may contribute to emotional distress	• Role-playing, reframing, reinforcing positive behavior

112. Exercise offers numerous psychological benefits for children, including enhanced self-esteem and confidence. Engaging in physical activity can help relieve stress, release emotions, and improve mood, ultimately reducing feelings of anxiety and despair. Regular exercise also promotes better sleep, leading to improved rest and overall well-being. Additionally, physical activity contributes to enhanced attention, concentration, and problem-solving abilities. Social skills are another area of improvement, as exercise helps children learn important teamwork and communication skills. Furthermore, exercise plays a crucial role in improving overall health, reducing the risk of obesity, diabetes, and heart disease among children.
113. During a patient's relocation to a new area, the PMHNP can provide valuable guidance and support. This assistance includes connecting the patient with appropriate healthcare providers, support groups, and community services available in the new location. The PMHNP can also assist in identifying and resolving potential challenges related to the transition, such as coping with the

emotional aspects of leaving friends and family behind or finding a new primary care physician. Referral to local mental health resources, such as therapists or counselors, can be recommended to help the patient manage the psychological aspects of the move effectively. Additionally, the PMHNP can collaborate with the patient to develop a comprehensive mental health management plan tailored to the transition period, addressing stress management and treatment adherence. In situations where immediate mental healthcare may be challenging to access, the clinician can consider prescribing up to 3 months of the patient's current medications if stability and treatment adherence are maintained to prevent medication discontinuation during the relocation process.

114. It is considered normal for children between the ages of 3 and 6 to engage in self-exploration and play with their genitals as part of their natural curiosity and development. The PMHNP can provide reassurance to parents that such behavior is a typical part of a child's development and should not be a cause for concern. However, it is essential to educate parents on setting appropriate boundaries and explaining to their children that touching their genitals in public or involving others in such activities is not acceptable behavior. The PMHNP can advise parents to address this issue gently, emphasizing the importance of open communication and age-appropriate discussions with their children about personal boundaries and privacy.
115. Breast growth and discomfort in 9–16-year-old males normally last 6 months. Monitor growth and discuss the patient's concern and psychological effects of this bodily transformation. PMHNPs should heed this worry and offer support and non-judgment. Boys go through puberty and breast growth, thus the PMHNP should reassure him. The PMHNP should clarify that these changes are typical and will pass naturally. She should also check for other physical issues and discuss the boy's health. In case of medical or mental health concerns, the PMHNP should recommend the kid for further examination and treatment.
116. Women have less alcohol dehydrogenase in their stomach lining, which breaks down alcohol. After drinking the same amount as men, women may absorb more alcohol. Because women have more body fat and less body water than men, their blood alcohol content may be higher. Women are more sensitive to alcohol's effects due to hormonal changes, making them more likely to experience its negative effects, such as decreased judgment and coordination.
117. 6 months; 2 years. These are general milestones that babies may attain at different ages. It is also crucial to remember that babies develop differently and may lose reflexes before regaining them.
118. Erectile dysfunction is treated with PDE-5 inhibitors. Inhibiting phosphodiesterase-5 relaxes penis smooth muscle and increases blood flow, causing an erection. PDE-5 inhibitors include Viagra, Cialis, and Vardenafil. PDE-5 inhibitors can interact with some drugs and create substantial side effects. For instance, PDE-5 inhibitors and nitrates like nitroglycerin can cause hazardous

blood pressure drops. Alpha blockers like doxazosin can lower blood pressure dangerously when taken with PDE-5 inhibitors.

119. Bulimia nervosa is an eating disorder characterized by recurrent episodes of binge eating, followed by compensatory behaviors to rid the body of the excess calories consumed during the binge, such as self-induced vomiting, laxative or diuretic use, fasting, or excessive exercise. It is essential to note that individuals with bulimia can have a normal BMI (Body Mass Index), and the disorder is not limited to individuals who are underweight or overweight.
120. Habeas corpus prohibits wrongful incarceration; It can bring a prisoner or detainee to court to determine their detention's legality. Habeas corpus protects against unlawful detention and guarantees due process in many countries.
121. TRUE. Healthcare practitioners should examine patients' medication knowledge and beliefs before training them. They can better comprehend the patient's perspective and customize their teaching to meet any misunderstandings or concerns. To improve patient education and ensure that they grasp the medication's advantages and hazards, doctors should analyze a patient's past knowledge or views.
122. Immunological system cells create cytokines; they signal the immunological response. Autoimmune illnesses cause inflammation and tissue damage when the immune system targets healthy cells.
123. Bedwetting, or enuresis, affects both children and adults. Adults with enuresis may be prescribed desmopressin (DDAVP). Synthetic desmopressin regulates fluid balance like vasopressin. Increased renal water reabsorption by desmopressin reduces urine output and involuntary urination.
124. The nurse-patient connection and patient privacy and confidentiality may be violated. Personal and medical information must be kept private by healthcare practitioners. This includes respecting the patient's privacy and not releasing personal information to third parties without authorization, unless there is a compelling cause to do so (e.g., to mitigate harm).
125. A black box warning is the FDA's most serious prescription drug warning. The black box at the top of the medication's prescribing information alerts doctors and patients about its hazards. A PMHNP should carefully study a new black box warning for a patient's prescription and weigh the risks and advantages of continuing it. If hazards outweigh benefits, the PMHNP may urge the patient to stop using the medicine or switch treatments. Alternatively, the PMHNP may urge the patient to continue the medicine with additional precautions or monitoring because the benefits outweigh the dangers. Whatever they propose, the PMHNP must communicate with the patient and explain why. The PMHNP should also promote patient queries and concerns.
126. When administering a drug "off label," a doctor must advise the patient that it is being used for a purpose not permitted by the FDA. The drug has been evaluated and verified safe and effective for one use, but is used for another. Side effects and consequences may manifest.
127. A PMHNP's reflective practice goal is to critically review and reflect on their practice to improve their knowledge, skills, and competences. Reflective

practice can help PMHNPs discover areas for improvement and understand how their activities affect patients and the healthcare system. Reflective practice can take several forms for hospital-based healthcare teams. A few examples:

- Journaling: Writing about experiences and thoughts might help one reflect on practice.
- Reviewing cases with colleagues might help one reflect on their practice and learn from others.
- Reflective practice involves researching a practice component and using the results to improve it.
- Reflective practice can be beneficial by discussing examples and receiving feedback from a supervisor or mentor.
- Engaging in continual learning and professional development can help PMHNPs keep up with the latest research and best practices and think on how to apply this information in their practice.

128. Mental status

MMSE (0–30)	SLUM (0–30)
Normal = 25–30Mild = 21–24 Moderate = 10–20 Severe = 0–9	Normal = 27–30 Mild = 21–26 Dementia = 0–20

Depression

HAM D (0–76)	PHQ-9 (0–27)	Beck (0–63)
Normal = 0–7 Mild = 8–13 Moderate = 14–18 Severe = 19–22 Very severe = >23	Normal = 0–4 Mild = 5–9 Moderate = 10–14 Moderate to severe = 15–19 Severe = 20–27	Normal = 0–9 Mild = 10–18 Moderate = 19–29 Severe = 30–63

Anxiety

HAM A (0–56)	GAD (0–23)
Mild = <17 Moderate = 18–24 Severe = >25	Normal = 0–4 Mild = 5–9 Moderate = 10–14 Severe = 15–21

Withdrawal

COWS (opioid)	CIWA (alcohol)
Normal = 0–4 Mild = 5–12 Moderate = 13–24 Moderate to severe = 25–35 Severe = >36 Start treatment at score >7	Normal = 0–9 Mild = 10–15 Moderate = 16–20 Severe = >21 Start treatment at score >8

129. Methadone, a synthetic opioid addiction treatment, can produce arrhythmias.
130. In general, patients who score "moderate" on the COWS scale should start opioid use disorder treatment with a moderate-to-high dose. This scenario may require buprenorphine, naltrexone, or methadone.
131.

COWS	CIWA
• Diarrhea • Nausea/vomiting • Abdominal cramps • Sweating • Tremors • Anxiety • Agitation • Piloerection (goosebumps) • Backache • Muscle cramps • Insomnia • Yawning • Runny nose • Restlessness	• Tremors • Sweating • Nausea/vomiting • Paroxysmal sweats • Anxiety • Agitation • Auditory disturbances • Visual disturbances • Headache • Tactile disturbances • Orientation and clouding of sensorium • Incoordination

132. The liver does not process disulfiram (Antabuse), an alcoholism treatment. Acetaldehyde dehydrogenase, which breaks down alcohol, is inhibited by disulfiram. Acetaldehyde accumulation in the body from disulfiram and alcohol can cause flushing, nausea, vomiting, and headache. These adverse effects may deter alcoholics.
133. Appreciative Inquiry (AI) is a strengths-based organizational development and change method. It holds that organizations and communities may be transformed by focusing on strengths rather than shortcomings or issues. AI is a discovery, debate, and action process that identifies and builds on an organization or community's strengths. It involves asking open-ended, positive questions to unearth and highlight the organization's or community's values, capacities, and successes, then leveraging this information to promote change and development. It believes that tales and narratives create organizations and communities and that shifting focus from problems to opportunities can lead to positive, long-term transformation.
134. Irvin D. Yalom's group psychotherapy theory emphasizes the therapeutic benefits of group support, feedback, and interpersonal learning for individuals. According to Yalom's theory, group therapy involves four essential elements: recognizing that group members share similar issues, sharing experiences and insights to promote self-understanding and empathy for others, helping fellow group members leading to personal growth and a sense of purpose, and engaging in interpersonal learning by examining and modifying one's own and others' behaviors. Yalom underscores the significance of creating a safe and supportive group environment, where participants can openly share their thoughts and emotions and collaboratively address their challenges. In this

framework, group dynamics and interactions play a crucial role in facilitating substantial life changes for individuals undergoing therapy.

135. Possible replies vary. Rights may include:
    - Access to care in the least restrictive setting
    - Right to dignity, respect, privacy, and confidentiality
    - Right to health and treatment information in their language and format
    - The right to professional, nondiscriminatory care
    - Treatment consent or refusal. Access to medical records and other care information
    - Right to know dangers, benefits, and treatment options
    - They can complain or get a second opinion if they're unhappy with their care
136. In the treatment of a first psychotic episode, atypical antipsychotic medications that combine serotonin and dopamine antagonism are commonly used to reduce the risk of extrapyramidal side effects (EPS). Some examples of intramuscular (IM) medications for this purpose include paliperidone, ziprasidone, and olanzapine. These medications are employed to manage acute psychosis, alleviate symptoms such as delusions, hallucinations, and disorganization, and typically produce relief within days to a week by blocking dopamine receptors in the brain.
137. The Recovery Model empowers mental health patients to take charge of their recovery and attain their full potential. It holds that everyone can recover, despite severity, and that it is a long-term process of personal growth. The Recovery Model stresses optimism, choice, and self-determination and recognizes each person's strengths and needs. It also acknowledges the role of social, environmental, and family, friend, and community support in recovery. Another difference is that the Recovery Model emphasizes strengths and potential rather than weaknesses or issues. It helps people overcome obstacles and achieve their goals rather than just managing symptoms.
138. The four-point QI approach helps healthcare organizations implement and evaluate QI. It has four parts:
    - Plan: This step involves identifying the issue, making goals, and creating a solution.
    - Do: Implement the QI plan and collect data to track progress and evaluate interventions.
    - Study: Data from the "Do" phase is studied to find trends, patterns, and opportunities for improvement.
    - Act: This phase entails making system modifications and improvements based on the "Study" phase's findings and then reassessing the results to determine their impact.
    - QI aims to enhance processes, cut costs, and boost productivity. They involve continuously assessing and improving processes and techniques to improve performance and results. Quality and safety in healthcare are improved via QI.

139. "Screening, Brief Intervention, and Treatment Referral" (SBIRT) is a comprehensive approach to identifying and addressing substance use issues, particularly in primary care settings. SBIRT involves several key steps: first, standardized tools are employed to screen individuals for substance use and related concerns. Next, those who screen positive for problematic substance use receive a brief intervention, which is a scheduled counseling session aimed at reducing their substance use and associated risks. Finally, individuals with more severe substance use disorders are referred to specialized treatment programs for further care and support. SBIRT is designed to rapidly identify and intervene with individuals who may be at risk of developing substance use disorders or who are already experiencing negative consequences from their substance use. It operates under the assumption that early detection and intervention can prevent the progression to more severe substance use disorders and lead to improved outcomes.
140. In cases where a patient makes threats to harm someone during a clinic visit, the PMHNP must prioritize the safety of all individuals involved. Depending on the specific circumstances and the level of risk perceived, the PMHNP should take appropriate actions, which may include contacting law enforcement promptly if they believe the patient poses a threat to the intended victim or others. If the whereabouts of the potential victim are known, the PMHNP should also reach out to them to advise taking necessary precautions. Collaborating with the patient and relevant stakeholders, such as therapists or case managers, is essential to develop a comprehensive safety plan. This plan may involve measures like imposing no-contact restrictions, obtaining temporary restraining orders, and making crisis referrals. Additionally, in cases where the threat is severe and the patient's mental health history suggests potential danger, the PMHNP should consider referring the patient for a psychiatric evaluation to determine the appropriate course of treatment. Prioritizing safety and following established protocols and ethical guidelines is paramount in such situations.
141. Rennie v. Klein
142. O'Connor v. Donaldson
143. Preoperational stage
144. Formal operational stage
145. Industry vs. inferiority

146.

Risk factors	Protective factors
• Suicide attempt in the past • Depression and other mental illnesses in the past • Chronic pain, for example, is a serious illness • Criminal/legal issues • Job/financial difficulties or loss • Impulsive or aggressive behavior • Use of drugs • Adverse childhood experiences, current or prior • A sense of helplessness • Victimization and/or perpetration of violence • Bullying • Suicide history in family/loved ones • Relationship breakdown • Relationships with a high level of conflict or violence • Isolation on a social level • Inadequate access to healthcare • Suicides are on the rise in the community as a result of acculturation stress • Violence in the community • Historical adversity • Discrimination • Stigma associated with seeking help and suffering from mental illness • People at risk have easy access to lethal suicide methods • Suicide depictions in the media are dangerous	• Effective problem-solving and coping abilities • Reasons to live (for example, family, friends, pets, etc.) • Cultural identity is strongly felt • Partner, friend, and family support • Connection to others connection to school, community, and other social institutions • Consistent and high-quality physical and behavioral healthcare • People at risk have less access to lethal suicide methods • Suicide has cultural, religious, or moral objections

Notes:

Notes:

Appendix B: PMHNP Interview Questions

1. How do you go about treating individuals who might not respond well to treatment or who find it hard to put their trust in medical professionals?

   Answer Example: In one instance, I worked with a patient named Sarah who had a history of bad experiences with medical professionals and was quite resistant to therapy. She had experienced trauma in the past, so at first she was reluctant to talk. I used a patient-centered strategy, letting her set the pace for our conversations in order to foster trust. I supported her sentiments, listened intently, and avoided rushing her into therapy. We worked together to create treatment goals and talked about the possible advantages of therapy as she started to feel more at ease. With time, our mutual respect and steady improvement strengthened trust, and Sarah started to take a more active role in her care.

2. Could you give an example of a moment in your practice when you had to handle a particularly difficult or complicated case?

   Answer Example: I once saw John, a patient, who had severe bipolar disorder and substance use disorder co-occurring. He had been in and out of treatment programs and had a history of numerous relapses. Our task was to concurrently treat his addiction and mental health problems. To give an integrated strategy, I worked closely with a professional therapist and an addiction specialist. Medication management, dual-diagnosis-focused individual therapy, and participation in a community support group were all part of John's treatment regimen. Because of the intricacy of his condition, the treatment team needed to communicate with each other frequently. As a result of our combined efforts, John's general well-being showed notable improvements.

3. How do you keep up with the latest advancements and best practices in the field of mental health and psychiatric nursing?

   Answer Example: I understand how important it is to stay current in our ever changing field. To give an example, I regularly attend pertinent conferences like the annual Psychiatric Nursing Symposium and actively participate in continuing education programs. I also subscribe to respectable psychiatric nursing

T. Stewart, *Psychiatric-Mental Health Nurse Practitioner Program Companion and Board Certification Exam Review Workbook*,
https://doi.org/10.1007/978-3-031-60894-0

journals, such as the *Journal of the American Psychiatric Nurses Association*. These experiences give me the chance to pick the brains of top specialists, participate in conversations about cutting-edge procedures, and apply evidence-based methods to my clinical work. In addition, I participate actively in the American Psychiatric Nurses Association (APNA), which provides me with access to a wealth of information as well as chances for networking and knowledge sharing.

4. Could you talk about your experience treating people who also have drug misuse disorders and mental health issues?

   Answer Example: Mark is a patient who came in with co-occurring alcohol use disorder and anxiety problems. Alcohol had been Mark's go-to self-medication for his anxieties, which made his mental health problems worse. We used integrated dual-diagnosis treatment in our method. In order to address his substance use and provide evidence-based therapies for his anxiety, I worked closely with an addiction specialist. Engaging Mark and examining his ambivalence towards change was made possible in large part by the use of motivational interviewing techniques. We worked on improving his coping mechanisms, preventing relapses, and harm reduction together. Mark was able to take charge of his anxiety and substance usage thanks to this all-encompassing strategy, which ultimately resulted in his long-lasting recovery.

5. How do you go about dealing with stigma and discrimination issues when you work with patients?

   Answer Example: Lisa, a patient I recently worked with, had been stigmatized by her family because of her schizophrenia diagnosis. She experienced prejudice at work in addition to in her personal social network. In order to address this, I started by establishing a therapeutic setting that was secure and judgment-free so that Lisa felt comfortable talking about her experiences. She received psychoeducation from me regarding the myths surrounding schizophrenia, and I made sure she understood that her diagnosis did not define who she was. In addition, we collaborated to create coping mechanisms for stigma, such as assertiveness education and creating a network of allies. In order to combat stereotypes in society, I also urged Lisa to get involved in neighborhood advocacy groups that raise awareness of mental health issues. Lisa's mental health improved overall, she experienced a decrease in self-stigma, and she gained confidence as a result of these interventions.

6. Could you talk about your experiences working with multidisciplinary teams to treat patients?

   Answer Example: Recently, I worked with an interdisciplinary team to treat a patient called Alex in a challenging case which required collaboration. Alex had a history of childhood trauma, severe depression, and self-harming inclinations. Our team included a social worker, a professional therapist, a trauma specialist, and a psychiatrist to provide complete care. To ensure continuity of care and to align our treatment strategies, regular team meetings were crucial.

Utilizing the skills of our group members, I also included trauma-focused cognitive-behavioral therapy (TF-CBT) into our strategy. We were able to give Alex individualized, evidence-based care that addressed both the short-term crisis and long-term rehabilitation by collaborating and exchanging information. Alex's safety and mental health significantly improved as a result of this cooperative approach.

7. In working with patients, how do you efficiently manage your time and prioritize your workload?

   Answer Example: Ensuring that every patient receives the right kind of care depends heavily on time management. I employ a system of prioritization that takes each case's complexity and urgency into account. Patients who are undergoing acute mental crises or who pose an immediate risk to their safety, for example, are given priority. At the same time, I keep my schedule flexible to deal with unanticipated situations and protect the standard of service. I also use electronic health records (EHRs) to expedite documentation so that I can spend more time talking with patients face-to-face. Following a well-planned timetable allows me to devote the appropriate time and resources to meeting each patient's specific needs while keeping my practice running smoothly.

8. Could you please elaborate on how you handle drug therapy and management for people with mental health issues?

   Answer Example: A crucial component of psychiatric-mental health nursing is medication management. I start by doing a thorough evaluation to ascertain whether each patient needs to take a certain prescription. I place a strong emphasis on shared decision-making with patients when I prescribe, making sure they are completely aware of the risks, benefits, and available options. Along with promoting honest discussion about any worries, I also instruct patients on drug adherence and any adverse effects. As part of continuing care, regular medication reviews and modifications are made as needed. In order to provide the greatest results for every patient, my method is in line with evidence-based guidelines and stresses a holistic viewpoint that takes into account both pharmaceutical and non-pharmacological interventions.

9. In what ways do you identify and manage your patients' risk of suicidal thoughts or self-harm?

   Answer Example: An essential component of psychiatric-mental health nursing is evaluating and treating suicidal ideation or self-harm. During the initial examinations, I ask straightforward and open-ended questions regarding the presence and intensity of suicidal ideation using a comprehensive suicide risk assessment form. I create a safety plan with coping mechanisms, emergency contacts, and a crisis hotline for patients who are at risk. For those who are experiencing a crisis, frequent follow-up appointments and close observation are crucial. I also work with a multidisciplinary team to guarantee that patients who are at risk receive a coordinated approach. My method places a strong emphasis on developing a therapeutic connection, communicating with empathy, and listening without passing judgment in order to promote trust and candor when talking about these delicate subjects.

10. What is your experience working with patients from different cultural backgrounds, and how do you make sure that your practice is culturally competent?

    Answer Example: I've had the honor of working with patients from a variety of ethnic backgrounds during my career, and I know that each of them has particular values, beliefs, and healthcare preferences. In order to guarantee cultural competency, I start by acknowledging my own prejudices and working hard to increase my understanding of other cultures. I aggressively endeavor to comprehend each patient's perspective without presumptions, with cultural humility. I work with interpreters when there are language obstacles to ensure that people can communicate effectively. Furthermore, when it is appropriate, I modify my treatment plans to accommodate patients' cultural preferences while always honoring their autonomy and choices. In order to continuously improve my work, I am dedicated to cultural competency and make an effort to attend training programs and stay updated about cultural quirks.

11. In what ways do you assist patients with their rehabilitation and the acquisition of coping mechanisms to effectively handle their mental health disorders?

    Answer Example: One of the main tenets of my work is helping patients along their road to recovery. I start by carefully evaluating their objectives, needs, and strengths. I work with the patient to create a customized treatment plan that highlights their strengths and strengthens their current coping mechanisms. I provide them evidence-based symptom management techniques and psychoeducation on their mental health condition. Encouraging patients to take an active role in their care, I stress the value of wellness activities, self-care, and connecting with support systems. In addition, I monitor their development on a regular basis and modify the treatment plan as necessary. By enabling patients to take charge of their mental health, I hope to support their recovery with resilience and independence.

12. Could you elaborate on how you educate and encourage patients to manage their mental health disorders on their own?

    Answer Example: The cornerstones of encouraging mental health self-management are patient education and support. I take a patient-centered approach, customizing talks and instructional materials to meet the unique requirements and preferences of each patient. I take the time to thoroughly explain in understandable terms their diagnosis, available treatments, and the reasoning for measures. Key information is frequently reinforced through the use of textual materials and visual aids. In order to make sure patients are actively participating in their education, I also encourage inquiries and candid conversation. I work with patients to jointly establish realistic goals and give resources for monitoring symptoms and advancement in order to promote self-management. Frequent follow-up appointments give the opportunity to evaluate the patient's comprehension and provide continuous support as they progress through their mental health journey.

13. How does your practice make sure that patients' confidentiality and privacy are respected?

    Answer Example: Upholding patient confidentiality and privacy is a top ethical duty. I strictly abide by the rules set out by the Health Insurance Portability and Accountability Act (HIPAA) and any other applicable laws. I hold the first evaluations and conversations in quiet, soundproof spaces to protect privacy. In addition, I inform patients of their rights and the restrictions on confidentiality, especially in cases where there are safety issues. Use of EHRs is restricted by password encryption and stringent access constraints. In addition, I keep lines of communication open with my patients, stressing the value of truthful disclosure and reassuring them that their information will be kept private to the extent permitted by law. In order to maintain compliance and protect patients' trust, I constantly evaluate and refresh my understanding of privacy laws and security measures.

14. Could you elaborate on your experience with traumatized individuals and how you tackle trauma in your treatment plan?

    Answer Example: Since many of my patients have suffered from various types of trauma, providing trauma-informed care is essential to my practice. One particularly noteworthy case concerned Maria, a victim of marital abuse. Acknowledging the delicate nature of her experiences, I established a secure and trauma-sensitive therapeutic environment where she felt empowered to take charge of her recovery. I started out by providing psychoeducation on trauma responses and emphasized that her reactions were typical reactions to unusual occurrences. Together, we were able to recognize stressors and create coping mechanisms. Crucially, I included CBT and evidence-based trauma-focused therapies like EMDR. Maria felt resilient and empowered during her recuperation, and she also acquired skills to control the effects of her trauma.

15. What is your methodology for diagnosing and treating those who suffer from severe and chronic mental illness?

    Answer Example: Individuals who suffer from serious and ongoing mental illnesses frequently need assistance and care from specialists. I approach their evaluation from a broad, multifaceted standpoint. A comprehensive psychiatric diagnosis, a review of their social and functional domains, and an investigation of their personal and family history are all included in my assessment. I work with a multidisciplinary team to create customized treatment regimens that could incorporate community-based assistance, psychological therapies, and pharmaceutical management. The main focus is on recovery-oriented care, which addresses each patient's specific issues and emphasizes their strengths and ambitions. To guarantee the greatest results and quality of life for these patients, I constantly monitor them and make modifications to their treatment plan.

16. Could you talk about your experiences treating people who have been identified as having personality disorders?

    Answer Example: I've worked with individuals who have been diagnosed with personality disorders, including BPD (borderline personality disorder). Sarah, one of the patients, has a history of impulsivity and self-harm, which are traits of BPD. Since there is evidence that DBT is useful for BPD, I used this method to create a structured treatment plan. Our main areas of focus were interpersonal effectiveness, distress tolerance, and emotion regulation. To further ensure Sarah felt safe and stable, I set clear boundaries and communicated with her on a regular basis. She showed tremendous improvement in her ability to control her symptoms and her interpersonal interactions over time. This event served as more proof of the value of treating people with personality disorders using a customized, evidence-based strategy.

17. In what ways do you include the family and support networks of your patients in their care and treatment?

    Answer Example: Providing patients with complete treatment requires working in tandem with their families and support networks. In a recent instance, I saw how important it was to include Alex's family in the therapy process. Alex was a young adult going through severe depression. In order to improve understanding and communication among the family, I started family therapy sessions. These meetings gave Alex and their loved ones a forum to talk about the effects of depression. I also taught the family the value of providing emotional support while honoring Alex's independence. Through the active involvement of the family in the therapy process, we were able to enhance coping mechanisms, fortify the support system, and eventually aid in Alex's healing.

18. Could you elaborate on your experience treating patients who have psychotic disorders, such as bipolar disorder or schizophrenia?

    Answer Example: I've worked with individuals who have been diagnosed with psychotic disorders, such as schizophrenia and bipolar disorder with psychotic aspects. Daniel, one of the patients, had auditory hallucinations and paranoid delusions. I used a combination of individual therapy and antipsychotic drug control. Creating a therapeutic alliance was essential because it gave Daniel the confidence to talk freely about his upsetting symptoms. We talked about his concerns and beliefs, progressively assisting him in reframing and challenging his misconceptions. A major part was performed by psychoeducation regarding the characteristics of psychosis and the significance of medication adherence. His psychotic episodes became less frequent and less intense over time, which helped his everyday functioning and general well-being.

19. In what ways do you handle crisis intervention and management in your professional life?

Answer Example: A key component of psychiatric-mental health nursing is crisis intervention. In one instance, I worked with Emily, a patient who had a history of self-harm and acute suicidal thoughts. In order to protect her safety, I took urgent action. This included closely monitoring her, removing any potential self-harming tools, and doing a full suicide risk assessment. In order to give Emily further support, I worked with a local crisis stabilization unit and a crisis helpline. DBT is one psychotherapeutic strategy that was used to assist her manage her discomfort. I underlined the value of having a safety plan that includes emergency contacts and coping mechanisms. Emily's crisis steadily diminished with continued crisis management and a multidisciplinary approach, allowing her to move on to a more stable stage of her care.

20. Could you elaborate on your experience treating people who struggle with eating disorders or issues related to their bodies?

    Answer Example: Individuals suffering from eating disorders need to receive specialized care that takes into account their mental and physical health. I've dealt with people with significant body image issues and anorexia nervosa, such as Sarah. I used a combination of CBT, nutritional counseling, and routine physical health monitoring. Building trust was essential since eating disorder patients frequently experience intense anxiety related to food and body image. I worked closely with a qualified dietician to make sure the treatment plan was thorough. In order to address the underlying psychological issues causing Sarah's eating disorder, I also offered individual therapy. Sarah's relationship with food and body image improved over time, demonstrating the value of a multidisciplinary, holistic approach to eating disorder therapy.

21. Regarding the transition from inpatient to outpatient care, or from one level of care to another, how do you assist patients?

    Answer Example: A patient's treatment journey is crucial during the transition between levels of care. I place a strong emphasis on coordination and communication between the patient, the healthcare team, and myself to ensure seamless transitions. I involve the patient in the decision-making process through thorough discharge planning. We talk about the transition's objectives, anticipated difficulties, and possible roadblocks. I make sure the patient is aware of all of the follow-up visits, medication schedule, and post-discharge support programs that are offered. I also give my patients skills and resources to assist them stay stable during the change. To improve the continuity of care, regular follow-up appointments and continuous communication are crucial for tracking improvement and addressing any new problems.

22. Could you talk about your experience offering patients remote mental health services, such as telepsychiatry?

    Answer Example: Telepsychiatry has grown in importance as a means of delivering mental healthcare, particularly to underprivileged groups. I've had success connecting with patients who are unable to receive in-person care due to obstacles such as distance or other difficulties through the use of telepsychiatry. Maria, a patient in a noteworthy instance, resided in a far-flung rural area. I provided Maria with thorough mental assessments and therapy sessions via telepsychiatry, making sure she got the care she needed in the convenience of her own home. I placed a strong emphasis on private and secure communication channels and created a clear virtual appointment calendar in order to preserve the therapeutic partnership. This experience demonstrated how telepsychiatry can improve access to mental health services without sacrificing the standard of care.

23. In what ways does your practice handle problems with treatment adherence?

    Answer Example: In the field of psychiatric-mental health nursing, treatment adherence is sometimes a concern. I tackle this problem by combining goal-setting that is collaborative, patient education, and continuing support. I spend time learning about the patient's views, worries, and possible obstacles to adherence during the initial assessment. We collaborate to develop a treatment strategy that takes into account their interests and values. I stress the value of being transparent about any worries or adverse effects associated with treatment. The purpose of routine follow-up visits is to evaluate the effectiveness of treatment and deal with any new problems. In order to improve adherence, I also closely collaborate with patients to create routines and reminders. Encouraging patients to take an active role in their care and make knowledgeable decisions about it is my aim.

24. In your practice, how do you handle socioeconomic determinants of health that could have an effect on a patient's mental health?

    Answer Example: Considering the significant impact that social determinants of health have on mental health, I use a patient-centered and holistic approach. I start by performing a comprehensive social assessment, looking into things like job security, social support networks, access to healthcare, and stable housing. For example, I worked with community resources to find temporary housing alternatives for a patient called James who was experiencing homelessness while pursuing long-term stability. When required, I also incorporate social work and case management services into the patient's care plan, addressing problems with food insecurity, transportation, and legal matters that could have an effect on their mental health. Through cooperative approaches to tackling socioeconomic determinants of health, my goal is to establish a nurturing atmosphere that fosters general well-being.

25. What motivated you to pursue a career in psychiatric-mental health nursing?

    Answer Example: A personal event had a significant impact on my path to becoming a PMHNP. A close family member experienced a mental health crisis a few years ago and found it difficult to get prompt, caring treatment. As I followed their path, I became aware of the significant influence mental health specialists can have on people and their families. My enthusiasm for mental health advocacy was sparked by this encounter, which also motivated me to seek a profession in psychiatric-mental health nursing. My motivation stems from the conviction that each person should have the ability to live a happy and fulfilled life and should have access to excellent mental healthcare. My own experience inspires me to offer compassionate, research-based care and to help lessen the stigma associated with mental health issues.

26. How do you keep abreast of the most recent advancements in the field of psychiatric-mental health nursing?

    Answer Example: Providing the best care possible requires staying up to date in the constantly changing field of psychiatric-mental health nursing. I take a diversified approach to staying current. This entails routinely participating in workshops, conferences, and continuing education classes that highlight the most recent findings and evidence-based procedures. I participate actively in professional associations, such as the APNA, which offers networking opportunities, publications, and resources. I also place a high priority on self-directed learning through reading peer-reviewed publications, taking part in online forums, and having conversations with mentors and coworkers. I make sure that my practice stays rooted in the most recent research and industry best practices in psychiatric-mental health nursing by integrating formal education with continuous self-directed learning.

27. Tell us about a situation in which you had to deal with a challenging or uncooperative patient. How did you respond to the circumstance?

    Answer Example: Empathy and a patient-centered approach are necessary when dealing with challenging or resistant patients. I once worked with a patient named John who was first reluctant to participate in treatment. He was reluctant to disclose his doubts regarding the efficacy of the treatment. I started by using non-judgmental communication and active listening to establish rapport and trust. I reassured him that his goals and preferences constituted the foundation of our collaboration and acknowledged his concerns. John eventually felt more understood and heard, which increased his willingness to take an active role in therapy. I modified the therapy strategy to fit his particular requirements and advantages. This encounter reaffirmed the value of tolerance, understanding, and adaptability while forming therapeutic relationships with difficult patients.

28. Regarding workload prioritization, how do you handle several patients with varying needs?

    Answer Example: I've learned how to prioritize my task when I have a lot of patients. I tackle each issue methodically, taking into account its intricacy and urgency. For instance, patients experiencing a crisis or those with serious safety issues are attended to right away to guarantee their stability and safety. At the same time, I set aside enough time for patients who need help with chronic diseases, medication management, or ongoing therapy. I keep my schedule open to meet unanticipated needs while making sure every patient gets the attention they require. To maintain a balanced workload while delivering high-quality treatment, it helps to use EHRs for documentation, manage your time well, and communicate clearly with the rest of the healthcare team.

29. How do you establish rapport and trust with your patients?

    Answer Example: The foundation of a therapeutic connection with patients is the development of trust and rapport. I start by paying attention to their worries and expressing respect and understanding for their experiences. I ask them open-ended questions to encourage them to be honest about their feelings and opinions. I also try hard to recall specifics from past conversations to show that I genuinely care about their welfare. Since openness is crucial, I make sure that patients are aware of the expectations, goals, and treatment plan. In addition, I uphold constant limits in order to establish a therapeutic setting that is predictable and safe. My method places a strong emphasis on teamwork and mutual decision-making, giving patients a sense of control and worth over their treatment.

30. What characteristics do you think are most crucial for a successful PMHNP?

    Answer Example: A PMHNP must possess a number of attributes. First and foremost, empathy and compassion are essential because they allow me to establish a very personal connection with patients and offer assistance when they are at their most vulnerable. Good communication techniques, such as attentive listening and concise explanations, promote trust and understanding between people. Given the variety and dynamic nature of mental health issues, adaptability is essential. My dedication to continuous education guarantees that I remain up to date with industry advancements and optimal methodologies. My ability to deliver tailored care that honors individuals' varied experiences and backgrounds is made possible by my cultural competence. Ultimately, I am guided in resolving difficult moral conundrums and upholding the greatest standards of care by resilience and a solid ethical foundation.

31. How do you allow patients to plan and make decisions about their own care?

    Answer Example: Person-centered care is oriented around the patient's engagement in treatment planning and decision-making. As I begin this process, I actively involve patients in talking about their goals, concerns, and preferences through a collaborative assessment. We create a treatment plan together that takes into account their skills and values. Patients can ask inquiries, share their preferences for treatments, and express any reluctance or worries. Medication selections, therapeutic modes, and treatment duration are all areas where shared decision-making is applicable. As their needs and priorities change throughout the course of the care journey, I often ask for input and modify the treatment plan. Encouraging patients to participate actively in their care and giving them a sense of agency and ownership over their recovery is my main objective.

32. How would one go about recognizing and removing possible obstacles to care, like a lack of transportation or insurance?

    Answer Example: To guarantee that all patients have fair access to mental health services, it is imperative to recognize and remove care barriers. I start with a thorough evaluation that looks into potential socioeconomic determinants of health, such as insurance status and mobility issues. When obstacles are found, I work with patients to create workable solutions. I link uninsured individuals, for example, to opportunities for low-cost mental health treatments or prescription assistance programs. When a patient is having trouble getting about, I help them find local transportation services or look into possibilities like telepsychiatry. Patient advocacy, putting patients in touch with neighborhood resources, and making sure that access to care is not impeded by financial or practical difficulties are all important aspects of my approach.

33. To what extent do your treatment techniques integrate evidence-based practices?

    Answer Example: My approach to psychiatric-mental health nursing is centered on the use of evidence-based approaches. Firstly, I make sure that I am up to date on the most recent research, guidelines, and best practices by participating in continuing education and professional development. I give priority to therapies when creating treatment plans that are in line with current clinical recommendations and have substantial empirical backing. To treat depression, for instance, I might prescribe medications that follow evidence-based guidelines or employ CBT. In addition, based on patient progress and the most recent research findings, I routinely evaluate therapy outcomes and modify approaches. Patients will receive the most cutting-edge, clinically proven treatments possible, thanks to my dedication to evidence-based practice.

34. In what ways do you handle consent and capacity difficulties in your practice?

    Answer Example: In ethical psychiatric-mental health nursing practice, consent and capacity issues are critical. In order to make decisions about a patient's care, I first perform a comprehensive evaluation of their ability to make decisions. When necessary, I ensure a thorough review by using standardized capacity assessment instruments. When a patient is judged to be capable of making decisions, I participate in shared decision-making, making sure they are well-informed about the advantages, disadvantages, and available options for treatment. I acquire informed consent from authorized representatives or guardians in situations where a patient's capacity is compromised, adhering to legal obligations and recognized ethical principles, all the while involving the patient as much as feasible. My method puts an emphasis on patient autonomy and upholds their right to make decisions regarding their care, given their capacity.

35. What is mental health and how is it addressed in your practice?

    Answer Example: A person's entire functioning and state of mind are greatly influenced by their mental health, which includes their emotional, psychological, and social well-being. As I recognize the connections between mental health, physical health, and social variables, I address mental health from a holistic perspective in my practice. I use in-depth assessments to determine mental health, taking into account a person's emotional state, cognitive abilities, coping strategies, and social support. I take a strengths-based approach that prioritizes mental health and resilience. I treat mental health by adjusting evidence-based treatments to the particular requirements and objectives of every patient. This can entail counseling, managing medications, changing one's lifestyle, and assistance in overcoming obstacles and difficulties. Furthermore, I collaborate with patients to create plans for improving their resilience and mental health, which is an essential component of overall health.

36. What kind of cooperation do you have with the other medical professionals that a patient sees, such as their therapist or primary care physician?

    Answer Example: Providing holistic treatment requires working together with the patient's other medical professionals. To guarantee care continuity, I place a high priority on efficient communication and information exchange. For instance, I frequently share updates with a primary care physician on a patient's mental health, any pertinent physical health concerns, and any changes to their medication. When patients are seeing a licensed therapist, I keep lines of communication open in order to coordinate treatment plans and objectives. Planning for shared care can be facilitated by multidisciplinary team meetings where applicable. I use a patient-centered approach that prioritizes the patient's general health. Working together with other healthcare professionals enables us to address the connection between mental and physical health and provide all-encompassing care tailored to the individual needs of each patient.

Index

T. Stewart, *Psychiatric-Mental Health Nurse Practitioner Program Companion and Board Certification Exam Review Workbook*, https://doi.org/10.1007/978-3-031-60894-0

Q

R

S

Kolibri 360 GmbH
Ferdinand-Jühlke-Straße 7
99095 Erfurt, Deutschland
produktsicherheit@kolibri360.de